PRESCRIPTION DRUG DIVERSION AND PAIN

Prescription Drug Diversion and Pain

HISTORY, POLICY, AND TREATMENT

Edited by

John F. Peppin, DO, FACP
DIRECTOR
CENTER FOR BIOETHICS, PAIN MANAGEMENT AND MEDICINE
FLORHAM PARK, NEW JERSEY, NJ
CLINICAL ADJUNCT PROFESSOR
MARIAN UNIVERSITY, COLLEGE OF OSETOPATHIC MEDICINE
INDIANAPOLIS, IN
CONSULTANT
HAMDEN, CT

John J. Coleman, MA, MS, PhD
ASSISTANT ADMINISTRATOR (RETIRED)
DRUG ENFORCEMENT ADMINISTRATION
FOUNDER AND PRESIDENT (RETIRED)
PRESCRIPTION DRUG RESEARCH CENTER LLC
CLIFTON, VA

Kelly K. Dineen, RN, JD, PhD
ASSISTANT PROFESSOR OF LAW
DIRECTOR, HEALTH LAW PROGRAM
CREIGHTON UNIVERSITY SCHOOL OF LAW
OMAHA, NE

Adam J. Ruggles, JD, MA
ATTORNEY AND BIOETHICIST
EVANSVILLE, IN

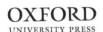
OXFORD
UNIVERSITY PRESS

OXFORD
UNIVERSITY PRESS

Oxford University Press is a department of the University of Oxford. It furthers
the University's objective of excellence in research, scholarship, and education
by publishing worldwide. Oxford is a registered trade mark of Oxford University
Press in the UK and certain other countries.

Published in the United States of America by Oxford University Press
198 Madison Avenue, New York, NY 10016, United States of America.

Library of Congress Cataloging-in-Publication Data
Names: Peppin, John F., editor. | Coleman, John J., Ph. D., editor. | Dineen, Kelly K., editor. | Ruggles, Adam J., editor.
Title: Prescription drug diversion and pain: history, policy, and treatment /
edited by John F. Peppin, John J. Coleman, Kelly K. Dineen, Adam J. Ruggles.
Description: New York, NY : Oxford University Press, [2018] | Includes bibliographical references.
Identifiers: LCCN 2018000838 | ISBN 9780199981830 (pbk.)
Subjects: | MESH: Analgesics, Opioid | Chronic Pain—therapy | Drug and Narcotic Control |
Prescription Drug Diversion—prevention & control | Opioid-Related Disorders—prevention & control | United States
Classification: LCC RC568.O45 | NLM QV 89 | DDC 615.7/822—dc23
LC record available at https://lccn.loc.gov/2018000838

9 8 7 6 5 4 3 2 1
Printed by Webcom, Inc., Canada

We dedicate this volume to the memory of two wonderful health professionals and human beings. This project has been plagued by sadness for most of the editors. Soon after starting this project, Dr. Howard Smith passed away suddenly. Howard was a wonderful man, dedicated to advancing the science and treatment of pain. He was gracious and was always willing to help others build their careers. He will be sorely missed. Dr. Kenneth L. Kirsh was a dear friend who spent his professional life trying to improve the lives of chronic pain patients. Soon after starting work on this volume, Ken was diagnosed with advanced cancer and was not able to continue with this project. He passed away in March 2017. He too was a wonderful person who will be missed by his friends, colleagues, family, and patients.

CONTENTS

CONTRIBUTORS

Timothy Atkinson, PharmD, BCPS, CPE
Clinical Pharmacy Specialist, Pain
  Management
Veterans Affairs Tennessee Valley
  Healthcare System
Murfreesboro, TN

Pravardhan Birthi, MD
Interventional Pain and PM&R Physician
CHI Health Saint Francis Pain and Physical
  Medicine Clinic
Grand Island, NE

Martin D. Cheatle, PhD
Associate Professor
Center for Studies of Addiction
Perelman School of Medicine
University of Pennsylvania
Philadelphia, PA

**Yvonne D'Arcy, MS, ARNP-C,
CNS, FAANP**
Pain Management and Palliative Care
  Nurse Practitioner
Ponte Vedra, FL

**Jeffrey Fudin, BS, PharmD, DAIPM
FCCP, FASHP, FFSMB**
Chief Executive Officer and Chief Medical
  Officer, Remitigate LLC
Delmar, NY
Clinical Pharmacy Specialist and
  Director, PGY2 Pharmacy Pain
  Residency (WOC)
Stratton VA Medical Center
Adjunct Associate Professor of Pharmacy
  Practice
Albany College of Pharmacy & Health
  Sciences
Albany, NY
Adjunct Assistant Professor of Pharmacy
  Practice
Western New England University College
  of Pharmacy
Springfield, MA

Kelly N. Gable, PharmD, BCPP
Associate Professor
Southern Illinois University Edwardsville
School of Pharmacy
Edwardsville, IL

Christopher M. Herndon, PharmD, BCPS, CPE, FASHP
Associate Professor
Southern Illinois University Edwardsville
School of Pharmacy
Edwardsville, IL

Hani Raoul Khouzam, MD, MPH, FAPA
Staff Psychiatrist
Chief of Salinas Outpatient Adult Services
Natividad Medical Center
Salinas, CA

Bill H. McCarberg, MD, FABPM
Neighborhood Healthcare (FQHC)
Elizabeth Hospice
San Diego, CA

Michael E. Schatman, PhD
Department of Public Health and
    Community Medicine
Tufts University School of Medicine
Boston, MA

Anand C. Thakur, MD
CEO/Medical Director
ANA Pain Management
Clinical Assistant Professor
Department of Anesthesiology
Wayne State University
Detroit, MI

DISCLOSURES

Pravardhan Birthi, Martin D. Cheatle, John J. Coleman, Kelly N. Gable, Christopher M. Herndon, Hani Raoul Khouzam, Michael E. Schatman: Potential conflicts of interest.

Timothy Atkinson: Axial Healthcare Inc. (Consultant); Daichii Sankyo (Advisory Board); Purdue Pharma (Epidemiology Advisory Board)

Yvonne D'Arcy: Purdue (Ad board, Speakers Bureau—non-branded materials), Ortho-McNeil (Speaking—non-branded), Egalet (Ad board), Practicing Clinicians Exchange (Speaking—Chronic Pain)

Kelly K. Dineen: My spouse is a full-time employee of Medtronic, Inc., which manufactures medical devices, including implantable devices for the treatment of chronic pain. I did not write about the use of devices for pain.

Jeffrey Fudin: Astra Zeneca (Speakers Bureau); Collegium (Consultant, Films); Daiichi Sankyo (Advisory Board); DepoMed (Advisory Board, Speakers Bureau); Endo (Consultant, Speakers Bureau); Iroko Pharmaceuticals (Speakers Bureau); Kashiv Pharma (Advisory Board); KemPharm (Consultant); Pernix Therapeutics (Speaker); Remitigate, LCC (Owner)

Bill H. McCarberg: Advisor: Pfizer, Collegium, DepoMed, Daiichi Sankyo, Pernix, Eaglet; Stock holdings: Johnson and Johnson, Biospecifics Technologies, Nektar Therapeutics, Galena, Collegium; Speaker's Bureau: Collegium

John F. Peppin: Janssen (Consultant); Ferring Pharmaceuticals (Consultant, Speaker); OneSource Regulatory (Consultant); YourEncore (Consultant)

Anand C. Thakur: DepoMed Pharmaceuticals (Speaker); Purdue Pharmaceuticals (Speaker); Kaleo Pharmaceuticals (Speaker); BDSI Pharmaceuticals (Speaker); Daiichi-Sankyo Pharmaceuticals (Speaker)

PREFACE

Chronic pain and the use of prescription opioids: There are very few topics today that can raise more emotional response than this combination, which just happens to be the central theme of this book. In today's world, opioids, like some of the people who use them and some who prescribe them, are being vilified because of what experts are calling an *epidemic* of opioid abuse. Described as "painkillers" and "narcotics" by the media, there is a growing sense that physicians who routinely prescribe these drugs for nonmalignant chronic pain are compromising professional norms, including that of the sacred Hippocratic Oath directive *to first do no harm*.

Chronic pain patients, many of whom are already beset by their medical problems, are further troubled and confused by the back-and-forth public debates over the safety and soundness of their treatment protocols. The topic of opioids is more divisive today than ever before.[1] Ideology rather than physiology becomes all too often the prevailing sentiment not only for practitioners, but also for pain patients, policymakers, public health and safety officials, and even members of the public. Views are often expressed in divisive pronouncements rather than arrived at through civil discourse.

Opioids indeed are controversial, but the complete story of their benefits and burdens remains untold. From time to time, data may be selected and interpreted to buttress a claim that, in turn, may be untrue or only partially true. There has been so much written in the medical literature for so many years on this topic that one should have no problem finding an authoritative source or two to reference a pet theory. Although concern for the long term use of opioids has existed for millennia, the wave of current fear gripping the nation no doubt has come about because of the increasing morbidity and mortality associated with their use in treating nonmalignant chronic pain.

Over just the last several years, a major shift has occurred in the literature over the long term use of opioids to treat chronic pain. The effect of this shift has been felt by patients who suddenly find their healthcare providers reluctant to continue chronic opioid therapy.

In the absence of suitable alternatives, many patients will likely bear the personal burden of this changing environment. Some will become dispirited and confused by the stereotypical accounts of opioid addiction that abound in the popular media.[2]

As we show in this book, essential data about opioid abuse, morbidity, and mortality are lacking and what little data we have are derived from flawed and obsolete government databases. Yet, these sources are relied upon for public policy development, resource allocation, and lawmaking. In the absence of sound data, ingrained cultural feelings about addiction can become a powerful driver of attitudes, even among pain specialists who, despite their professional training and experience, may be influenced by such bias in their prescribing practices.

Most would agree that the modern era of chronic pain treatment began in earnest the mid-1990s with the introduction of an extended-release form of oxycodone called OxyContin®. It was aggressively marketed as the answer to millions of untreated or undertreated chronic pain patients. OxyContin offered benefits that shorter acting immediate-release opioids lacked. Professional medical groups and organizations representing the interests of pain patients heralded the new drug. With their support, in 2000, congress enacted a statute declaring the decade beginning in 2001 as the "Decade of Pain Control and Research."

Lurking beneath the growing euphoria at the time was a growing concern by state and federal officials over increasing reports of overdoses and deaths attributed to the misuse of OxyContin, particularly in places like Maine, Ohio, and parts of Appalachia. By the end of the Decade of Pain Control and Research, the government was geared up and ready to transition to a decade of drug control. In this book, we explain in detail when, how, and why this happened.

A basic aim of this book is to inform healthcare professionals and others about some of the essential aspects of chronic pain treatment, particularly in an time of changing attitudes about the long term use of opioid therapy. Opioids are not, and never have been, a panacea for treating pain; they are just one of several tools available for use in specific instances and with specific patients. Much has changed in the pain field since this book was first envisioned, and much is expected to change over the coming years.

It is the hope of the authors and publisher that readers employed in the fields of law enforcement, medicine, regulatory policy and enforcement, pharmacy, drug treatment, and academia, as well as interested members of the general public, will benefit from the expertise and candor of the authors. This volume cannot begin to cover all of the important issues surrounding prescription opioids and chronic pain; rather, it is meant to be a starting point, a roadmap of sorts for professionals and non-professionals interested in the modern era of pain treatment and how we arrived at where we are today.

As mentioned in the dedication page, the editors would like to offer their sincere condolences to the families of Drs. Kenneth L. Kirsh and Howard Smith, two dedicated and skilled individuals with whom we began this project and who untiringly worked for the betterment of pain patients.

John F. Peppin, John J. Coleman, and Kelly K. Dineen

REFERENCES

1. http://health.usnews.com/health-news/blogs/eat-run/2015/04/08/the-problem-with-opioids-for-chronic-pain. Accessed May 10, 2017.

2. Peppin JF. Marginalization of patients with chronic pain on chronic opioid therapy. *Pain Physician.* 2009;12:493–498.

PRESCRIPTION DRUG
DIVERSION AND PAIN

CHAPTER 1

OPIOID MEDICATIONS

Old Wine in New Bottles

Timothy Atkinson, John J. Coleman, and Jeffrey Fudin

OPIOID HISTORY

An *opiate*, as defined by the United Nations Office of Drugs and Crime, is a substance naturally derived from the poppy plant, including raw opium, several psychoactive substances (thebaine, papaverine, and noscapine), morphine, codeine, and the semisynthetic heroin.[1] In contrast, the term *opioid* is broad and includes everything from the naturally occurring opiates (e.g., opium, morphine, codeine, etc.) to the synthetic or semisynthetic opioids used medically for the treatment of pain (e.g., fentanyl, hydrocodone, hydromorphone, methadone, oxycodone, oxymorphone).[1]

The appropriate use of opium and its derivatives and the distinction between their medical and recreational (or nonmedical) use are problems not unique to modern times. Booth (1996) reports that as early as 3400 BC opium poppies were cultivated in Mesopotamia by the Sumerians, who referred to it in their writings as the "joy plant."[2] The Ebers Papyrus (2000 BC) contains over 700 recipes using opium, while Assyrian medical tablets (700 to 601 BC) list opium in 42 of 115 vegetable remedies.[2] The prominent use of opium in spiritual life is evident as well and is clearly evident in the portrayal of many Greek and Roman gods wearing or holding opium poppies.[3] In the hands of priests, opium was a powerful agent to relieve grief, worry, and regret while producing a seemingly spiritual euphoria for the user.[2]

As demand for opium increased so did its influence on international trade and policy. For centuries, opium was traded as a commodity along the Silk Road from the Middle East, India, and China across the continent to Europe.[4] In the 17th century, in response to increasing opium demand in England, the East India Company was formed, and it dominated opium trade and production in Southeast Asia for nearly two centuries.[2] During this time, Great Britain fought two "opium wars" with China for the continued right to import and sell opium in China.[5]

Medical use of opium has been a polarizing issue for centuries, with many physicians both praising and condemning its use. As early as the third century BC, Greek physicians Erasistratus and Diagoras opposed opium use.[2] Erasistratus promoted complete abstinence while Diagoras went even further, declaring it would be better to suffer pain than become dependent upon opium.[2] Galen, living in the first and second centuries AD, claimed that opium cured nearly every known ailment.[2] Galen also published findings on the toxic side effects of opium and, importantly, his writings show that he understood the concept of tolerance.[2] There were other physicians of the time who believed opium should be used sparingly and judiciously and only within controlled environments.[2] This was the position of Hippocrates (460–357 BC), the "father of medicine," who described opium as useful for the treatment of headaches, cough, asthma, pain, and melancholy.[2]

Thus, from the earliest times to the present, opium has played a significant role in medicine. At the end of the 19th century, Sir William Osler, first physician-in-chief of Johns Hopkins Hospital and one of four original faculty members at its medical school, referred to opium as "God's Own Medicine."[2] Despite these testimonials, concerns for opium's adverse side effects have always shared equal concern among practitioners. In 1940, speaking before the 91st annual session of the American Medical Association (AMA), noted surgeon Lyndon E. Lee, Jr., MD, cautioned members in the use of opioids, even for end-of-life care:

> The use of narcotics in the terminal cancer patient is to be condemned if it can possibly be avoided. Morphine and terminal cancer are in no way synonymous. Morphine usage is an unpleasant experience to the majority of human subjects because of undesirable side effects. Dominant in the list of these unfortunate effects is addiction.[6]

However, definitions of addiction have changed dramatically since Dr. Lee's time. The American Society of Addiction Medicine now defines addiction as follows:

> Addiction is a primary, chronic disease of brain reward, motivation, memory and related circuitry. Dysfunction in these circuits leads to characteristic biological, psychological, social and spiritual manifestations. This is reflected in an individual pathologically pursuing reward and/or relief by substance use and other behaviors. Addiction is characterized by inability to consistently abstain, impairment in behavioral control, craving, diminished recognition of significant problems with one's behaviors and interpersonal relationships, and a dysfunctional emotional response. Like other chronic diseases, addiction often involves cycles of relapse and remission. Without treatment or engagement in recovery activities, addiction is progressive and can result in disability or premature death.[7]

Whether in the third century BC, 1940, or today, physicians have always had to weigh the therapeutic benefits of opium against its known risk of addiction and dependence.

US LEGISLATIVE HISTORY

The modern medical use of opium began in Germany in 1806 with the publication of experiments describing *Principium somniferum*, or morphine.[2] For the first half of the 19th century, physicians mainly administered opium to relieve pain, cough, or diarrhea.[2] Morphine was marketed as early as 1817 for analgesia and as a cure for alcohol and opium addiction.[2] The intravenous administration of morphine became possible in the 1850s with the invention of the hypodermic needle, and the rapid onset of action and ease of use quickly made intravenous morphine the analgesic gold standard for many healthcare professionals.[2,5]

The second half of the nineteenth century brought with it the highest rate of opiate use in American history. Numerous opium-containing concoctions were pitched for a wide variety of ailments, often promoted with exaggerated claims while failing to disclose their potentially toxic ingredients.[8] The American Civil War was the first major conflict in which morphine in powdered form was available and used as a battlefield analgesic.[9] Musto describes how medics, employing the new technology of the hypodermic syringe, unsparingly administered morphine to wounded soldiers, many of whom would bring their addiction home with them after the war.[9]

Following the Civil War, the use of opiates in so-called patent medicines sold by street peddlers, mail-order suppliers, and local druggists added to the problem of addiction.[8,10] Physicians of the time often overprescribed opiates for relatively simple ailments such as menstrual symptoms, children's colic, or infants' teething pain.[11] This practice, according to Kandall, contributed to middle-class white women becoming the largest group of addicted individuals.[11] By the 1890s, some were expressing concern about the rising levels of opiate addiction, and "inebriety hospitals," modeled on insane asylums, were opened with the intention of treating addiction as a medical problem.[4]

Early opiate addiction treatment consisted of experimental regimens that, in retrospect, were sometimes brutal and ineffective. Musto describes the "Towns Cure," named for Charles B. Towns, a wealthy stockbroker who despite his lack of formal medical training had a profound interest in "curing" opiate addiction. In 1909, Towns convinced a nationally prominent physician, Dr. Alexander Lambert (later president of the AMA), to endorse his treatment program. The Towns Cure consisted of denying addicts narcotics while aggressively treating their symptoms of withdrawal with strong laxatives and other drugs. This "cure" became the standard of care for the treatment of opiate addiction until the 1920s, when Lambert and others recognized the symptoms and significance of psychological dependence resulting from the use of narcotics, and the need to address the addict's drug cravings to achieve long-term remission.[9]

The popularity of the Towns Cure notwithstanding, the patent medicine industry wasted no time getting into the business of detoxification and opiate addiction treatment. Samuel Hopkins Adams, a noted investigative journalist for *Collier's Weekly*, wrote a series of articles called "The Great American Fraud" in which he exposed fraudulent claims by the patent medicine industry, including those by the "fakers claiming to cure the drug habit."[8] Adams purchased 16 different patent medicines being advertised as "cures" for morphinism or opium addiction.[8] All 16 were found to contain morphine.[8] Describing the purveyors of these bogus cures, Adams wrote:

> At the bottom of the noisome pit of charlatanry crawl the drug habit specialists. They are the scavengers, delving amid the carrion of the fraudulent nostrum business for their profits. The human wrecks made by the opium and cocain [*sic*] laden secret patent medicines come to them for cure, and are wrung dry of the last drop of blood.[8]

Adams' writings were credited with raising public awareness of the problem of patent medicines that, in turn, influenced Congress to pass the Pure Food and Drug Act of 1906.[9,12] While this act did not prevent sales of dangerous drugs containing opiates and cocaine, it did require accurate labeling of all contents for medicinal products sold in interstate commerce.[9]

In 1898, the Bayer Company began marketing a cough suppressant featuring a new ingredient called "heroin."[5] Fewer obvious side effects led to the assumption that heroin was not addictive.[5] Heroin's effectiveness as a pain reliever and cough suppressant were soon overshadowed by its abuse potential. Heroin's increased potency over morphine, its availability over the counter or from street peddlers, and its ease of use made it a natural target for recreational drug abusers who crushed and snorted or solubilized and injected the drug.[4] By 1910, heroin abusers were mostly working-class young men.[4]

In 1909, the first international opium conference was held in Shanghai, China, to discuss worldwide control of opium.[13] While not reaching consensus on control, the meeting nonetheless raised international awareness of the problem of opiate addiction, particularly as it affected China.[13] In 1914, a second opium conference was held at The Hague, Netherlands, where participants agreed to reduce opium production and restrict nonmedical use of the drug.[2,13] US attendees, elected by their fellow members to preside over both conferences, were embarrassed by having to propose international controls that were not yet adopted by the United States.[2]

Public opinion in the United States supported a proposed federal law to regulate the sale of narcotic drugs.[14,15] With support from Congress and President Woodrow Wilson, the Harrison Narcotics Tax Act of 1914 was enacted into law.[16] This act provided "for the registration of, with collectors of internal revenue, and to impose a special tax on all persons who produce, import, manufacture, compound, deal in, dispense, sell, distribute, or give away opium of coca leaves, their salts, derivatives, or preparations, and for other purposes."[17] Oddly, the act treated coca leaves as a narcotic.[17] The act permitted "the sale, dispensing, or distributing of any of the aforesaid drugs by a dealer to a consumer under and in pursuance of a written prescription issued by a physician, dentist, or veterinary surgeon registered under this Act."[17] Thus, for the first time, narcotic drugs could be dispensed or sold only upon presentation of a valid prescription issued by a practitioner registered under the act.

Perhaps the most controversial aspect of the Harrison Act was a relatively short provision that in later years would prove to have enormous legal significance. Restrictions placed on regulated drugs, according to Section 2, Subparagraph (a), of the act, did not apply "To the dispensing or distribution of any of the aforesaid drugs to a patient by a physician, dentist, or veterinary surgeon registered under this Act *in the course of his professional practice only*"[17] [emphasis added].

Although the scandals involving the patent medicine industry may have raised public support for regulation of narcotics, the Harrison Act's real target was the prescribers and dispensers of medicinal narcotics, whom some viewed as purveyors of addiction.[18] In just the first 4 months following the passage of the act, federal authorities charged 257 physicians and 40 dentists with violating the law.[19] Included among them was Dr. Jin Fuey Moy of Pittsburgh, who was convicted of prescribing 1/16 of an ounce of morphine sulfate to Willie Martin, an addict.[19] Dr. Moy's conviction mobilized the medical community, and in 1915, his case was appealed to the US Supreme Court.[19] There, on June 5, 1916, by a vote of 7–2, the Justices sided with Dr. Moy and his supporters, ruling that it was unlawful for the government to interfere with what amounted to the lawful practice of medicine.[20,21]

In 1919, the Supreme Court revisited the Harrison Act by accepting two new drug cases. In the first, Dr. Charles T. Doremus of San Antonio was charged with providing 500 tablets of morphine to a known addict.[19] Although a district court had ruled that the federal law was unconstitutional because it usurped the police powers of the state, the Supreme Court disagreed and declared the Harrison Act constitutional.[22]

The second case involved W. S. Webb, MD, and a pharmacist named Jacob Goldbaum, both from Memphis.[19] They were charged with routinely supplying addicts with large quantities of morphine.[19] In upholding their convictions, the Supreme Court found that, contrary to the Harrison Act's requirement, Webb and Goldbaum were not acting in the course of their professional practice only.[19,23] In reversing its earlier decision in Dr. Moy's case, the Court held that a physician might not prescribe "for the purpose of providing the user with morphine sufficient to keep him comfortable by maintaining his customary use."[23]

While the Treasury Department's strategy for addressing the problem of addiction was to focus on errant physicians and pharmacists, some in Congress had a different view of addicts. Representative Stephen G. Porter of Pittsburgh, chairman of the House Committee on Foreign Affairs and a staunch supporter of strict drug control, viewed addiction as a disease: "A person who is addicted to drugs is sick. He or she is the victim of a disease and should be placed where treatment can be given. You can't cure a sick person by sending that person to jail."[24]

Convinced that the bogus "cures" offered by the patent medicine industry were doing more harm than good, in 1929 Congress enacted legislation proposed by Porter to establish two "narcotic farms" run by the US Public Health Service as prison-hospitals dedicated to finding a cure for drug addiction.[25] The Porter Narcotic Farm Act, as it was called, mandated that the care of those confined to the farms "shall be designed to rehabilitate them, restore them to health, and where necessary train them to be self-supporting and self-reliant."[25,26]

The first narcotic farm was opened in 1935 on 1,000 acres of farmland just outside of Lexington, Kentucky.[27] By all accounts, it was a novel approach to addiction research.[27] Male and female convicts arrested for drug offenses did time alongside volunteers who checked themselves in for rehabilitation.[27] The treatment regimen followed the then-standard approach to treating psychological disorders with discipline and compassion in a healthful, rural setting, where patients could receive vocational therapy and group or individual psychotherapy, attend religious services, participate in indoor and outdoor recreation, and perform physical labor by working on a real farm.[27] The media enjoyed covering the narcotic farm, alternating between describing it as "A New Deal for the Drug Addict" and "A Million Dollar Flophouse for Junkies."[27]

In 1938, the second farm was opened in Fort Worth, Texas.[27] For several decades these two prison-hospitals would be the only research centers in the world devoted solely to finding a cure—or at least effective treatment—for drug addiction.[27] Although they never succeeded in fully achieving this goal, the scientific research performed at these unique facilities eventually led to the first protocols using methadone drug therapy in the treatment of opiate addiction.[27] By 1949, methadone was the preferred medication for detoxification at the Lexington narcotic farm.[27] In the 1960s, Drs. Vincent Dole and Marie Nyswander of the Rockefeller Medical Research Institute were credited with pioneering the general use of methadone to treat opiate addiction.[28] Although it had been used as an experimental protocol since the late 1940s, the first statutory approval of "maintenance treatment" (referring to the use of methadone for opioid addiction treatment) occurred in the Narcotic Addict Treatment Act of 1974.[29]

In 1930, with the demise of the Bureau of Prohibition on the horizon, President Herbert Hoover established the Federal Bureau of Narcotics within the Department of the Treasury and appointed Harry J. Anslinger, a former Bureau of Prohibition agent and counselor officer with the Department of State, as its first commissioner.[30] Anslinger's responsibilities included representing the United States at the League of Nations' Opium Advisory Committee, where he quickly gained an international reputation for being tough on drug crimes.[13] With the end of World War II, the League of Nations was replaced by the United Nations (UN), and in 1946, the responsibilities of the former Opium Advisory Committee were transferred to a newly formed but similarly designed UN Commission on Narcotic Drugs. Anslinger maintained his position as a US representative to the commission.[13]

On the domestic front, Anslinger was a well-known public figure whose strong views on drug control and repertoire of exciting drug cases made him a popular after-dinner speaker and a frequent guest on radio and TV.[30] In a 1948 movie, *To the Ends of the Earth*, that dramatized the work of his agents, Anslinger appeared in a cameo role as himself to explain the importance of international drug control.[31] In 1951, Anslinger's public support helped Congress to pass the Boggs Act, which included the first mandatory minimum sentences for drug offenses.[4] Anslinger would continue to be an influential figure on the national and international drug scene until his retirement in 1962 at age 70.[19]

The Controlled Substances Act (CSA) of 1970 was passed in response to an alarming increase in drug abuse during the 1960s.[19] The CSA classified drugs in five "schedules" according to their medical usefulness and abuse potential. Responsibility for enforcing the CSA was assigned to the newly created Bureau of Narcotics and Dangerous Drugs, the successor agency to Anslinger's Federal Bureau of Narcotics, which was abolished by executive order in 1968.[32]

To carry out the provisions of the CSA, Congress gave the Attorney General and the Secretary of Health, Education, and Welfare statutory authority to assess the abuse potential of drugs and other substances. Five "schedules" or classification categories for controlled substances, including regulated pharmaceutical drugs, were established, and specific, detailed criteria addressing abuse potential, medical usefulness, and psychological and physiological dependence were included to differentiate substances for control purposes.[33]

Schedule I and II controlled substances, according to the CSA criteria, have "high potential for abuse" but differ as to their currently accepted medical use in treatment in the United States.[34] Schedule I substances lack accepted safety for use under medical supervision, whereas Schedule II substances have "a currently accepted medical use in treatment in the U.S. or a currently accepted medical use with severe restrictions."[34] Substances in Schedules III, IV, and V are approved for medical use and have descending abuse potential.[34]

The CSA regulates approximately 1.6 million "registrants," comprising physicians, pharmacies, wholesale distributors, packagers, reverse distributors, manufacturers, teaching institutes, researchers, hospitals, and other handlers of controlled substances.[35] Rules are designed to ensure the security of the regulated drugs and to prevent diversion from legitimate to illegitimate channels.[36] Understandably, the rules are stricter and enforced more frequently when the substances in question pose a greater threat to public health and safety.[36] For example, the CSA expressly prohibits the refilling of Schedule II prescriptions.[37] In 2007, in response to numerous requests from prescribers and patients, the Drug Enforcement Administration (DEA) issued a Final Rule allowing "practitioners to provide individual patients with multiple prescriptions, to be filled sequentially, for the same schedule II controlled substance, with such multiple prescriptions having the combined effect of allowing a patient to receive up to a 90-day supply of that controlled substance."[38] The rule contained a number of additional requirements that must be met by the prescriber.[38] The easing of the statutory prohibition on refilling Schedule II prescriptions was hailed by patients and practitioners; of the 264 public comments received in response to DEA's proposed rule, 88.5% (231) were in favor of the change.[38]

Under the CSA, prescription refills for substances in Schedules III and IV may be authorized five times for up to 6 months and they may be transmitted to the dispensing pharmacy by phone, facsimile, or electronic prescribing.[39] State controlled substance laws may differ from federal ones in the sense that they may be stricter, but never less severe. For example, hydrocodone-containing products were designated under state law as Schedule II controlled substances in New York more than a year before the federal law was amended in October 2014 to reclassify all hydrocodone products to Schedule II.[40,41]

OPIOID-RELATED MORBIDITY AND MORTALITY

According to the Centers for Disease Control and Prevention (CDC), Opioids— prescription and illicit—are the main driver of drug overdose deaths.[42] Opioids were involved in 33,091 deaths in 2015, and opioid overdoses have quadrupled since 1999.[43] Between 2013 and 2014, the age-adjusted rate of death involving methadone remained unchanged; however, the age-adjusted rate of death involving natural and semisynthetic opioid pain relievers, heroin, and synthetic opioids other than methadone (e.g., fentanyl), increased 9%, 26%, and 80%, respectively.[44] The sharp increase in deaths involving synthetic opioids other than methadone, in 2014 coincided with law enforcement reports of increased availability of illicitly manufactured fentanyl, a synthetic opioid; however, illicitly manufactured fentanyl generally is not distinguished from prescription fentanyl in death certificate data.[44]

The CDC's data for drug-related deaths are based on a review of death certificates completed by funeral directors, physicians, medical examiners, and coroners.[45] Studies of these data have revealed several limitations, not the least of which is the ambiguity often found in death certificates filed before postmortem toxicology tests are completed.[46] A certificate in which the attending authority writes "suspected drug overdose" or "drug overdose" as the cause of death lacks specificity as to the drug(s) that caused or contributed to the death.[46] It is estimated that one in four drug-related deaths cannot be categorized according to the specific drugs involved because of this limitation.[46] Thus, it is likely that the totals given by the CDC for annual drug-related deaths attributed to opioids or to any other specific class of substances represent an undercount.[47]

Patients taking opioids may accidentally die of drug interactions.[48] In approximately 29% of opioid-related deaths, victims were found to have consumed benzodiazepines, which can heighten central nervous system depression when combined with opioids, thus resulting in reduced respiratory drive—something that can prove fatal in some patients.[49] Other medication classes that are present in higher numbers in opioid-related deaths include antidepressants (13.4%), antiepileptic and antiparkinsonian drugs (6.8%), and antipsychotic and neuroleptic agents (4.7%).[49]

Methadone accounts for only 2% of prescriptions for opioids but consistently results in over 30% of opioid-overdose deaths, more than twice the amount of any other opioid.[50] There were nearly six times as many methadone overdose deaths in 2010 as there were in 1999, mostly driven by an increase in the number of prescriptions written for pain.[51] While methadone's multiple mechanisms of action can be useful in the treatment of chronic pain, it often is prescribed by practitioners unfamiliar with its complicated features—including its variable and extensive distribution into tissues, its long half-life, QTc prolongation that may result in dangerous cardiac arrhythmias, variations in dose conversions, and a myriad of potential drug interactions that can increase methadone's absorption to dangerous levels.[52–54] Recent reports point to an underappreciated but clinically significant interaction with P-glycoprotein that may contribute to fatal overdoses resulting from medications that are generally considered safe to administer with methadone.[55]

Methadone is the preferred option by many insurers based solely on cost and is prescribed frequently by primary care physicians for headaches (17%), although efficacy is lacking for this indication.[51] More alarming is the fact the CDC's finding that nearly a third of methadone prescriptions were dispensed to patients who had received no opioids at all in the prior 30 days.[51]

PAIN COMMUNITY

The number of patients being treated for various chronic pain conditions, including cancer survivors and patients with lower back pain, has increased significantly over the last 15 years.[56] At the same time, the number of prescriptions for opioids has dramatically increased, as has their misuse.[57] According to a government survey of persons 12 years or older who admitted to using pain relievers nonmedically in 2011, 54.2% reported that they obtained their most recently used drug from a family member or friend for free, 18.1% said they obtained the drug from one doctor, and 3.9% said they obtained the drug from a street dealer or stranger.[58] In a follow-up question asking where the respondents believed that their family member or friend obtained the drug, approximately 81% believed that the relative or friend obtained the drug from just one doctor.[58]

Opioids diverted for nonmedical purposes come primarily from prescriptions issued by individual practitioners, usually primary care physicians.[58] However, there is evidence that thefts from hospital and pharmacy drug supplies, as well as in-transit thefts from manufacturers and distributors, may also be a significant source of diverted opioids.[59] As previously mentioned, at least one government survey found that friends and family members represent the single greatest source of abused pain medications.[58] Since 2006, national strategies to reduce prescription drug abuse have called for educating patients and their families as to the importance of quickly and safely disposing of unneeded medications.[60] In addition, since 2010, state and federal law enforcement agencies have collaborated on collecting unused or outdated prescription drugs from the public.[61] According to the DEA, the National Prescription Drug Take-Back Day collection by state and federal law enforcement agencies at 5,500 sites across the nation in April 2017 resulted in the removal of a record 900,386 pounds of unwanted medicines.[61]

WHY PRESCRIPTIONS FOR OPIOIDS HAVE INCREASED

In 1998, the Federation of State Medical Boards of the United States released Model Guidelines for the Use of Controlled Substances for the Treatment of Pain; these guidelines were revised and expanded in 2004.[62] They urged state medical boards to encourage physicians to view the undertreatment of pain as inappropriate care and provided guidance for performing a patient evaluation, preparing a treatment plan, obtaining a patient's informed consent, preparing and executing an agreement with the patient covering the proposed treatment, and conducting a periodic review of the patient's case.[63] The guidelines also provided assurance of support to pain physicians prescribing controlled substances for a legitimate medical purpose, provided the physician maintains proper and complete medical records.[63] State medical boards were also encouraged to cooperate with state attorneys general to evaluate state rules and regulations to identify regulatory restrictions that might impede the use of opioids in pain management.[63]

Following widespread acceptance and implementation by state medical boards, the Joint Commission on Accreditation of Healthcare Organizations (JCAHO) approved new standards for pain management in 2000.[64] Because JCAHO (in 2007 the group shortened its name to the Joint Commission) is the accrediting body for hospitals and long-term care and behavioral health facilities, these institutions were expected to adopt the new standards for treating pain or risk losing their accreditation.[65]

Not surprisingly, the increased awareness of untreated pain over the course of the last several decades was accompanied by an increase in the number of prescriptions for pain relievers.[66] The US Food and Drug Administration (FDA) reports that the number of outpatient opioid prescriptions dispensed from US retail pharmacies increased from 174.1 million in 2000 to 256.9 million in 2009, a 67.7% increase.[67] On an average day in the United States, the Department of Health and Human Services reports, more than 650,000 opioid prescriptions will be dispensed, 3,900 people will initiate nonmedical use of prescription opioids, 580 people will initiate heroin use, and 78 people will die from an opioid-related overdose (based on 2014 data).[68]

However, there are hints in the current data stream that the epidemic of prescription opioid abuse has reached its apex and may be starting to decline.[69] In April 2016, QuintilesIMS, an industry information company, released an analysis of the US healthcare market that showed an 8.5% increase in drug spending in 2015 over 2014.[69] Total prescriptions dispensed in 2015 reached 4.4 billion, up 1% over the previous year.[69] Importantly, the report noted that for 2015, "Among those therapy areas that declined, narcotic drugs saw a 16.6% drop in the number of prescriptions dispensed."[69]

QuintilesIMS's information is corroborated by government data for prescription opioids dispensed for medical use by the nation's pharmacies. By law, reports of bulk transactions and commercial distributions of controlled substances must be reported to the DEA where they are maintained in a database called the Automation of Reports and Consolidated Orders System (ARCOS).[70] The volume of opioids, for example, distributed by manufacturers and distributors to retail pharmacies in the United States is considered a reliable measure of their outpatient dispensing for medical use.[71] According to ARCOS data, between 2014 and 2016, the volume of oxycodone distributed to pharmacies for retail dispensing to patients declined 4.2% (from 54,322,092.80 grams to 52,050,579.29 grams); hydromorphone declined 11.8% (from 1,521,232.39 grams to 1,342,091.34 grams); hydrocodone declined 20.3% (from 35,885,092.97 grams to 28,615,716.36 grams); methadone declined 24.6% (from 4,473,779.04 grams to 3,372,211.67 grams); morphine declined 11.8% (from 19,603,645.48 grams to 17,287,250.62 grams); and fentanyl declined 13.5% (from 405,193.38 grams to 350,397.31 grams).[72] Codeine, the only prescription opioid whose retail distribution volume increased (+23.5%) during the period, also is the only opioid in this list still available as a Schedule III narcotic drug combined with a nonnarcotic ingredient.[34,72]

CHRONIC PAIN

According to the Institute of Medicine's (IOM) 2011 report on pain, 100 million Americans suffer from chronic pain.[73] Pain costs the United States as much as $635 billion each year in medical treatment costs and lost productivity, which is more than the cost of heart disease, cancer, and diabetes combined.[73] Pain is consistently the most common reason people consult a physician as well as the primary reason for delayed recovery, and it severely burdens the workers' compensation system.[73] The IOM report stated that pain represents a national healthcare challenge for which a cultural transformation is needed to prevent, assess, treat, and understand all pain types.[73] The IOM report concluded that, given pain's societal burden in terms of lives, dollars, and social consequences, finding new and improved treatments for it should be a national priority.[73]

As noted in the IOM report, the use of opioids for treating cancer pain or pain in the palliative care setting has long been accepted in medical practice.[73] In 1986, the World Health Organization introduced a three-step analgesic ladder that called for the oral administration of drugs in the following order: nonopioids (e.g., aspirin and paracetamol); then, as necessary, mild opioids (e.g., codeine); then, strong opioids (e.g., morphine), until the patient is free of pain.[74,75] The appropriateness of using opioid therapy for nonmalignant chronic pain, however, is still a subject of considerable debate among healthcare professionals.[76,77] In general, there seems to be consensus that opioids are overprescribed and that providers need more education about pain management strategies, particularly as they apply to different types of pain.[78]

Several addiction risk assessment tools are available to help professionals determine the risk of abuse associated with prescribing and maintaining chronic opioid therapy.[79] They can be used to assess pretreatment risks as well as during ongoing treatment to carefully monitor for aberrant signals.[79] Opioid prescribers are encouraged to proactively and periodically assess patients for degree of pain relief, level of psychosocial and physical functioning, extent of medication side effects, and the presence of potentially problematic substance use-related behavior.[79-81]

Attempting to ensure that the benefits of a drug outweigh its risks, the FDA may require a sponsor to develop and obtain approval for a Risk Evaluation and Mitigation Strategy (REMS).[82] The t reformulation of OxyContin, for example, with an abuse-deterrent extended-release delivery system resulted from the FDA's guidance that encouraged sponsors of long-acting opioids to address abuse risks through a class-wide REMS.[83,84] In 2013, the FDA used its authority under the REMS provisions of the Federal Food, Drug, and Cosmetic Act (as amended by the FDA Amendments Act of 2007) to withdraw OxyContin's original New Drug Application (NDA) from the Orange Book, thus invalidating any Abbreviated New Drug Applications that might be submitted by sponsors seeking approval for generic versions of the original (i.e., abusable) form of OxyContin.[83]

While the federal government is involved in regulating and approving the commerce in controlled substances, state governments via medical boards and professional societies have primary responsibility for regulating and setting standards for medical practice, including medication use.[85] Most federal drug regulations require compliance with state regulations as a condition for federal compliance.[86] As noted above, state laws may be stricter than federal laws when it comes to regulating controlled substances but they cannot, at least in theory, be less strict than the federal laws.[85]

CONCLUSION

Centuries of opioid experience worldwide have evolved as a circle of life from both a therapeutic and a regulatory perspective. Ongoing and future efforts will likely improve pharmaceutical formulations to mitigate abuse risk from mechanical manipulation. Additionally, additional receptor and subreceptors may be identified that will enhance analgesia without producing a reinforcing euphoric effect. New molecular entities that provide pain relief as well as new and improved non-pharmacological treatments for chronic pain are likely to replace the centuries-old opiates and their semi-synthetic derivatives and analogs still considered first line therapy for moderate to severe chronic pain. For now, however, there are no simple solutions to the opioid crisis. Enacting stronger regulatory controls has not reduced opioid-related morbidity and mortality. Just as the early opiate treatment protocols discussed in this chapter were unproductive until researchers identified the importance of the psychological dependency factor, finding a solution to today's opioid abuse problem will likely require that we broaden the scope of our current analyses.

REFERENCES

1. United Nations, Office of Drugs and Crime. World Drug Report. 2011. http://www.unodc.org/documents/data-and-analysis/WDR2011/World_Drug_Report_2011_ebook.pdf. Accessed May 10, 2017.

2. Booth M. *Opium: A History*. New York: St. Martin's Griffin; 1996.

3. Hays J, Mitchel J, Target Health Global. *Short History of Opioids* (official blog of Target Health, Inc.). 2017. http://blog.targethealth.com/short-history-of-opioids/. Accessed May 9, 2017.

4. Acker C. International overview. In: Korsmeyer P, Kranzler H, eds. *Encyclopedia of Drugs, Alcohol, and Addictive Behavior*. Vol. 3. New York: Macmillan Reference USA; 2009:183–189.

5. Acker C. International overview. In: Korsmeyer P, Kranzler H, eds. *Encyclopedia of Drugs, Alcohol, and Addictive Behavior*. Vol. 3. New York: Macmillan Reference USA; 2009:178–183.

6. Lee LE. Medication in the control of pain in terminal cancer. *JAMA*. 1941;116(3):216–220.

7. American Society of Addiction Medicine. Public Policy Statement: Definition of Addiction: Short Definition of Addiction. 2017. http://www.asam.org/quality-practice/definition-of-addiction. Accessed May 11, 2017.

8. Adams SH. The scavengers. *Collier's Weekly*. New York: P. F. Collier and Son; 1906.

9. Musto DF, ed. *Drugs in America*. New York: New York University Press; 2002.

10. Smith EL. *Patent Medicine: The Golden Days of Quackery*. Lebanon, PA: Applied Arts Publishers; 1973.

11. Kandall SR. *Substance and Shadow: Women and Addiction in the United States*. Cambridge, MA: Harvard University Press; 1999.

12. US Food and Drug Administration. Federal Food and Drugs Act of 1906. 2009. https://www.fda.gov/RegulatoryInformation/LawsEnforcedbyFDA/ucm148690.htm. Accessed May 13, 2017.

13. McAllister WB. *Drug Diplomacy in the Twentieth Century: An International History*. London and New York: Routledge Press; 2000.

14. New anti-drug law is in effect today. *New York Times*. July 1, 1914: 8.

15. Washington Correspondent, Chicago Record-Herald. Lack of efficient federal laws handicap war on drug habit in this country: fighting the opium evil. *Washington Post*. May 26, 1912.

16. Musto DF. The history of legislative control over opium, cocaine, and their derivatives. In: Hamowy R, ed. *Dealing with Drugs: Consequences of Government Control*. Lexington, MA: D. C. Heath and Company; 1987.

17. US Congress. Harrison Narcotic Tax Act. 1914. http://www.druglibrary.org/schaffer/history/e1910/harrisonact.htm. Accessed May 8, 2017.

18. Marshall E. Uncle Sam is the worst drug fiend in the world. *New York Times*. March 12, 1911.

19. Jonnes J. *Hep-Cats, Narcs, and Pipe Dreams: A History of America's Romance with Illegal Drugs*. New York: Scribner; 1996.

20. Ruckman PS Jr. Jin Fuey Moy in the Supreme Court. 2011. http://www.pardonpower.com/2011/01/jin-fuey-moy-in-supreme-court.html. Accessed May 8, 2017.

21. *U.S. v. Jin Fuey Moy*, No. 525; Argued December 7, 1915, Decided June 5, 1916. http://caselaw.lp.findlaw. com/scripts/getcase.pl?navby=case&court=US&vol=241&page=394#Scene_1. Accessed September 21, 2016.

22. *United States v. Doremus*, 249 U.S. 86 (US Supreme Court 1919).

23. *Webb v. United States*, 249 U.S. 96 (US Supreme Court 1919).

24. Calls drug traffic a world problem: Representative Porter says here that no one nation can suppress it. *New York Times*. February 13, 1930.

25. Baumohl J. Porter Narcotic Farm Act. In: Kleiman MAR, Hawdon JE, eds. *Encyclopedia of Drug Policy*. Los Angeles: SAGE Publications; 2011.

26. US Congress. Seventieth Congress, Session II, Chs. 80–82; "Chap. 82: An Act to establish two United States narcotic farms for the confinement and treatment of persons addicted (etc.) . . ." 1929. http:// legisworks.org/congress/70/publaw-672.pdf. Accessed May 13, 2017.

27. Campbell ND, Olsen JP, Walden L. *The Narcotic Farm*. New York: Abrams; 2008.

28. Newman RG. "Maintenance" treatment of addiction: to whose credit, and why it matters. *Int J Drug Policy*. 2009;20(1):1–3.

29. Substance Abuse and Mental Health Services Administration, Center for Substance Abuse Treatment. *Medication-Assisted Treatment for Opioid Addiction in Opioid Treatment Programs*. Treatment Improvement Protocol (TIP) Series 43. HHS Publication No. (SMA) 12-4214. 2005. http://store.samhsa.gov/shin/ content//SMA12-4214/SMA12-4214.pdf. Accessed May 8, 2017.

30. McWilliams JC. *The Protectors: Harry J. Anslinger and the Federal Bureau of Narcotics, 1930–1962*. Cranbury, NJ: Associated University Presses; 1990.

31. "To the Ends of the Earth" (1948); Harry J. Anslinger (appearing as Commissioner H. J. Anslinger). 2017. http://www.imdb.com/title/tt0040887/?ref_=nm_flmg_act_1. Accessed May 13, 2017.

32. Drug Enforcement Administration. *Drug Enforcement Administration: A Tradition of Excellence, 1973– 2008*. Arlington, VA: DEA; 2008.

33. Coleman JJ. *Reducing Prescription Drug Abuse by Design*. PhD dissertation; School of Public Policy, George Mason University. UMI (ProQuest); 2007.

34. Controlled Substances Act. Title 21, US Code, Sect. 812; Schedules of Controlled Substances, 1970. http://uscode.house.gov/search/criteria.shtml. Accessed May 8, 2017.

35. Drug Enforcement Administration, Office of Diversion Control. Registrant Population—Summary. 2017. https://apps.deadiversion.usdoj.gov/webforms/jsp/odrReports/odrRegSummaryReport.jsp. Accessed May 10, 2017.

36. US House of Representatives. *Committee on Interstate and Foreign Commerce Report on Comprehensive Drug Abuse Prevention and Control Act of 1970; Rept. 91-1444 (Part 1)*. Washington, DC: US Congress; 1970.

37. Controlled Substances Act. Title 21, US Code, Sect. 829(a); Prescriptions: Schedule II Substances. 1970. http://uscode.house.gov/search/criteria.shtml. Accessed May 8, 2017.

38. Federal Register. Rules and Regulations: Issuance of Multiple Prescriptions for Schedule II Controlled Substances (FR Doc E7-22558; vol. 72, No. 222). 2007. https://www.gpo.gov/fdsys/pkg/FR-2007-11- 19/pdf/E7-22558.pdf. Accessed May 8, 2017.

39. Controlled Substances Act. Title 21, US Code, Sect. 829(b); Prescriptions: Schedule III and IV Controlled Substances. 1970. http://uscode.house.gov/search/criteria.shtml. Accessed May 10, 2017.

40. Drug Enforcement Administration. Federal Register (79 FR 49661): Schedules of Controlled Substances: Rescheduling of Hydrocodone Combination Products from Schedule III to Schedule II; Final Rule. 2014. http://www.ncbi.nlm.nih.gov/pubmed/25167591. Accessed May 8, 2017.

41. New York State Department of Health. Changes to Controlled Substance Schedules Section 3306 of the Public Health Law: Schedule II Additions (hydrocodone). 2013. https://www.health.ny.gov/ professionals/narcotic/laws_and_regulations/. Accessed May 10, 2017.

42. Centers for Disease Control and Prevention. Press release: Opioids drive continued increase in drug overdose deaths: drug overdose deaths increase for 11th consecutive year. 2013. https://www.cdc.gov/media/releases/2013/p0220_drug_overdose_deaths.html. Accessed May 3, 2013.

43. Rudd RA, Seth P, David F, Scholl L. Increases in drug and opioid-involved overdose deaths—United States, 2010–2015. *MMWR Morb Mortal Wkly Rep.* 2016;65(5051):1445–1452.

44. Rudd RA, Aleshire N, Zibbell JE, Gladden RM. Increases in drug and opioid overdose deaths—United States, 2000–2014. *MMWR Morb Mortal Wkly Rep.* 2015;64(Dec. 18).

45. Centers for Disease Control and Prevention, National Vital Statistics System. Mortality Data. 2016. https://www.cdc.gov/nchs/nvss/deaths.htm. Accessed May 13, 2017.

46. Jones CM, Mack KA, Paulozzi L. Research letter: pharmaceutical overdose deaths, United States, 2010. *JAMA.* 2013;309(7):657–659.

47. Warner M, Trinidad JP, Bastian BA, Minino AM, Hedegaard H. Drugs most frequently involved in drug overdose deaths: United States, 2010–2014. *Natl Vital Stat Rep.* 2016;65(10):1–15.

48. Pergolizzi JV. Quantifying the impact of drug–drug interactions associated with opioids. *Am J Manag Care.* 2011;17(Suppl 11):S288–292.

49. Jones CM, Mack KA, Paulozzi LJ. Pharmaceutical overdose deaths, United States, 2010. *JAMA.* 2013;309(7):657–659.

50. Centers for Disease Control and Prevention. Vital signs. Prescription painkiller overdoses: Use and abuse of methadone as a painkiller. 2012. https://www.cdc.gov/vitalsigns/pdf/2012-07-vitalsigns.pdf. Accessed May 10, 2017.

51. Centers for Disease Control and Prevention. Vital signs. Risk for overdose from methadone used for pain relief—United States, 1999–2010. *MMWR Morb Mortal Wkly Rep.* 2012;61(26):493–497. https://www.cdc.gov/mmwr/preview/mmwrhtml/mm6126a5.htm?s_cid=mm6126a5_w. Accessed May 10, 2017.

52. Fudin J, Marcoux MD, Fudin JA. A mathematical model for methadone conversion examined. *Practical Pain Management.* 2012;12:46–51.

53. Zorn KE, Fudin J. Treatment of neuropathic pain: the role of unique opioid agents. *Practical Pain Management.* 2011;11(4):26–33.

54. Fudin J. Opioid pain management: balancing risks and benefits. CE Program of the University of Connecticut School of Pharmacy and Drug Topics. *Drug Topics.* 2011;Sept.:46–58.

55. Fudin J, Fontenelle DV, Fudin HR, Carlyn C, Hinden DA, Ashley CC. Potential P-glycoprotein pharmacokinetic interaction of telaprevir with morphine or methadone. *J Pain Palliat Care Pharmacother.* 2013;27(3):261–267.

56. Freburger JK, Holmes GM, Agans RP, et al. The rising prevalence of chronic low back pain. *Arch Intern Med.* 2009;169(3):251–258.

57. Paulozzi LJ, Weisler RH, Patkar AA. A national epidemic of unintentional prescription opioid overdose deaths: how physicians can help control it. *J Clin Psychiatry.* 2011;72(5):589–592.

58. Substance Abuse and Mental Health Services Administration. *Results from the 2011 National Survey on Drug Use and Health: National Findings.* NSDUH Series H-44, HHS Publication No. (SMA) 12-4713. Rockville, MD; 2012. http://www.samhsa.gov/data/NSDUH/2k11Results/NSDUHresults2011.pdf. Accessed May 10, 2017.

59. Joranson DE, Gilson AM. Drug crime is a source of abused pain medications in the United States. *J Pain Symptom Manage.* 2005;30(4):299–301.

60. Office of National Drug Control Policy. Synthetic Drug Control Strategy: A Focus on Methamphetamine and Prescription Drug Abuse. 2006. https://www.justice.gov/archive/olp/pdf/synthetic_strat2006.pdf. Accessed May 17, 2016.

61. Drug Enforcement Administration. DEA Collects Record-Setting Amount of Meds at Latest National Rx Take-Back Day. 2017. https://www.dea.gov/divisions/hq/2017/hq050817a.shtml. Accessed May 13, 2017.

62. Model Policy for the Use of Controlled Substances for the Treatment of Pain. *J Pain Palliat Care Pharmacother*. 2005;19(2):73–78.

63. Federation of State Medical Boards of the United States I. Model policy for the use of controlled substances for the treatment of pain. *J Pain Palliat Care Pharmacother*. 2005;19(2):73–78.

64. Phillips DM. JCAHO pain management standards are unveiled. *JAMA*. 2000;284(4):428–429.

65. The Joint Commission. Facts About the Joint Commission. 2017. https://www.jointcommission.org/about_us/fact_sheets.aspx. Accessed May 13, 2017.

66. Centers for Disease Control and Prevention. Prescribing Data. 2016. https://www.cdc.gov/drugoverdose/data/prescribing.html. Accessed May 13, 2017.

67. Food and Drug Administration, Office of Surveillance and Epidemiology. Outpatient Prescription Opioid Utilization in the U.S., years 2000–2009. 2010. https://www.fda.gov/downloads/AdvisoryCommittees/CommitteesMeetingMaterials/Drugs/AnestheticAndLifeSupportDrugsAdvisoryCommittee/UCM220950.pdf. Accessed May 10, 2017.

68. Department of Health and Human Services. The Opioid Epidemic: By the Numbers. 2016. https://www.hhs.gov/sites/default/files/Factsheet-opioids-061516.pdf. Accessed May 9, 2017.

69. QuintilesIMS (formerly known as IMS Health). News Release: IMS Health Study: U.S. Drug Spending Growth Reaches 8.5 Percent in 2015. 2016. http://www.imshealth.com/en/about-us/news/ims-health-study-us-drug-spending-growth-reaches-8.5-percent-in-2015. Accessed May 9, 2017.

70. Drug Enforcement Administration. Automation of Reports and Consolidated Orders System (ARCOS); Background. 2012. http://www.deadiversion.usdoj.gov/arcos/index.html. Accessed May 13, 2017.

71. Joranson DE, Ryan KM, Gilson AM, Dahl JL. Trends in medical use and abuse of opioid analgesics. *JAMA*. 2000;283(13):1710–1714.

72. Drug Enforcement Administration, Office of Diversion Control. ARCOS Retail Drug Summary Reports. 2016. https://www.deadiversion.usdoj.gov/arcos/retail_drug_summary/index.html. Accessed May 9, 2017.

73. Institute of Medicine. *Relieving Pain in America; A Blueprint for Transforming Prevention, Care, Education, and Research*. Washington, DC; 2011.

74. World Health Organization. Cancer Pain Relief. 1986. http://apps.who.int/iris/bitstream/10665/43944/1/9241561009_eng.pdf. Accessed May 10, 2017.

75. World Health Organization. WHO Pain Relief Ladder. 2006. http://www.who.int/cancer/palliative/painladder/en/. Accessed Nov. 13, 2006.

76. Catan T, Perez E. A pain-drug champion has second thoughts. *Wall Street Journal*. Dec. 17, 2012. http://www.wsj.com/articles/SB10001424127887324478304578173342657044604. Accessed March 31, 2016.

77. Ansari H, Kouti L. Drug interaction and serotonin toxicity with opioid use: another reason to avoid opioids in headache and migraine treatment. *Curr Pain Headache Rep*. 2016;20(8):50.

78. Food and Drug Administration, Center for Drug Evaluation and Research. FDA Blueprint for Prescriber Education for Extended-Release and Long-Acting Opioid Analgesics. 2017. https://www.fda.gov/downloads/Drugs/DrugSafety/InformationbyDrugClass/UCM515636.pdf. Accessed May 13, 2017.

79. Zacharoff K, Pujol L, Corsini E. PainEDU.org: A pocket guide to pain management. 2010. https://www.painedu.org/index.asp. Accessed June 13, 2013.

80. Rice JB, White AG, Birnbaum HG, Schiller M, Brown DA, Roland CL. A model to identify patients at risk for prescription opioid abuse, dependence, and misuse. *Pain Med*. 2012;13(9):1162–1173.

81. White AG, Birnbaum HG, Schiller M, Tang J, Katz NP. Analytic models to identify patients at risk for prescription opioid abuse. *Am J Manag Care*. 2009;15(12):897–906.

82. Food and Drug Administration. Questions and Answers: FDA Approves a Risk Evaluation and Mitigation Strategy (REMS) for Extended-Release and Long-Acting (ER/LA) Opioid Analgesics. 2012. http://www.fda.gov/Drugs/DrugSafety/InformationbyDrugClass/ucm309742.htm. Accessed May 13, 2017.

83. Federal Register, Vol. 78, No. 75/Thursday, April 18, 2013/Notices (p. 23273). Department of Health and Human Services; Food and Drug Administration Notice: Determination That the OXYCONTIN (Oxycodone Hydrochloride) Drug Products Covered by New Drug Application 20–553 Were Withdrawn From Sale for Reasons of Safety or Effectiveness. 2013. https://www.gpo.gov/fdsys/pkg/FR-2013-04-18/pdf/2013-09092.pdf. Accessed March 18, 2017.

84. Okie S. A flood of opioids, a rising tide of deaths. *N Engl J Med.* 2010;363(21):1981–1985.

85. Donovan KJ, Fudin J. How changing hydrocodone scheduling will affect pain management. *Practical Pain Management.* 2013;13(5):69–74.

86. Office of the Federal Register. *Code of Federal Regulations: Title 21, Food and Drugs; Part 1300 to end.* Washington, DC: USGPO; 2016.

CHAPTER 2

LEGAL REGULATION OF PRESCRIPTION OPIOIDS AND PRESCRIBERS

Kelly K. Dineen and Adam J. Ruggles

INTRODUCTION

Healthcare is estimated to account for nearly 20% of the US economy by 2025.[1] It also is one of the most heavily regulated industries at the federal, state, and even local levels. The professional behavior of individual healthcare providers is also regulated directly and indirectly through myriad legal mechanisms. Providers (including physicians, advanced practice nurses, physician's assistants, and others with prescriptive authority) are compelled to comply with statutory requirements that govern entry and fitness to practice;[2] conflicts of interest, business relationships, and billing;[3] privacy and confidentiality laws;[4] prescribing;[5] and many other aspects of care. The ubiquitous regulatory environment in healthcare often leaves providers wary of the law.

The desire to avoid legal entanglement altogether is a powerful driver of provider behavior—one such example would be the trends in overtreatment motivated by the wish to avoid malpractice suits.[6] The fear of legal entanglement is particularly strong in the realm of prescribing medications with the potential for abuse (controlled substances), such as opioids and other medications commonly used in the treatment of pain. In the realm of opioid prescribing, the stakes for providers are especially high. Opioids occupy a unique and shifting space between useful medical tool and agent of harm—they are also plagued by historical and cultural factors that continue to jeopardize evidence-based approaches to both patient care and legal regulation.[7]

In 2006, the US Drug Enforcement Agency (DEA) dismissed providers' fears of legal scrutiny as not grounded in fact; however, legal scrutiny around prescribing opioids has increased in recent years, with increases in actions against prescribers in civil, criminal, and regulatory settings.[8] Providers' fears of legal scrutiny around prescription opioids are also amplified because of the nexus with federal and state drug laws, which criminalize the distribution of controlled substances outside of the usual practice of medicine, a context-dependent and easily manipulated standard. Nonetheless, law enforcement actors are increasingly scrutinizing medical practice around opioids, with a fourfold increase in DEA actions against physicians between 2011 and 2014.[8] This compounds the typical sources of legal scrutiny for providers, such as state health professional licensure boards.[5] A single event of misprescribing or adverse patient outcome can lead to multiple legal actions—from state licensure boards, federal agencies, federal and state criminal charges, and civil and malpractice lawsuits.[9]

Recent concerns about the harms of opioids have magnified these fears for many providers, with some reports that physicians have recently refused continued prescriptions even to patients for whom the medications were providing benefit (therapeutic opioids).[10,11] Others have removed opioids from their toolbox completely.[12] This is concerning—refusal to provide treatment that is both beneficial and legal because of provider self-interest is contrary to the goals of medicine and the ethical obligations of providers.[13] As a matter of professional ethics, providers have a fiduciary duty to their patients,[14] which requires them to prioritize the overall well-being of their patients over any other interest. Neglect of treatable pain or any other condition without countervailing beneficent justifications fails to show respect for the patient and is fundamentally unethical.[15]

At the same time, care and caution when prescribing opioids and other controlled substances is warranted.[9] There have been serious concerns in recent years about indiscriminate and nonmedical use of opioids and the related, sometimes deadly harms.[16] At least in part, some of the overtreatment may be a result of a desire to avoid malpractice charges.[17] At least some of the responsibility for those harms sits at the feet of physicians and other prescribing providers.[9]

However, the widespread blame that providers face for "creating" addiction after prescribing opioids may be increasing patient avoidance.[18,19] This is not a new phenomenon—widespread blame of physicians for addiction was common in the early 20th century.[20] Coupled with fears of harming patients and fears of legal scrutiny, providers may be less willing than ever to prescribe even therapeutic opioids.[13] Regulatory and legal constraints; the historical context of pain and addiction treatment; the deeply embedded cultural stigmas against people with pain, addiction, or both; and many other factors make caring for patients for whom opioids are appropriate a significant challenge for providers.

Appropriate prescribing is highly complex and its evaluation requires a careful analysis of contextual, patient-centered information.[21,22] These medications are neither good nor bad absent context, despite the public tendency to oversimplify their use and mischaracterize their utility. Similarly, applicable law and rates of enforcement are prone to distortions. These laws are also embedded in a larger historical and cultural context of misunderstanding and stigma around pain and addiction. Healthcare providers, administrative officials, and law enforcement officers are not immune from the impact of these distortions and oversimplifications. Each of these groups can benefit from a basic understanding of the current regulation of prescription opioids and other controlled substances coupled with factual information about evidence-based treatment of pain and addiction.

This chapter provides a brief overview of the history of opioid prescribing law. The current regulatory and legal framework for prescribing opioids and other controlled substances is also reviewed. Definitions for types of inappropriate prescribing are offered. Also addressed are the various legal entanglements that a provider may face for inappropriately prescribing opioids or after a bad patient outcome related to opioids. The authors offer suggestions for appropriate legal scrutiny of opioid prescribing.

PRESCRIPTIVE AUTHORITY

Basic prescriptive authority is a function of state law. Entry to practice for healthcare professionals is governed by state professional boards, such as boards of medicine and boards of nursing.[23] These boards are agencies created by state legislatures to protect citizens by regulating entry to practice through licensure and ensuring continued basic professional competence through investigation of complaints and licensee discipline.[24,25] As described by the Federation of State Medical Boards, their purpose, in part, is to protect the public from "unprofessional, improper, incompetent, unlawful, fraudulent and/or deceptive practice" by licensees.[26] Boards tend to hold licensees to a higher standard of conduct than those in the general population, in recognition that licensure is a privilege with associated professional ethical obligations.[27]

Once licensed by a state board, a variety of providers are granted some level of basic prescriptive authority; these include physicians, advanced practice nurses (APRNs),[28] physician assistants,[29] dentists,[30] and others depending upon state law. Physicians have the most liberal and consistent prescriptive authority across the United States. Licensed medical doctors and doctors of osteopathy may prescribe any medication legally marketed in the United States, provided they have complied with the regulatory requirements discussed below. APRNs have full prescriptive authority in many states, meaning that the state allows them to prescribe any medication to their patients, including Schedule II medications.[31] Some states have more restrictive rules for APRNs that, for example, limit controlled substance prescribing.[31,32] Physician assistants are required to practice under the supervision of a physician; however, like APRNs, their prescriptive authority varies by state.[29]

Providers must also comply with additional requirements to prescribe controlled substances within the parameters allowed by their state professional licensure boards. The licensing boards control the relevant healthcare professional practice and general medication prescribing, whereas state and federal law enforcement agencies are gatekeepers for controlled substances prescribing. At the federal level, providers must apply for a certificate of registration (COR) from the DEA, which allows them to prescribe controlled substances within the limits of their state licensure.[33] The federal regulation of controlled substances is "designed to work in tandem with state controlled substance laws."[34] Typically, providers must also register to prescribe controlled substances with either their state drug enforcement agency (also known as narcotics bureaus) or state board of pharmacy, depending on state law.[35] In those cases, the provider must demonstrate compliance with the state before a COR will be issued by the DEA.[36] Therefore, to prescribe to the fullest extent allowed by state professional boards, providers must comply with at least three requirements: (1)

professional licensure, (2) federal registration with the DEA for COR, and (3) state registration. Those who wish to prescribe controlled substances for the treatment of addiction face additional regulatory hurdles.

HISTORICAL RESTRICTION OF OPIOID ACCESS FOR MEDICAL USE AND SEGREGATING ADDICTION TREATMENT FROM HEALTHCARE

Prior to 1914, drugs for medical use were generally available without a prescription from pharmacists, usually upon the recommendation of a pharmacist or physician. A few states had established requirements for opium and similar drugs before 1900;[37] however, the first federal law that established prescription-like requirements for medical use of opioids was enacted in 1914 in response to concerns about addiction at the beginning of the 20th century.[38] The Harrison Narcotic Tax Act of 1914 required, among other things, patient recordkeeping requirements and prescriptions for narcotics that exceeded a certain dosage.[39,40] The act also introduced legal language permitting medical use of opioids when prescribed by a physician to a patient in "the course of his professional practice only."[41] This language has since pervaded laws implicating prescribing, including the Controlled Substances Act (CSA).[42]

The Harrison Act also ushered in the criminal prosecution of physicians for prescribing opioids outside the "course of professional practice." Immersed in the culture of prohibition,[43] the Narcotics Division of the Treasury Department—charged with enforcing the Harrison Act—shut down then-existing addiction treatment centers that offered medical maintenance of addiction with regular opioid administration. The Narcotics Division did so after adopting the position that medical maintenance of addiction, an early version of medication-assisted treatment (MAT), was not within the practice of medicine and therefore the centers were illegally distributing drugs.[44]

In 1919 the Supreme Court affirmed this interpretation of the Harrison Act, declaring that prescribing regular doses of opioids for managing addiction was not the "legitimate practice of medicine."[45,46] In 1920, the American Medical Association adopted a resolution against medical maintenance.[44] The same year, the Supreme Court reversed a lower court's dismissal of the criminal prosecution of a physician for prescribing opioids to a known "dope fiend" and "not for the treatment of any disease."[47] Thus, two ideas that linger today were reinforced by the highest US court: (1) misprescribing physicians are criminally blameworthy for addiction and (2) addiction is not a medical problem or within the professional scope of medicine.

It is unsurprising that we continue to struggle with law and policy that segregates treatment of addiction—now known as substance use disorders—from the traditional practice of medicine.[48] Legal enactments for the last 100 years reinforced the separation. In 1962, Maurer and Vogel explained

Most physicians simply want to get the addict out of their office as quickly as possible, which is understandable. On the whole medical men tend to view addiction as a police problem rather than a medical problem largely because they do not have the facilities or even the knowledge at the present time to handle it otherwise. Furthermore, the law in the main justifies this medical attitude.[49]

A multilayered regulatory structure has consistently separated opioid prescribing for addiction treatment from all its other uses; moreover, it reflects and reinforces cultural misconceptions that addiction treatment is unusual and particularly dangerous and that healthcare providers engaged in such care require heightened surveillance.[44] Although recent efforts have eased some restrictions,[50] the ability of providers to prescribe opioids as part of MAT for addiction is far more limited and labor intensive than any other prescribing practice, despite ample evidence of its effectiveness.[51,52] Who provides MAT and how, where, and to how many patients, are all still strictly regulated by the federal government in ways that dramatically exceed other regulatory controls around prescribing.[53] In what follows, we describe the legal and regulatory frameworks for prescription opioids and other controlled substances in contexts other than addiction treatment.

FEDERAL DRUG SAFETY AND ACCESS

The Pure Food and Drug Act of 1906 was the first comprehensive federal food and drug safety law. It prohibited interstate commerce of drugs that were adulterated, effectively requiring quality consistency of the active ingredient and accurate labeling of the container.[54] It was reactive in nature—drugs did not yet require approval before they were marketed nor were there any requirements related to efficacy. Instead, there were penalties, such as seizure of the noncompliant goods already on the market. The US Food and Drug Administration (FDA) was created in 1930, and in 1938 the Federal Food, Drug and Cosmetic Act (FDCA) was enacted. The FDCA designated the FDA as the enforcement agency for the act; it also required manufacturers to submit a premarketing application with evidence of drug safety to the FDA, upon which the FDA could act to prevent marketing if the drug presented safety concerns.[55] The foundation of modern drug safety regulation was introduced by the Drug Amendments of 1962,[56] which mandated that manufacturers demonstrate both safety and substantial evidence of effectiveness of new drugs as well as myriad other requirements for drug safety.[55] Manufacturers or others who market drugs without complying with the FDA requirement are liable for introducing a misbranded drug into interstate commerce, which carries significant monetary penalties and incarceration.[57]

PRESCRIPTION-ONLY STATUS AND MODERN REGULATION OF DRUGS FOR MEDICAL USE

The Durham-Humphrey Amendments of 1951 created a prescription-only status for drugs based on whether the drug was safe for use without professional supervision.[58]

Today, prescription-only status denotes a drug that "because of its toxicity or other potentiality for harmful effect, or the method of its use, or the collateral measures necessary to its use, is not safe for use except under the supervision of a practitioner licensed by law to administer such drug."[59] In practical effect today, new drugs begin as prescription-only status.[60]

Despite the FDA's considerable authority, the FDA does not directly regulate provider prescribing practices. It is primarily a consumer protection agency and acts to ensure marketed drugs meet safety, consistency, and effectiveness standards. Drug approval and marketing requires specific labels and labeling with indications for use, dosing, and other information for the prescriber.[61] While the manufacturer must adhere to the labeling and other approval criteria or face penalties from the FDA, the same is not true for individual prescribers generally.[59] While prescribing practices are strongly influenced by drug labeling, prescribers are not required to adhere strictly to those parameters. In fact, it is common and within the standard of care in many instances to prescribe drugs "off-label"—meaning prescribing an approved drug in a way that is outside the label and labeling, including deviations from listed indication, dose, or age ranges.[61]

CONTROLLED SUBSTANCES, CONSUMER PROTECTION, AND LAW ENFORCEMENT

Opioids and other substances with both a medical use and potential for abuse sit at the intersection of consumer protection and law enforcement regulation. The criminal justice approach to drug control found new strength in the Comprehensive Drug Abuse and Prevention Control Act of 1970, also known as the CSA,[62] under which the Harrison Act and other drug laws were consolidated. The CSA is a federal criminal drug law that prohibits illegal drug manufacturing and distribution; it is enforced by the DEA,[63] a unit of the Federal Bureau of Investigation within the Department of Justice. States have their own versions of the CSA that mirror the federal CSA and govern intrastate and interstate illegal drug manufacturing and distribution.[64] State CSAs may be more, but not less, restrictive than the federal CSA.

The DEA places drugs into one of five schedules under the CSA based on (1) whether there is a currently accepted medical use and (2) the degree to which the drug carries the potential for abuse, misuse, and physical and psychological dependence.[65] Schedule I drugs have no acceptable medical use and a high potential for abuse.[66] The only access by providers to Schedule I drugs is through highly restrictive programs for research use.[67] Schedules II through V drugs have medically acceptable uses but also carry the potential for abuse, misuse, and dependence. Those with the highest risks of abuse, misuse, and dependence are in Schedule II; drugs with progressively less potential for abuse, misuse, and dependence are in Schedules III, IV, and V, respectively.[68] Most opioids are Schedule II drugs, including drugs such as morphine, oxycodone and oxycodone combination products, hydrocodone and hydrocodone combination products, methadone, and meperidine.[69,70] Other drugs that may be useful for the treatment of pain and anxiety but subject to misuse are Schedule III drugs such as codeine combination products,[71] and Schedule IV drugs including benzodiazepines such as lorazepam (Ativan), diazepam (Valium), and alprazolam (Xanax).[72]

Drug scheduling at the federal level also includes regulatory limits on requirements such as whether original prescriptions are required, the permissibility of partial prescription fills, limits on quantity or supply, and whether prescriptions may be transmitted electronically or by phone.[73] These limits set the floor for each state—states are free to create more restrictive laws but may not loosen the federal restrictions. States historically have followed the federal schedules closely; however, in response to the opioid crisis, many states have significantly restricted laws in this area.[74] States may create or amend their laws either through their own controlled substances act, by changing the medical or other health professional practice acts, or through regulations promulgated by the state professional boards. For example, Indiana recently passed a law limiting opioid prescriptions to opioid-naïve patients to 7 days, with certain limitations.[75] These laws are changing quickly, so providers are urged to familiarize themselves with the laws of their own states.

Each drug in Schedules II through V is both a prescription drug and an illicit drug. Whether a particular drug is medicinal or illicit is entirely dependent upon the context. On one hand, this seems obvious. Nevertheless, when prescribers' practices are scrutinized, the quality of the judgment of this context by law enforcement or professional boards can make or break a prescriber's career.

CONSUMER PROTECTION

When the FDA approves or reviews drugs with a medical benefit and the potential for abuse, it is required by law to make a recommendation on the appropriate classification or schedule for the drug.[76,77] In the specific language of the law, "at the time a new-drug application is submitted . . . for any drug having a stimulant, depressant, or hallucinogenic effect on the central nervous system, it appears that such drug has an abuse potential, such information shall be forwarded by the Secretary to the Attorney General."[78] The FDA is also consulted for any proposed rescheduling of drugs, although the DEA retains ultimate responsibility.[62]

The FDA also has power to provide enhanced warnings and impose special requirements on drugs for safety, which it has increasingly done for opioids. In 2007, the FDA Amendments Act strengthened the FDA's ability to require a Risk Evaluation and Mitigation Strategy (REMS) as a condition of drug approval or to impose a REMS upon receipt of new safety information of an already approved drug.[79,80] REMS may take a variety of forms and often include special medication guides for patients, heightened safety warnings and labeling, and mandated provider education.[81,82] A relevant example is the existing REMS for long-acting and extended-release opioids, the purpose of which the FDA describes as "to reduce serious adverse outcomes resulting from inappropriate prescribing, misuse, and abuse of extended-release or long-acting (ER/LA) opioid analgesics while maintaining patient access to pain medications."[82] Continued compliance is a statutory requirement and failure to comply is grounds for misbranding charges,[83] the penalties for which include imprisonment and significant civil monetary penalties.[84]

The FDA can also issue requirements for new and enhanced warnings on already approved drugs on the basis of new safety information.[85] In 2016, the FDA issued a long-overdue notice of enhanced warning requirements on the dangers of combining opioids with benzodiazepines or central nervous system depressants, such as alcohol.[86] These concerns are paramount and too often ignored in general discussions of the dangers of opioids. In fact, the significant majority of overdose deaths involving prescription opioids involve the concomitant use of benzodiazepines or alcohol.[87,88] As we discuss below, guidance around prescribing has been too slow to acknowledge the disproportionate dangers of certain opioids, such as methadone, and the dangers of concomitant use of alcohol or benzodiazepines.[13]

LAW ENFORCEMENT

Under the federal CSA, it is "unlawful for any person to *knowingly or intentionally* . . . manufacture, distribute, or dispense . . . a controlled substance."[89] Each state has its own version of the CSA under which violators may face charges.[90] Providers who prescribe controlled substances for a valid medical purpose are exempted from the ban on distribution. To avoid liability under the CSA, providers must have a current COR *and* issue a valid written prescription for a controlled substance, "for a legitimate medical purpose . . . in the usual course of . . . professional practice."[91,92]

Courts have explained these requirements many times in the context of criminal cases against prescribers. The possession of a valid COR is necessary for the exemption to apply but not sufficient alone to avoid prosecution.[93] The meanings of "legitimate medical purpose" and "usual course of professional practice" are also carefully examined. In 2014, the Fourth Circuit explained that the prosecution must show that a provider "distributed or dispensed a controlled substance, knowingly or intentionally, and his actions were not for legitimate medical purposes in the usual course of professional practice or were beyond the bounds of medical practice."[94] According to the Supreme Court, "the prescription requirement is better understood as a provision that ensures patients use controlled substances under the supervision of a doctor so as to prevent addiction and recreational abuse. As a corollary, the provision also bars doctors from peddling to patients who crave the drugs for those prohibited uses."[95]

INAPPROPRIATE PRESCRIBING PRACTICES AND THE MISPRESCRIBER

Despite abundant cultural and social commentary on the failings of providers around opioid prescribing, there is very little discourse about carefully defining misprescribing. There is also shockingly scant research on the characteristics of providers who misprescribe.

Although most providers are careful prescribers, inappropriate prescribing can take a variety of forms. There are an extremely small number of prescribers who deliberately use their prescribing privileges in ways that are unambiguously outside the clinical context, such as writing prescriptions for nonexistent patients or self-prescribing to supply an untreated substance use disorder.[9] However, the majority of misprescribing in the clinical context requires careful description. We divide the most common conceptions of inappropriate prescribing into four categories: (1) qualitative overprescribing, (2) quantitative overprescribing, (3) multi-class misprescribing, and (4) underprescribing. These distinctions are critical because the reasons behind them and the corrective measures differ for each.

Some providers prescribe opioids to patients for whom there is little evidence of potential or continued benefit,[96] which we refer to as *qualitative overprescribing*. If the patient suffers harm from qualitative overprescribing, such as subsequent development of an opioid use disorder or overdose, the provider may face legal action.

Perhaps more commonly, providers prescribe a higher number of pills than most patients are likely to use—resulting in large amounts of leftover pills.[97,98] This may be the result of a provider not keeping up with prescribing standards or as a deliberate effort to reduce the need for follow-up prescriptions or patient visits, particularly when patients travel long distances to see the provider.[13,99] This is a dangerous practice precisely because these leftover pills are ripe for diversion; in fact, they are the source of most nonmedical use of prescription opioids.[100] We call this *quantitative overprescribing*. Although this is a dangerous practice for the general public, quantitative overprescribing is rarely met with legal scrutiny unless it is associated with criminal diversion of the leftover pills.

Perhaps the most overlooked and dangerous type of misprescribing occurs when opioids are prescribed along with benzodiazepines or to patients who have inconsistent or heavy alcohol consumption. We call this *multi-class misprescribing*. Multi-class misprescribing is remarkably dangerous precisely because the majority of opioid-related deaths consistently occur in individuals with benzodiazepines, alcohol, or both in their system.[101–103] A recent study found that individuals prescribed both opioids and benzodiazepines were 10 times more likely to die of an overdose.[103] Of course, use of both opioids and benzodiazepines may be appropriate in particular situations; however, it should be undertaken with heightened caution, monitoring, and patient education. Multi-class misprescribing is increasingly associated with legal scrutiny, especially because of the increased risk of an adverse patient event.

Often lost in discussions of inappropriate prescribing is the reality that some providers may refuse to prescribe controlled substances to patients for whom they are appropriate and would provide benefit. We call this *underprescribing*. Unfortunately for patients who suffer as a result, the US legal system has little appetite for penalizing providers who neglect treatable pain.

CHARACTERISTICS OF MISPRESCRIBERS

There is little empirical evidence on individual traits of providers who misprescribe. What data exist are from retrospective review of legal action against prescribers, including malpractice actions,[104] licensing board discipline,[105] and criminal charges.[106] The 4D model, describing misprescribers as either dated, duped, disabled, or dishonest, was adopted by the American Medical Association decades ago and is still used by many regulatory and law enforcement agencies.[107–109] Dated providers are described as "so out of date on current practice standards . . . they inappropriately prescribe."[108] A duped provider "inadvertently supplies drugs to a drug abuser because the physician has been deceived by a drug abuser posing as a patient."[107] Disabled prescribers may divert controlled substances for their own use because of their own substance use disorder or exhibit poor judgment.[107] Those prescribers who use their access for personal gain are described as dishonest.[107]

The 4D model is both over- and under-inclusive and does not reflect what evidence exists in the literature. One of the authors of this chapter has recently criticized the model on a number of grounds.[9] First, the categories do not consistently focus on prescriber behavior. For example, the duped category reflects patient behavior. Worse yet, it feeds the demonstrably false idea that competent providers can avoid being fooled by a patient fabricating pain to obtain opioids. In fact, research from the field of lie detection confirm that even trained professionals do little better than chance in accurately detecting dishonesty.[9] Second, the dishonest category does not accurately reflect the level of corruption involved when providers use their prescribing privileges for personal gain. Third, the dated category inappropriately focuses on age or time in practice, when it should focus on competence. Finally, the disabled category is misleading in name—no one should be presumed to be a misprescriber by virtue of a disability. Instead, the prescriber's behavior in misprescribing is a more appropriate focus.

For these reasons and others detailed in a previous article, a new model was proposed that we share here. A 3C model should replace the 4D model. The 3C model of misprescribers includes individuals who are (1) careless, (2) corrupt, and (3) compromised by impairment. The careless category includes those who neglect the standard of care or those who fail to include standard-of-care patient monitoring. The most careful prescriber can be fooled on occasion; in contrast, duped providers are only included in the careless category if basic precautions would have easily revealed the duplicity. The careless category also better reflects someone who is not up to date on standard practices or neglects those practices. The corrupt category is more appropriate because dishonest is too gentle a term to describe the behavior of manipulating the privilege of prescribing. Finally, compromised by impairment reflects more than the existence of a disorder—it reflects a failure *because of a disorder*, such as a substance abuse disorder.

This 3C model is supported by a 2016 retrospective mixed-methods analysis of 100 cases of misprescribing. The study revealed that those sanctioned were predominantly men (88%) who practiced in solo or small practice environments of low oversight and accountability (97% of cases reviewed).[110] Based on their review, the authors developed three explanatory typologies that explained 93% of their cases, all of which include a small practice environment with little oversight. The first is the financially motivated misprescriber with self-centered personality traits. This fits squarely within the corrupt category. The second are impaired prescribers with their own substance use disorder, which fits within the compromised by impairment category. The third is physicians with poor skills or judgment,[110] which matches the careless category.

This information should guide regulatory agencies, law enforcement, and others involved in investigating and punishing misprescribing. Because of the fear of legal scrutiny among providers and the incredibly fact-intensive nature of misprescribing cases, it is essential that the frameworks for approaching misprescribing are accurate, consistent, and reliable. Moreover, one incident of misprescribing can result in countless legal actions, which can effectively destroy a wrongly accused provider's career and personal life.

REMEDIES FOR MISPRESCRIBING

Even one incident of misprescribing can create myriad legal difficulties for a provider; this is particularly true if it was related to an adverse patient outcome or media attention. In fact, even appropriate prescribing may give rise to investigations and cases against providers if the patient is injured or dies. Misprescribing can result in additional legal and quasi-legal entanglements, including, but not limited to, civil lawsuits (including malpractice), state board actions, criminal charges, hospital peer review, actions by insurers for reimbursement or breach of contract, censure from professional associations, exclusion from federal and state programs, and others. Below we review the most common of these and explain the legal standards involved in each.

MEDICAL MALPRACTICE AND RELATED TORT LAW CLAIMS

Medical malpractice cases are civil lawsuits brought by a patient or a patient's family member alleging professional negligence by the provider that caused harm. They are typically brought for harms suffered because of opioid-related overdose morbidity or mortality; however, a growing trend in malpractice is suits alleging that prescribers caused addiction.[111] Because they are brought by the patient or surviving family, these actions typically follow qualitative overprescribing or multi-class misprescribing with an adverse outcome. They can also follow careful prescribing that nonetheless resulted in patient harm.

Adverse verdicts do not correlate perfectly to substandard care; instead they tend to reflect factors such as the severity of the patient harm, the level of sympathy engendered by the plaintiff,[112] and even the degree to which the patient likes the provider.[113] The fact that a provider has settled a case or has a reported adverse verdict is not evidence of poor care alone; it is only a rough indicator of provider quality. Patterns tend to be more reliable.

To succeed in a medical malpractice case, a patient/plaintiff alleging harm must demonstrate all of the following by the preponderance of the evidence (more likely than not): (1) the provider had a duty to the patient, (2) that duty was breached by (3) a deviation from the standard of care that (4) caused the harm and (5) associated financial losses.[114] Anytime there is a patient–provider relationship, duty is established; breach is established by proving the provider deviated from the standard of care, typically defined as the range of practices of similarly situated providers caring for similar patients.[115]

The standard of care is often difficult to determine and always includes a range of acceptable options.[115] In the context of opioid prescribing, multiple factors are often included in determining whether prescribing was conducted within the standard of care. These include (1) whether doses were excessive in the context of the patient's history; (2) the degree and type of patient education, including warnings of dangers such as polysubstance use; (3) the existence, frequency, and thoroughness of the history and physical; (4) the prudent use of specialty referrals; (5) the adequacy of recordkeeping; and (6) the degree to which the prescriber considered patient and family concerns as well as patterns of patient behavior.[116]

A 2011 study examined medical records from opioid overdose malpractice cases from 2005 to 2009 and determined that 75% of the cases were related to physician errors.[104] The authors categorized the errors as follows: (1) starting opioid-naïve patients on excessive and dangerous doses of drugs, (2) inaccurately converting doses when changing opioids, (3) authorizing dose escalations too rapidly, and (4) failing to screen for comorbidities. Twenty-five percent of the cases were attributable to patient behaviors outside the control of the prescriber, such as self-medication, self-escalation of doses, and polysubstance abuse.

While prescribers must act carefully within the standard of care, this does not mean they must provide the highest or most vigilant level of care.[117] For example, a 2010 case from the Supreme Court of Connecticut held that a physician did not breach the standard of care for opioid prescribing simply because he did not contact the patient's reported previous providers and pharmacies.[118] Conversely, one significant deviation from the standard of care can create liability.[104] Therefore, as we noted above, the existence of an adverse malpractice verdict does not indicate overall competency, a fact acknowledged by state medical boards, who traditionally regard patterns of malpractice liability as much more concerning than single incidents.[119]

The harm commonly involved in opioid prescribing cases is related to the medical sequela of survived overdose. However, a recent trend in medical malpractice cases is for the harms of "causing" addiction.[111] For example, the West Virginia Supreme Court held in 2015 that such cases were allowed under a comparative negligence standard—meaning the jury could decide to what extent the prescriber and the patient were to blame for the addiction.[120] Finally, if the patient dies from an overdose, providers may face wrongful death civil lawsuits. Generally, wrongful death suits require the patient's surviving family member to prove that the provider had a duty to the patient and breached that duty (by deviating from the standard of care), that the breach caused the patient's death, and that financial losses resulted.

Providers who are defendants in civil suits overwhelmingly settle their cases for a variety of practical reasons, including overall cost of defense, the ability to negotiate what is disclosed by the parties, and sometimes the ability to shield the individual identity of the provider.[121] Sometimes the provider's attorney can prevent disclosure to the National Practitioner Data Bank completely. Nevertheless, providers increase their ability to reach a favorable settlement if existing evidence, such as patient records, reveals careful prescribing. Careful practice also may help decrease the risk of repeated civil suits, which itself carries an increased risk of further malpractice actions.[121] Those who are careless, corrupt, or compromised by impairment can expect repeated legal entanglements beyond professional negligence.

PROFESSIONAL BOARD DISCIPLINE

In addition to civil lawsuits, providers may face investigation and discipline from their state professional board. The purpose of state professional licensure boards is to protect citizens from incompetent or substandard healthcare practice. In addition to creating educational, behavioral, and practice standards for initial licensure, they also investigate reports of poor practice and sanction providers through various mechanisms. Disciplinary actions are reactive in nature, but state boards typically can negotiate a variety of remedies, from mandatory education to conditional licensure, suspension, or even revocation.[122]

Professional board investigations and disciplinary actions often involve misprescribing,[123] specifically qualitative overprescribing and multi-class misprescribing most commonly. Misprescribing is one of the most common complaints to medical boards[124] and represents a significant percentage of the 41% increase in investigations and discipline between 2004 and 2014.[8] Investigations and disciplinary actions can arise from several sources, including citizen complaints to the state board, reports of criminal charges, disciplinary actions by a hospital, or notification of reports to the National Practitioner Data Bank.[27,125] Given the degree to which opioids attract media coverage and the overwhelming focus on the negative impact of opioids, it is unsurprising that state boards receive complaints from citizens and others about misprescribing. Some of these reports or complaints are elective (e.g., citizen or patient complaints) and some are mandatory (e.g., hospitals reporting adverse actions), depending upon the nature of the violation and the particular state law. There is also variation in what kinds of disciplinary actions state boards are required to share with boards in other states.[124]

At the conclusion of a state board investigation, the board will decide how to proceed. Options range from finding no violations to informal resolutions or agreements with the licensee (such as alternative to discipline programs) to moving forward with a formal administrative hearing.[124,126] In the case of an administrative hearing, the case is heard before a judge and includes presentation of evidence by both the board and the defendant.[126] The standard by which a board must prove a violation by the licensee varies by state but is typically either preponderance of the evidence (more likely than not) or clear and convincing evidence.[127] Avoiding a formal hearing is usually advantageous to the provider.

Prescribing-related morbidity or mortality that receives media coverage is more likely to attract attention from state boards. While malpractice verdicts and settlements are generally acted upon by state boards when they become a pattern, certain criminal convictions create automatic revocations of state licensure.[128] Criminal investigations alone frequently lead to state board scrutiny.[129] Further, in states where criminal convictions do not automatically revoke licensure, providers usually face revocation of their COR from the DEA for convictions involving controlled substances.[130] This is also true of state authorizations to prescribe controlled substances, leaving a provider technically able to provide care but unable to prescribe any of the many drugs with medical use in Schedules II through V.

CRIMINAL ACTIONS

The use of controlled substances in Schedules II through V can be viewed as compliance with medical treatment or a criminal act, depending upon the context. On either side of this reality are prescribing healthcare providers and law enforcement officers, who are faced with evaluating when prescribing falls outside medical practice.[131] Both groups have the ultimate goal of improving the health and safety of citizens, but their missions sometimes collide. One of us has previously described this tension as follows:

> Law enforcement inhabits a professional space in which drugs (including abused prescription drugs) are the enemy: dangerous, deadly, and harmful. Physicians inhabit a professional space in which prescription drugs are useful tools, often helpful, and rarely deadly. These professional spaces converge at controlled substances, most of which have simultaneous potential for causing great harm and for providing great benefit, depending on the particular circumstances and context. It is interpreting those circumstances where the cultural collision is most profound.[9]

Drug enforcement agencies at the federal and state levels sometimes investigate prescribers, and the extent to which they do so has increased significantly in recent years.[8,132] At the federal level, providers are most often charged with violating the CSA; sometimes they are charged with misdemeanor or felony misbranding violations of the FDCA.[133] If convicted and the prescription caused a death, misprescribers face an enhanced penalty of a minimum of 20 years in prison.[134] At the state level, they may also be charged with violations of the state controlled substances law. Moreover, providers may face criminal charges for the death of a patient, such as manslaughter or negligent homicide.[8] While civil suits and professional board actions threaten financial and professional damage or even personal ruin, criminal charges additionally threaten the loss of the most basic liberties through imprisonment.

In criminal proceedings, the government, through a prosecutor, brings the legal action against the defendant alleging violation of particular state or federal laws. For example, a federal attorney general will prosecute a prescriber under the CSA if the underlying evidence collected by federal law enforcement officers supports the charges. In order to secure a conviction, the prosecutor must prove every element of a crime beyond a reasonable doubt. Typically, criminal laws include elements of both a particular mental state (*mens rea*) and a particular criminal action (*actus rea*). The common mental states are purposely or intentionally, knowingly or willfully, recklessly, and negligently.[135,136] The *mens rea* requirement is particularly controversial in prescribing cases.[131]

As previously explained, under the CSA, it is "unlawful for any person to *knowingly or intentionally* . . . manufacture, distribute, or dispense . . . a controlled substance."[137] The *mens rea* requirement is knowingly; the *actus rea* is distributing, dispensing, possessing, or manufacturing controlled substances.[138] Prescribers are distributing or dispensing when they prescribe opioids. However, they are exempt under the statute from criminal liability when they issue a prescription for a "legitimate medical purpose in the usual course of professional practice."[139] Therefore, to secure a conviction, the government must prove that the prescriber (1) knowingly prescribed a controlled substance, (2) without a legitimate medical purpose, (3) outside the course of professional practice.[94]

In *United States v. Katz*, the Court explained the knowingly element, stating that defendant prescribers must have "actual knowledge of the illegal activity or deliberately failed to inquire about it before taking action to support it."[140] Prosecution and convictions under the CSA are rarely controversial when the defendant prescriber has actual knowledge of a criminal endeavor. These types of misprescribers fall squarely within the corrupt category and criminal remedies are appropriate.

However, the knowingly requirement can also be met if the defendant prescriber deliberately failed to inquire about illegal activity before prescribing. This is justified by the legal theory of willful blindness, under which the deliberate avoidance of inquiry—often described as putting your head in the sand—is interpreted as the knowing or reckless *mens rea* of the particular crime. Several federal courts have upheld convictions of prescribers under a theory of willful blindness, which is met if the provider ignores repeated warnings and red flags and fails to conduct basic screenings.[141] The knowing act of ignoring obvious information substitutes for actual knowledge of criminal activity.

When a theory of willful blindness is advanced to meet the *mens rea* requirement in prescribing cases, evidence of standard of care (normally a civil standard) is typically used to demonstrate that the defendant (1) missed warning signs that providers would not miss unless they did so deliberately and (2) failed to conduct screenings that providers routinely conduct. Advocates for prescribers criticize this approach as essentially criminalizing malpractice. This approach is also criticized because the *mens rea* and *actus rea* collapse into one another. This is because standard-of-care evidence is also used to show that the interaction was not part of the legitimate practice of medicine and outside the course of professional practice. In other words, evidence of prescribing below the standard of care is used to prove criminal behavior, the appropriate remedy for which is malpractice.

In fact, there are a number of well-publicized criminal prosecutions of physicians—although not typically convictions—that demonstrate the dangers of this approach.[142] It is not clear just how far below the standard of care prescribers must fall to be outside the legitimate practice of medicine. Even the DEA has acknowledged the definitional difficulties, saying

> Throughout the 90 years that this requirement has been a part of U.S. law, the courts have recognized that there are no definitive criteria laying out precisely what is legally permissible, as each patient's medical situation is unique and must be evaluated based on the entirety of the circumstances. DEA cannot modify or expand upon this longstanding legal requirement through the publication or endorsement of guidelines.[143]

In 2014, a federal appellate court explained that "there are no specific guidelines concerning what is required to support a conclusion that an accused acted outside the usual course of professional practice. Rather, the courts must engage in a case-by-case analysis."[94]

Despite the imprecise nature of these inquiries, the facts of most criminal convictions of prescribers support the idea that while standard-of-care evidence is used, the deviations are far beyond substandard care. The Court in *United States v. Feingold* explained that simply falling below the standard of care (a bad doctor) is not enough; instead, the defendant must act "as a 'pusher' whose conduct is without a legitimate medical justification."[144] In 2014, another federal court explained that falling below the standard of care was not enough. Once jurors decide that the defendant practiced below the standard of care, they must decide if the behavior was simply negligent or if it went far beyond negligent to a place in which the doctor had become a "criminal drug dealer."[145]

Investigators and prosecutors should carefully evaluate the evidence with the assistance of both credible prescribing experts and state boards. In most cases of misprescribing, such as by those who are careless or compromised, malpractice or state board discipline is more appropriate. The penalties of a criminal investigation and prosecution alone are overwhelming to the accused and government resources are better expended on corrupt prescribers.

CONCLUSION

This chapter can only present broad concepts related to opioid prescribing law and regulation. Opioids occupy a unique space at the intersection of law and healthcare—they are steeped in US historical and cultural tradition, including the structural and legal separation of medicine and addiction; the criminalization of addiction; individualistic attitudes about the nature of suffering, pain, and addiction; and deeply held stigma against the people who live with those disorders. Prescribers are both part of this culture and caught in the crossfire of a current environment disposed to black-and-white solutions over the nuance that the complexity of opioid use and abuse requires. Opioid prescribing is an area of practice that threatens perhaps the most diverse pathways for legal scrutiny—federal and state civil, criminal, and administrative proceedings are possible. Weighing this reality against the professional and ethical fiduciary obligation to patients is a task that requires thoughtful engagement on the subject. Moving forward, we urge policymakers to carefully examine the evidence around opioids and use precise language around misprescribing. We have suggested four kinds of misprescribing in this chapter: qualitative overprescribing, quantitative overprescribing, multi-class prescribing, and underprescribing. It is also imperative that research around the characteristics of misprescribers continues to inform prevention and rehabilitative efforts. We have provided an alternative framework to the current 3D model. We hope this chapter provides prescribers, administrators, law enforcement officials, and policymakers a window into the complexity of the issue and compels careful, contextual study of opioid-related issues before any actions are taken.

REFERENCES

1. Keehan SP, Stone DA, Poisal JA, et al. National health expenditure projections, 2016–25: price increases, aging push sector to 20 percent of economy. *Health Affairs* 2017;3(36):553–563.

2. Federation of State Medical Boards, *2016 Annual Report: Building Value.* https://www.fsmb.org/Media/Default/PDF/Publications/FSMB_2016_Annual_Report.pdf. Accessed June 20, 2017.

3. US Department of Health & Human Services, Office of the Inspector General. A Roadmap for New Physicians: Fraud and Abuse Laws. https://oig.hhs.gov/compliance/physician-education/01laws.asp. Accessed June 20, 2017.

4. US Department of Health & Human Services. Health Information Privacy, The HIPAA Privacy Rule. https://www.hhs.gov/hipaa/for-professionals/privacy/index.html. Accessed June 20, 2017.

5. Webster LR, Grabois M. Current regulation of opioid prescribing. *Phys Med Rehab.* 2015;7:S236–247.

6. Johnson SH. Regulating physician behavior: taking bad law claims seriously. *St. Louis University Law Journal.* 2009;53:973–988.

7. Johnson SH. Legal and ethical perspectives in pain management. *Anesthesia Analgesia* 2007;105(1):5–7.

8. Yang YT, Larochelle MR, Harrajee RL. Managing increasing liability risks related to opioid prescribing. *Am J Med*. 2017;130(3): 249–250.

9. Dineen KK, DuBois JM. Between a rock and a hard place: can physicians prescribe opioids to treat pain adequately while avoiding legal sanction? *Am J Law Med*. 2016;42(1):7–52.

10. Hofman J. Patients in pain, and a doctor who must limit drugs. *New York Times*. March 16, 2016. https://www.nytimes.com/2016/03/17/health/er-pain-pills-opioids-addiction-doctors.html. Accessed July 15, 2017.

11. Zara C. Treated like addicts. *Vice News*. October 24, 2016. https://news.vice.com/story/opioids-chronic-pain. Accessed June 20, 2017.

12. Schattman ME. A glimmer of hope in American pain medicine? *J Pain Res*. 2016;9:509–513.

13. Dineen KK. Addressing prescription opioid abuse concerns in context: synchronizing policy solutions to multiple complex public health problems. *Law Psychol Rev*. 1 (2016).

14. Joffee S, Truog R. Consent to medical care: the importance of fiduciary context. In: FG Miller, A. Wertheimer, eds., *The Ethics of Consent: Theory and Practice*. 2010: 347–374.

15. Dubois JM. *Ethics in Mental Health Research*. New York: Oxford University Press; 2008.

16. Jones CM, Mack KA, Paulozzi LJ. Research letter: pharmaceutical overdose deaths, 2010. United States. *JAMA*. 2013;309(7):657–659.

17. Hermer LD, Brody H. Defensive medicine, cost containment, and reform. *J Gen Internal Med*. 2010;25(5):470–473.

18. Fry E. Here's who Americans blame most for the opioid epidemic. *Fortune*. June 21, 2017.

19. Kennedy-Hendricks A, et al. Primary care physicians' perspectives on the prescription opioid epidemic. *Drug Alcohol Depend*. 2016;165(1).

20. Herrick WR. *Second Annual Report of the Narcotic Drug Control Commission*, State of New York. J. B. Lyon Co.; 1920:1–41.

21. Peppin JF, et al. The complexity model: a novel approach to improve chronic pain care. *Pain Med*. 2015;16:653–666.

22. Cheatle, MD, Gallagher RM, O'Brien CP. Low risk of producing an opioid use disorder in primary care by prescribing opioids to prescreened patients with chronic noncancer pain. *Pain Medicine* 2017; https://doi.org/10.1093/pm/pnx032.

23. Sawicki NN. Character, competence, and the principles of medical discipline. *J Health Care Law Policy*. 2010;13:285.

24. Meyer DJ, Price M. Peer review committees and state licensing boards: responding to allegations of physician misconduct. *J Am Acad Psychiatry Law Online*. 2012;40(2):193–201.

25. National Council of State Boards of Nursing. *About Boards of Nursing*. https://www.ncsbn.org/about-boards-of-nursing.htm. Accessed July 15, 2017.

26. Federation of State Medical Boards. *Essentials of a State Medical and Osteopathic Practice Act* (2015) at 3. http://www.fsmb.org/Media/Default/PDF/FSMB/Advocacy/GRPOL_essentials.pdf.

27. Bal AK, Bal BS. Medicolegal sidebar: state medical boards and physician disciplinary actions, *Clin Orthop Rel Res*. 2014;472(1):28–31.

28. National Council of State Boards of Nursing. *Consensus Model for APRN Regulation*. https://www.ncsbn.org/Consensus_Model_for_APRN_Regulation_July_2008.pdf.

29. Herman J. Prescriptive authority update 2017. *Contemp Clinic*, June 3, 2017. http://contemporaryclinic.pharmacytimes.com/journals/issue/2017/june2017/prescriptive-authority-update-2017. Accessed July 31, 2017.

30. American Dental Association. *Statement on the Use of Opioids in the Treatment of Dental Pain*. http://www.ada.org/en/about-the-ada/ada-positions-policies-and-statements/statement-on-opioids-dental-pain. Accessed August 1, 2017.

31. American Association of Nurse Practitioners. *State Practice Environment*. https://www.aanp.org/legislation-regulation/state-legislation/state-practice-environment. Accessed August 1, 2017.

32. 20 Mo. C.S.R. 2200-41.000.

33. 21 C.F.R.§1301(2014).

34. US Department of Justice. *DEA Practitioner Manual* (2006), at 4. https://www.deadiversion.usdoj.gov/pubs/manuals/pract/pract_manual012508.pdf. Accessed July 23, 2017.

35. Barnes MC, Arndt G. The best of both worlds: applying federal commerce and state police powers to reduce prescription drug abuse. *J Health Care Law Policy*. 2013;16:271.

36. US Department of Justice, Drug Enforcement Agency, Division of Diversion Control, Instructions for Application Form 224, Section 4. http://www.deadiversion.usdoj.gov/drugreg/reg_apps/224/224_instruct.htm. Accessed August 10, 2017.

37. Morgan P. The legislation of drug law. In: J Weismann, RL Dupont. *Criminal Justice and Drugs: The Unresolved Connection*. New York: Kennikat Press; 1982.

38. Courtwright DT. *Dark Paradise: A History of Opiate Addiction in America*. Cambridge, MA: Harvard College; 2001.

39. Harrison Narcotic Tax Act, Pub. L. 223, Stat.785 (1914) (later codified at 26 U.S.C. § 4701 et. seq.).

40. Terry CE. The Harrison Anti-Narcotic Act. *Am J Pub Health*. 1915;5(6):518.

41. Harrison Narcotic Tax Act, §2 (a).

42. Controlled Substances Act of 1970, Pub. L. 91-513, 84 Stat. 1236 (1970) (codified at 21 U.S.C. § 801 et. seq.).

43. Stanley LL. Morphinism. *J Am Institute Criminal Law Criminology*. 1915;6(4):586–593.

44. Institute of Medicine. *Federal Regulation of Methadone Treatment*. Washington, DC: National Academies Press; 1995.

45. *Webb v. United States*, 249 U.S. 96 (1919).

46. King R. The Narcotics Bureau and the Harrison Act: jailing the healers and the sick. *Yale Law Journal*. 1953;62:736.

47. *United States v. Doremus*, 249 U.S. 86 (1919).

48. Merrill JO. Policy progress for physician treatment of opiate addiction. *J Gen Internal Med*. 2002;17(5):361–368.

49. Maurer D, Vogel VH. *Narcotics and Narcotic Addiction*. Springfield, IL: Charles C. Thomas; 1962:19.

50. US Department of Health & Human Services. Medication assisted treatment for opioid use disorders. 81 Federal Register 44711. July 8, 2016. https://www.federalregister.gov/documents/2016/07/08/2016-16120/medication-assisted-treatment-for-opioid-use-disorders. Accessed August 17, 2017.

51. Volkow ND, et al. Medication assisted therapies—tackling the opioid overdose epidemic. *N Engl J Med*. 2014;370(22):2063–2066.

52. Potter JS, et al. The multi-site opioid addiction treatment study: 18-month outcomes. *J Substance Abuse Treatment*. 2015;48:62–69.

53. Davis CS, Carr DH. The law and policy of opioids for pain management, addiction treatment, and overdose reversal. *Industrial Health Law Rev*. 2017;14:1.

54. Pure Food and Drug Act of 1906 (P.L. 59-384, 34 Stat. 768) (1906).

55. Federal Food, Drug, & Cosmetic Act, Pub. L. No. 111-31, 52 Stat. 1040 (1938)(codified as amended at 21 U.S.C. §301 et seq.) (2017)).

56. Drug Amendments of 1962, Pub. L. 87–781, 76 Stat. 780 (Oct. 10, 1962).

57. 21 U.S.C. § 352(y).

58. US Food & Drug Administration. *A History of Drug Regulation in the United States*, at 7. http://www.fda. gov/downloads/AboutFDA/WhatWeDo/History/ProductRegulation/PromotingSafeandEffectiveDru gsfor100Years/UCM114468.pdf. Accessed August 19, 2017.

59. 21 U.S.C. 353(b)(2016).

60. Hutt PB, Merrill RA, Grossman CA. *Food and Drug Law: Cases and Materials*. 4th ed. Foundation Press; 2013.

61. U.S. Department of Health and Human Services, Food & Drug Administration, *Understanding Unapproved Uses of Approved Drugs Off-Label*, May 17, 2017. http://www.fda.gov/forpatients/other/offlabel/default. htm. Accessed August 2, 2017.

62. Comprehensive Drug Abuse and Prevention & Control Act of 1970, 21 U.S.C. §801 et. seq.

63. US Department of Justice, Drug Enforcement Agency. DEA Fact Sheet. https://www.dea.gov/docs/ DEA_Factsheet_june2016.pdf. Accessed August 21, 2017.

64. Uniform Law Commission. Uniform Controlled Substances Act. http://www.uniformlaws.org/Narrative. aspx?title=Why%20States%20Should%20Adopt%20UCSA. Accessed July 27, 2017.

65. 21 U.S.C. § 812.

66. 21 C.F.R.§ 1308.11.

67. 21 C.F.R.§§1301.32.

68. 21 U.S.C. § 812(b).

69. 21 C.F.R.§1308.12.

70. US Department of Justice, Drug Enforcement Administration. *Schedules of Controlled Substances: Rescheduling of Hydrocodone Combination Products from Schedule III to Schedule II*, 79 Federal Register 163, 49661 (August 22, 2014) (amending 21 C.F.R. 1308).

71. 21 C.F.R.§ 1308.13.

72. 21 C.F.R.§ 1308.14.

73. 21 C.F.R.§ 1306.

74. American Academy of Pain Medicine. *State Legislative Updates*. http://www.painmed.org/advocacy/ state-updates/. Accessed August 26, 2017.

75. Indiana Senate Enrolled Act 226, Creating Indiana Code § 1. IC 25-1-9.7, http://iga.in.gov/legislative/ 2017/bills/senate/226#document-b9523207. Accessed August 21, 2017.

76. 21 U.S.C. §§811(f) & 812.

77. US Department of Health & Human Services, Food and Drug Administration, Center for Drug Evaluation and Research. *Manual of Policies and Procedures*, 4200.3 Rev. 1, March 6, 2017. https:// www.fda.gov/downloads/aboutfda/centersoffices/officeofmedicalproductsandtobacco/cder/ manualofpoliciesprocedures/ucm073580.pdf. Accessed August 1, 2017.

78. 21 U.S.C. §§811(f).

79. Food and Drug Administration Amendments Act, P.L. 110-85, 121 Stat. 823 (2007).

80. 21 U.S.C. § 355-1(a)(2)(2017).

81. 21 U.S.C. § 355-1(f)(2017).

82. US Department of Health & Human Services, Food and Drug Administration, *Approved REMS for Extended Release and Long Action Opioid Analgesics*, last updated June 2015, http://www.fda.gov/downloads/ Drugs/DrugSafety/PostmarketDrugSafetyInformationforPatientsandProviders/UCM311290.pdf. Accessed July 30, 2017.

83. 21 U.S.C. § 333.

84. 21 U.S.C. § 352(y).

85. 21 U.S.C. §355(o)(4).

86. US Department of Health & Human Services, Food & Drug Administration, *Response Letter from FDA CDER to Baltimore Department of Health*, August 31, 2016, https://www.regulations.gov/document?D=FDA-2016-P-0689-0003. Accessed August 2, 2017.

87. Jones C, McAninch J. Emergency department visits and overdose deaths from combined use of opioids and benzodiazepines. *Am J Prev Med*. 2015;49(4):493–501.

88. Park T, Saitz R, Ganoczy D, Ilgen M, Bohnert A. Benzodiazepine prescribing patterns and deaths from drug overdose among U.S. veterans receiving opioid analgesics: case-cohort study. *BMJ* 2015;350:h2698.

89. 21 U.S.C. § 846.

90. Barnes MC, Sklaver SL. Active verification and vigilance: a method to avoid civil and criminal liability when prescribing controlled substances, *DePaul J Health Care Law*. 2013;15:93.

91. 21 C.F.R. § 1306.04.

92. 21 U.S.C. §§ 353(b), 802(21), & 829(b).

93. *United States v. Moore*, 423 U.S. 122 (1975).

94. *United States v. Boccone*, 556 Fed.Appx. 215, 228 (4th Cir. 2014).

95. *Gonzales v. Oregon*, 546 U.S. 243, 274 (2006).

96. Alford DP. Opioid prescribing for chronic pain: achieving the right balance through education. *N Engl J Med*. 2016;374(4):301–303.

97. Hill MV, et al. Wide variation and excessive dosage of opioid prescriptions for common general surgical procedures. *Ann Surg*. 2017;265:4.

98. Maughan BC, et al. Unused opioid analgesics and drug disposal following outpatient dental surgery: a randomized controlled trial. *Drug Alcohol Depend*. 2016;168:328–334.

99. Keilman J. Doctors consider consequences of new Vicodin rules. *Chicago Tribune*. October 6, 2014.

100. Cicero TJ, et al. Multiple determinants of specific modes of prescription opioid diversion. *J Drug Issues*. 2011;41(2):283–304.

101. Foreman J. *A Nation in Pain: Healing Our Biggest Healthcare Problem*. New York: Oxford University Press; 2014:126–127.

102. US Department of Health & Human Services, Substance Abuse & Mental Health Services Administration. *Drug Abuse Warning Network, 2011: National Estimates of Drug Related Emergency Department visits (DAWN Drug Related Visits Study)*. HHS Publication No. (SMA) 13-4760, DAWN Series D-39 (2013).

103. Dasgupta N, Funk MJ, Proescholdbell S, Hirsch A, Ribisl KM, Marshall S. Cohort study of the impact of high-dose opioid analgesics on overdose mortality. *Pain Med*. 2016;17:85–98.

104. Rich BA, Webster LR. A review of forensic implications of opioid prescribing with examples from malpractice cases involving opioid-related overdose. *Pain Med*. 2011;12:S59–65.

105. Khaliq AA, et al. Disciplinary action against physicians: who is likely to get disciplined? *Am J Med*. 2005;118:773–777.

106. Heumann M, et al. Prescribing justice: the law and politics of discipline for physician felony offenders. *Boston University Public Interest Law Journal*. 2008;17:1.

107. Wesson DR, Smith DE. Prescription drug abuse: patient, physician, and cultural responsibilities in addiction medicine [special issue]. *West J Med*. 1990;152:613–616.

108. Longo LP, et al. Addiction: Part II. Identification and management of drug seeking patients. *Am Fam Physician*. 2000;61:2121–2128.

109. Voth EA. Prescribing controlled substances reconsidered. *J Global Drug Policyy Practice*. 2008;2:1.

110. Dubois, JM, Chibnall JT, Anderson, EE, et al. A mixed method analysis of reports on 100 cases of improper prescribing of controlled substances. *J Drug Issues*. 2016;46:4.

111. Messenger T. St. Louis jury sends $17.6 million message in opioid abuse verdict. *St. Louis Post Dispatch*. June 28, 2016. http://www.stltoday.com/news/local/columns/tony-messenger/

messenger-st-louis-jury-sends-million-message-in-opioid-abuse/article_b7628f83-0e94-5bc7-a2a8-38a12ab6d7d6.html. Accessed July 2, 2017.

112. Stelfox HT, et al. The relation of patient satisfaction with complaints against physicians and malpractice lawsuits. *Am J Med.* 2005;118:1126–1133.

113. Federation of State Medical Boards. *U.S. Medical Regulatory Trends and Actions*, 1-82, 7 (May 2014).

114. Bal GS. An introduction to medical, alpractice in the United States. *Clin Orthop Rel Res.* 2009;467(2):339–347.

115. Johnson SH. Customary standards of care. *Hastings Center Report* 2013;43(6):9–10.

116. Zitter JM. Physician's liability for patient's addiction to or overdose from prescription drugs. ALR 6th 2009; 44: 391.

117. Brushwood D. Debunking myths of negligence in pain management practices. *J Pain Palliat Care Pharmacother.* 2007;21(1):47–52, 48.

118. *Dallaire v. Hsu*, 2010 WL2822494 (Sup. Ct. of Connecticut 2010).

119. FSMB. *U.S. Regulatory Trends.*

120. *Tug Valley Pharmacy* et al. *v. All Plaintiffs*, 2015 W.Va. LEXIS 673 (2015).

121. Studdert DM, Bismark MM, Mello MM, et al. Prevalence and characteristics of physicians prone to malpractice claims. *N Engl J Med.* 2016;374:354–362.

122. Thompson JN, Robin LA. State medical boards. *J Legal Med.* 2012;33(1):93–114.

123. Gilson A. State medical board members' attitudes about the legality of chronic prescribing to patients with noncancer pain. *J Pain Symptom Manage.* 2010;40(4)599–612.

124. Federation of State Medical Boards, U.S. Medical Regulatory Trends and Actions, 2016. http://www.fsmb.org/Media/Default/PDF/FSMB/Publications/us_medical_regulatory_trends_actions.pdf. Accessed July 30, 2017.

125. US Department of Health & Human Services. *National Practitioner Data Bank Guidebook.* https://www.npdb.hrsa.gov/resources/aboutGuidebooks.jsp?page=APreface.jsp. Accessed July 1, 2017.

126. National Council of State Boards of Nursing. *Board Proceedings.* https://www.ncsbn.org/672.htm. Accessed August 2, 2017.

127. Bricklin P, Bennett B, Carroll W. Understanding licensing board disciplinary proceedings. American Psychological Association. http://www.apapracticecentral.org/ce/state/disciplinary-procedures.pdf. Accessed August 15, 2017.

128. Mo.Rev.Stat. § 334.103.1.

129. Kim CJ. The trial of Conrad Murray: prosecuting physicians for negligent overprescribing. *American Criminal Law Review.* 2014;51:517.

130. 21 U.S.C. §§ 824.

131. Hoffmann D. Treating pain versus reducing drug diversion and abuse. *St. Louis Univ J Health Law Policy.* 2008;1:231.

132. Joseph T. Rannazzisi, Deputy Asst. Director, Drug Enforcement Agency, US Department of Justice, *Statement for the Record: Responding to the Prescription Drug Abuse Epidemic*, US Senate Caucus on International Narcotics Control (July 18, 2012). http://www.dea.gov/pr/speeches-testimony/2012-2009/responding-to-prescription-drug-abuse.PDF.

133. 21 U.S.C. §§ 331, 333.

134. *Burrage v. United States*,134 S. Ct. 881(2014).

135. Model Penal Code § 2.02.

136. US Court of Appeals, Chapter 5: Mental States, http://www.ca3.uscourts.gov/sites/ca3/files/Chapter%205%20Rev%20Jan%202014.pdf. Accessed August 22, 2017.

137. 21 U.S.C. § 846.

138. 21 U.S.C. § 811.

139. 21 C.F.R. § 1306.04.

140. *United States v. Katz,* 445 F.3d 1023, 1031 (8th Cir. 2006).

141. *United States v. Florez,* 368 F.3d 1042, 1044 (8th Cir. 2004).

142. Silvergate H. *Three Felonies a Day.* New York: Encounter Books; 2011.

143. US Department of Justice, Drug Enforcement Agency. *Dispensing Controlled Substances in the Treatment of Pain,* 71 Federal Register 172, 52715-52723 (September 6, 2006).

144. *United States v. Feingold,* 454 F.3d 1001, 1007 (9th Cir. 2006).

145. *United States v. MacKay,* 20 F.Supp.3d 1287, at 1297 (D.Utah 2014).

CHAPTER 3

MONITORING PRESCRIPTIONS, THIRD-PARTY HEALTHCARE PAYERS, PRESCRIPTION BENEFIT MANAGERS, AND PRIVATE-SECTOR POLICY OPTIONS

John J. Coleman

INTRODUCTION

According to the Centers for Disease Control and Prevention (CDC), the abuse of prescription drugs, particularly opioids, has reached *epidemic* levels in the United States.[1] In 2015, there were 91 deaths each day, on average, from opioid-related overdoses (this figure includes prescription opioids and heroin).[1] The number of overdose deaths involving prescription drugs each year now exceeds the number of deaths from heroin and cocaine combined.[2] After increasing steadily since the 1990s, the death rate from the most common prescription opioids—oxycodone, hydrocodone, morphine, and methadone—declined slightly in 2012, only to rise again in 2013, 2014, and 2015.[3,4] In 2015, of the 52,404 drug overdose deaths reported in the United States, 33,091 (63.1%) involved an opioid. Nearly 13,000 of these deaths involved heroin.[4,5]

Besides causing overdose deaths, prescription opioid abuse is a major cause of hospital emergency department (ED) visits. Between 2004 and 2011, ED visits involving prescription opioids almost tripled, from 198,126 visits in 2004 to 556,551 visits in 2011.[6] Oxycodone, hydrocodone, methadone, and morphine were the top four categories of opioids involved in ED visits.[6] Between 2004 and 2011, the percentage of ED visits involving oxycodone

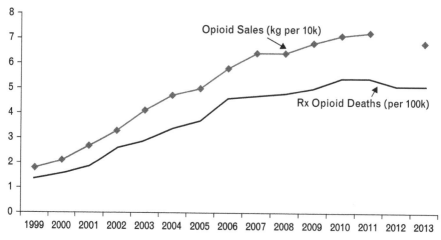

Source: CDC's National Vital Statistics System & DEA's Automation of Reports and Consolidated Orders System (ARCOS).

FIGURE 3.1 Opioid sales and prescription opioid overdose deaths in the United States, 1999–2013
Source: CDC (courtesy of Dr. Len Paulozzi)[10]

increased from 17.6 to 56.2 per 100,000 persons (219.3%).[6] The percentage involving hydrocodone increased from 15.9 to 31.2 per 100,000 persons (96.2%), the percentage involving methadone increased from 14.0 to 24.3 per 100,000 persons (73.6%), and the percentage involving morphine increased from 5.1 to 12.3 per 100,000 persons (141.2%).[6]

Comparing annual bulk sales of prescription opioids with deaths from their misuse, researchers from the CDC and Duke University School of Medicine discovered a close, almost parallel, relationship between the two, suggesting that the rate of fatal opioid overdose deaths is closely associated with, if not a direct correlate of, the rate of opioid sales[7,8] (Fig. 3.1).

MONITORING BULK DISTRIBUTIONS OF CONTROLLED SUBSTANCES

By law, manufacturers and wholesale distributors of controlled substances must report their bulk sales to the US Drug Enforcement Administration (DEA).[9,10] These reports are collected by DEA and archived in a database called ARCOS ("Automation of Reports and Consolidated Orders System"). ARCOS data show that distributions of several popular prescription opioids to pharmacies throughout the United States reached their peak in 2011 or 2012 and began to decline thereafter[11] (Fig. 3.2).

Contributing to this decline was the rescheduling of hydrocodone combination products in October 2014.[12] As of this date, all hydrocodone products were moved from Schedule III to Schedule II, a classification that increased regulatory controls on their prescribing and dispensing.[12] By October of the following year, prescriptions for hydrocodone products had

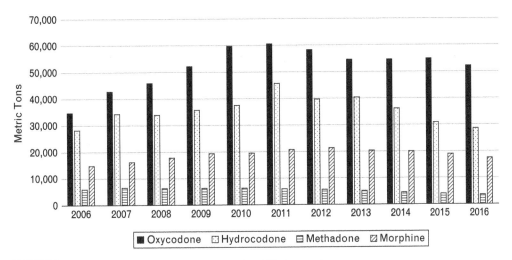

FIGURE 3.2 Volume of selected opioids distributed to US pharmacies

Source: DEA ARCOS[150]

declined 22%.[13] This decline was attributed to the elimination of automatic refills previously allowed when hydrocodone combination products were in Schedule III.[13]

Tracking bulk distributions of controlled substances to pharmacies provides a dependable measure of the volume of such drugs prescribed and dispensed for medical purposes.[14] Keeping track of these distributions is important because the lawful dispensing of controlled substances in the retail pharmacy setting remains a significant venue for drug diversion.[15] Although most dispensed drugs are properly obtained and used by legitimate patients, the total volume of drugs dispensed, particularly opioids, is so large, that even a relatively small percentage of fraudulent patients can account for a sizable quantity of diverted drugs.[16,17]

DEA reports that in 2013, drug manufacturers sold 16.2 billion dosage units of opioids to hospitals, pharmacies, and other authorized customers.[17] This was down 5.8% from the peak year of 2011, when 17.2 billion dosage units of opioids were sold.[17]

"Doctor shoppers," defined as persons visiting multiple doctors, posing as legitimate patients and feigning symptoms to obtain controlled substances by fraud, account for a sizable volume of diverted drugs.[16] In 2008, researchers studied 146.1 million opioid prescriptions written by 908,000 prescribers for 48.4 million patients.[16] They identified 135,000 patients as possible doctor shoppers ("extreme group"), based on the number of similar prescriptions they obtained from multiple prescribers during a 10-month period.[16] On average, each of the 135,000 patients obtained 32 opioid prescriptions from 10 different prescribers.[16]

Although the 135,000 suspected doctor shoppers accounted for a relatively small percentage of the total number of patients in the study—less than one-third of one percent—collectively they received about 4% of all opioids dispensed, or about 11.1 million grams, estimated to be the equivalent of approximately 5.4 million grams of morphine.[16] This, the researchers estimated, would have provided patients in the extreme group an average of 109 morphine equivalent milligrams per day for every day in 2008.[16]

PHARMACY THEFTS

Pharmacy thefts also constitute an important source of diverted drugs.[18] By law, all DEA registrants, including hospitals and pharmacies, must file written reports of thefts (and losses) of controlled substances as soon as discovered to the nearest DEA office.[19] Between 2009 and 2012, registrants reported 63,088 thefts of controlled substances to DEA.[20] Of this number, pharmacies accounted for 41,645 thefts (66%), followed by hospitals/clinics, with 12,265 thefts (19%).[20] Although commercial shipments of pharmaceuticals, including controlled substances, are occasionally targeted by professional cargo thieves, in recent years the use of covert GPS tracking devices in bulk drug shipments has greatly reduced the frequency of these crimes.[21]

In-house drug thefts from hospitals, including hospital pharmacies, have increased significantly within the past decade as street prices have climbed sharply for diverted prescription opioids and benzodiazepines. Most drug thefts in the clinical setting appear to be committed by healthcare professionals assigned to pharmacy or patient care facilities.[22]

HOSPITALS/CLINICS

In 2014, investigative reporters for *USA Today* reviewed more than 200 state and federal prosecutions involving drug diversion by healthcare providers.[23] Thirty cases (15%) involved persons stealing drugs for personal use.[23] Most cases (85%) involved doctors, nurses, and other hospital employees stealing and diverting drugs for profit, sometimes using prescription schemes in the commission of their crimes.[23]

An audit in 2014 of Beth Israel Medical Center in New York City uncovered irregularities in the inventory records of the hospital's central pharmacy.[24] An investigation resulted in the arrest of the pharmacy services director, who was charged with a number of criminal violations, including the theft of nearly 200,000 oxycodone tablets over a 5-year period.[24]

The street price for opioids is high, reaching a national average (in 2012) of $1 per milligram for hydrocodone and oxycodone tablets.[25] In the Beth Israel Medical Center case, media and police reports placed the street value of the stolen oxycodone tablets at $5.6 million.[24] The actual loss to the hospital, however, was reported to be about $212,000.[24] By this calculation, a single oxycodone tablet costing the hospital about $1.06, according to the police estimate, was worth as much as $28 on the street.[24]

Healthcare providers who steal drugs pose substantial risks to their employers as well as to the patients in their care.[26] In 2013, a traveling medical technician was sentenced to prison for infecting at least 45 patients with hepatitis C by contaminating their fentanyl syringes.[27] One patient died from the disease.[27] The technician had been employed by 10 hospitals in 8 states over a period of 4 years.[27] Following his arrest, the hospitals where he had worked had to notify thousands of patients of possible exposure to hepatitis C and provide them with expensive follow-up testing and care.[27] Besides facing a number of civil suits filed on behalf of harmed and potentially harmed patients, the hospitals received a good deal of adverse media coverage and a loss of public confidence in their healthcare services.[27,28]

THE HIDDEN COSTS OF OPIOID DIVERSION

More than 80% of the prescription opioid market is dominated by just two drugs, oxycodone and hydrocodone.[29] These also happen to be the most frequently abused opioids, according to government mortality and morbidity records.[30,31] US Food and Drug Administration (FDA) data show that between 2007 and 2011, retail pharmacies in the United States dispensed 560.6 million prescriptions for hydrocodone combination products and 251.4 million prescriptions for oxycodone products (immediate release [IR], extended release [ER], and combination).[a] By comparison, in the same period, only 33 million prescriptions for morphine products (IR and ER), and 10.6 million prescriptions for hydromorphone products were dispensed.[32]

Methadone, a popular and frequently abused opioid, was not included in the FDA analysis. Methadone, like buprenorphine, is indicated for treating opiate addiction as well as for treating pain but Schedule II methadone, unlike Schedule III buprenorphine, must be administered to patients receiving it for treatment of opiate addiction and cannot lawfully be prescribed for that purpose.[33]

Besides the social and health costs, the economic cost that prescription drug abuse imposes upon private and public insurance payers is significant. A 2009 Government Accountability Office (GAO) study examined reimbursement records for Medicaid beneficiaries in five states for fiscal years 2006 and 2007 and identified potentially fraudulent claims totaling more than $63 million submitted by 65,000 patients identified as likely doctor shoppers.[34] The latter were defined as claimants who had visited six or more doctors for the same controlled substance(s) within the 2-year study period.[34] To prevent this type of aberrant drug-seeking behavior, at least 20 states have laws requiring patients who are being prescribed controlled substances to disclose to the prescriber if they have obtained controlled substances from another prescriber within a specified period, typically within the past 30 days.[35]

The previously mentioned GAO report acknowledged that, by itself, merely obtaining controlled substances from multiple prescribers is not evidence of fraud or doctor shopping.[34] Even so, when GAO investigators recalibrated their search algorithm to identify claimants visiting multiple prescribers per month—a more probable fraud signal—they discovered that 400 of the 65,000 first-tier claimants had visited 21 to 112 different doctors and as many as 46 different pharmacies over the 2-year study period to acquire the same or similar controlled substances.[34]

A study of drug overdose deaths in Washington state by researchers from the CDC found that almost half (45.4%) of the 1,668 opioid-related overdose deaths between 2004 and 2007 involved Medicaid enrollees.[36] Patients with chronic pain often have comorbidities that are exacerbated by problematic use of opioids.[37] Overall, the cost of prescription opioid abuse is significant among such patients and represents billions of

---

a. In October 2014, hydrocodone combination products were reclassified as Schedule II controlled substances, meaning, among other things, that prescriptions for them no longer could be refilled automatically, if authorized, up to five times within six months.[12]

dollars a year in largely hidden economic costs.[38] Birnbaum et al. in 2011 estimated the total societal costs of prescription opioid abuse at $55.7 billion.[39] This total represented $25.6 billion in workplace costs, $25.0 billion in healthcare costs, and $5.1 billion in criminal justice costs.[39] These were estimates attributed solely to opioid abuse and did not include costs attributed to the abuse of other popular classes of prescription drugs, including stimulants and benzodiazepines.[39]

FLORIDA FIGHTS BACK

Strategies for addressing prescription drug abuse differ widely in cost and content: some emphasize tighter regulatory controls on medication access, while others focus on prosecuting wrongdoers, including rogue healthcare providers accused of diverting drugs.[40] Several states, notably Florida, Ohio, Kentucky, and Washington, have adopted drug control strategies that combine regulatory and law enforcement measures.[41–44]

Florida presents a good model for showing how comprehensive legislative reforms coupled with targeted policy initiatives reduced drug diversion and abuse. In 2010, drug-related overdose deaths in the state reached a peak of 9,001, of which 6,550 (72.8%) involved prescription opioids.[45] The following year, the state legislature declared a public health emergency and enacted sweeping legislation aimed at curbing *pill mills*—loosely defined as businesses posing as pain clinics selling controlled substances in bulk to persons pretending to be chronic pain patients.[46] The legislation prohibited physicians from dispensing controlled substances from their offices, required pain clinics to meet new standards for ownership and management, and required wholesale drug distributors to perform due diligence on customers and report to the state orders received for more than 5,000 dosage units of any controlled substance within a 1-month period.[46] In addition, pharmacies were required to report dispensing data for controlled substances to the state's Prescription Drug Monitoring Program (PDMP) within 7 days.[46]

Florida's new rules were accompanied by harsh penalties, some of which converted previously minor civil infractions to third-class criminal felonies punishable by fines and/or prison.[46] The impact of Florida's legislation was swift and impressive: within the first 6 months, nearly half of the estimated 1,000 pill mills in the state ceased operation.[47] By the end of 2012, opioid-related overdose deaths in Florida had declined 27% (from 13.6 to 9.9 per 100,000 persons).[48] Benzodiazepine-related overdose deaths declined 28.4% (from 6.9 to 5.0 per 100,000 persons).[48] Paradoxically, heroin-related overdose deaths increased 122.4% (from 0.3 to 0.6 per 100,000 persons).[48] However, compared with the number of deaths involving prescription opioids (2,042), the actual number of heroin-related overdose deaths (108) remained relatively small.[48] By the end of 2012, some 18 months after the new law took effect, the overall drug overdose death rate in Florida had declined 17.7% (from 17.0 to 14.0 per 100,000 persons).[48,49]

The closure of pill mills and the end of office dispensing of controlled substances in Florida increased the burden on pharmacies to meet the needs of patients on chronic opioid therapy.[50] According to media accounts, fear of harsh penalties for mistakenly filling fraudulent prescriptions—one of the new criminal law violations—caused some pharmacists to refuse to accept new patients, even those presenting valid prescriptions.[50,51] State officials, otherwise pleased with the law's results, expressed confidence that problems like this would resolve themselves in time as patients and providers adjust to the new rules.[52]

PRESCRIPTION DRUG MONITORING PROGRAMS (PDMP)

Monitoring the prescribing of drugs had its beginning in the spring of 1910 when the New York state legislature enacted a law permitting pharmacists to dispense cocaine to patients upon presentation of a physician's prescription.[53] The law required that the pharmacist retain and produce the prescription on demand to state inspectors. Failure to comply with this requirement could subject the pharmacist to a jail sentence of not more than 1 year and a fine of not more than $1,000, or both.[53]

The modern PDMP dates from 1939, when California adopted a "triplicate prescription program" requiring the use of state-issued three-part forms for prescribing regulated medications.[54] One copy of the completed prescription was to be forwarded to the state, a second copy was to be maintained in the patient's medical record, and the original was to be given to the patient to have filled.[54] In 1943, the territory of Hawaii adopted a similar program.[54] Between 1958 and 1988, five more states adopted PDMPs.[54] In the 1990s, using computer-based systems for the first time, seven more states established PDMPs.[54] Since then, all states have approved and/or adopted PDMPs. Today's PDMP is designed to collect data electronically from dispensing pharmacies rather than from prescribers.[54] Although all PDMPs share the same goal of preventing drug diversion and abuse, they may differ in their functional design and operation.[54]

In 2002, with the growing crisis of prescription opioid abuse looming, Congress appropriated funds to encourage the development of state PDMPs and directed the Department of Justice to manage what was called the Harold Rogers Prescription Drug Monitoring Program (HRPDMP), named for the Kentucky representative who spearheaded the legislation.[55] Federal grants were made available to states to weigh the feasibility of establishing a PDMP.[55] Generous startup grants were awarded to states enacting laws authorizing PDMPs.[55] Known popularly as "Rogers grants" and reauthorized annually by Congress, more than $48 million has been spent on this program since 2002.[55,56]

Rogers grants were welcomed by states needing to address the growing problem of prescription drug abuse but lacking sufficient resources or the political wherewithal to establish a PDMP on their own.[54] In 2005, additional PDMP funding was made available through the National All Schedules Prescription Electronic Reporting Act (NASPER).[56] Although HRPDMP and NASPER share a common goal, they have key differences in how each interfaces with state authorities. HRPDMP was the creation of Congress and its management by the Bureau of Justice Assistance gave it the imprimatur of the law enforcement community. NASPER, on the other hand, is the brainchild of the American Society of Interventional Pain Physicians (ASIPP), a group of physicians whose members advocated for an expanded use of the PDMP beyond simply collecting and storing prescription data.[56] In pressing for passage of NASPER, ASIPP members sought a national program modeled after a successful PDMP in Kentucky. The official name of the Kentucky PDMP is the Kentucky All Schedules Prescription Electronic Reporting Program (KASPER).[57] By August 2005, when NASPER was signed into law, besides the support of ASIPP, it had the support of the American Society of Anesthesiologists, the American Medical Association, and the American Association of Nurse Practitioners.[56]

After passage of NASPER, the PDMP program developed quickly as states eagerly sought federal grants to adopt programs endorsed by public safety *and* public health experts.[58] By the end of 2017, all states and the District of Columbia had approved PDMPs.

PDMP PRIVACY

In 1996, Congress enacted the Health Insurance Portability and Accountability Act (HIPAA).[60] The Act amended the Internal Revenue Code of 1986 to: improve the portability and continuity of health insurance coverage; combat waste, fraud, and abuse in health insurance and healthcare delivery; and address other issues.[60] Section 264 of the act required the Secretary of the Department of Health and Human Services (DHHS) to submit to Congress detailed recommendations on standards with respect to maintaining the privacy of individually identifiable health information.[60]

The Secretary's response was published in 2003 and immediately became known as the HIPAA Privacy Rule.[60] Although the rule preempts any state law that is contrary to it, the Secretary may exempt its application if, for example, a state law permitting the sharing of individually identifiable health information is deemed necessary to prevent fraud and abuse in the provision of healthcare, or is needed and intended to regulate the distribution, dispensing, or control of any drug defined as a controlled substance by federal or state law.[61,62]

To qualify for a HIPAA exemption, state laws authorizing PDMPs must meet at least one of the aforementioned criteria.[62] To help the states meet this requirement, the National Alliance of State Model Drug Laws (NASMDL) provided a draft model state law for PDMPs that, among other things, included privacy provisions satisfying state and federal requirements.[63,64] NASMDL is a nonprofit private organization and successor to the President's Commission on Model State Drug Laws.[63,64]

In 1972, New York's PDMP was challenged in court over privacy claims asserted on behalf of medical records being stored in a third-party computerized database.[65] The case eventually reached the US Supreme Court, which held, in essence, that the threat of an unlawful disclosure of patient information from a health record—principal grounds asserted by the plaintiffs—was insufficient to overcome a legitimate need of the state to prevent drug diversion.[65] In reaching its decision, the Court noted that other computerized databanks are properly used to maintain massive government files, including those used to collect taxes, distribute welfare and social security benefits, and so forth.[65]

Individual privacy violations continue to be litigated on a case-by-case basis when and if an unauthorized release or compromise of PDMP data occurs. In Tennessee, for example, a police officer who requested that a local pharmacist perform a PDMP check on a superior whom the officer believed was acting suspiciously was terminated from the department upon discovery of the unauthorized access/use of the PDMP data.[66] A state court of appeals upheld the officer's firing.[66]

In 2014, the confidentiality of state PDMP data was upheld by a federal district court in Oregon that ruled against the use of administrative subpoenas by DEA to obtain PDMP information.[67] The court found that in order to access PDMP data lawfully, the state statute required "a valid court order based on probable cause for an authorized drug-related investigation of an individual."[67] A DEA administrative or office subpoena issued without judicial oversight, the court said, did not satisfy this requirement.[67]

All states and the District of Columbia have detailed rules governing access to PDMP information.[63] Most states require some form of judicial process in criminal cases (e.g., affidavit of probable cause, search warrant, subpoena) and/or a written request from an authorized agency official or prosecutor pursuant to an active investigation or prosecution.[58] Two states (Virginia and Oklahoma) permit law enforcement disclosures only in response to a grand jury subpoena/request.[58]

The model PDMP statute proposed by NASMDL and adopted in whole or in part by most states devotes an entire section, amounting to more than two pages, to define the parameters for access and use of PDMP data. Despite these privacy concerns—or perhaps as a result of them—after more than a decade of operation, only a handful of cases involving unlawful access or disclosure of PDMP data have been reported.[68]

THE CHANGING PDMP

Early PDMPs were intended to identify prescribers suspected of diverting controlled substances.[53] Understandably, the first PDMPs were established in populous states like New York and California where, contrary to law, medicalized drug addiction was prevalent.[53,54] The first PDMPs required the use of state-issued, serialized paper forms for prescribing medications containing opium and cocaine and their derivatives—known today as *controlled substances*.[69]

The early PDMPs were inefficient because of the cost and time needed to hand-process thousands of paper forms each month.[53,54] This, however, changed dramatically with the development of microprocessors capable of quickly collecting, sorting, archiving, and retrieving vast amounts of data.[70]

Today's PDMP relies exclusively on electronic records automatically transmitted to a secure state computer directly from dispensing pharmacies.[70] As of April 2017, there were 71,665 pharmacies in the United States with active DEA registrations.[71] Most use specialized software to record sales of prescription drugs for insurance, regulatory, and inventory purposes.[72] The software isolates dispensing data for controlled substances that, in turn, are uploaded electronically to the state's PDMP on a schedule determined by state law or regulation.[72] Currently, only one state (Oklahoma) requires real-time reporting. Fifteen states require reporting within 24 hours, while five states require reporting within 72 hours. Twenty-six states require reporting within 7 days, and one state (Hawaii) requires reporting monthly.[58] These reporting schedules in force as of 2016 are expected to change to real time as systems are upgraded and modernized.[58]

As previously mentioned, NASMDL has actively promoted PDMPs on a national basis, receiving grants from the Office of National Drug Control Policy and other federal agencies for its work in preparing and disseminating a model statute to meet state and federal requirements.[73] Most states have used some form of the NASMDL model, adjusted as necessary to meet local requirements, such as data reporting timeframes.[74]

States choosing to use the NASMDL model statute are not obliged to adopt *all* the recommended provisions, and many, for example, have chosen *not* to include the form of payment in their data collection/reporting requirements.[74] This eliminates the ability of the PDMP to track cash payments for prescriptions of controlled substances—a potential signal of doctor shopping by persons seeking to avoid leaving traceable records.[16]

As of June 30, 2015, 35 states permit practitioners to access the PDMP for their patients' records.[58] At least six states have provisions mandating that prescribers, under certain circumstances, check a patient's PDMP record *before* commencing treatment with controlled substances and/or during specified intervals when long-term treatment with controlled substances is expected or indicated.[58]

As state officials become familiar with PDMPs, they are finding new uses for the rich data they collect. For example, six states (Washington, Montana, North Dakota, Utah, Arizona, and Ohio) currently permit PDMP access by worker's compensation specialists, two states (Washington and Wisconsin) permit access by Department of Corrections officials, and two states (North Dakota and Kentucky) permit access by probation/parole officers.[58] Most PDMPs, under limited circumstances, permit access by patients as well as parents of minor children.[58] Thirteen states permit access by mental health/substance abuse professionals, or officials representing peer review committees or quality improvement committees of hospitals.[58]

Besides allowing access to PDMP data for these purposes, some states that use the NASMDL model permit anonymized PDMP data to be used for statistical, research, public policy, and educational purposes.[74] This is important to ensure not only integrity in the PDMP process itself, but also to evaluate individual state programs, identify best practices, ascertain educational and training needs for prescribers and dispensers, and provide statistical information for public dissemination on the volume and types of controlled substances dispensed in the state.[74]

The medical community's embrace of the PDMP program, although improved over the past two decades, remains problematic.[75] Since 2002, there have been more than 200 articles in the medical literature published on prescription monitoring programs.[76] Some are statistical in nature and exist as a result of state laws permitting access to PDMP anonymized data for research purposes.[76] Some provide useful analyses and methods for identifying potential doctor shoppers.[76] Others test a hypothetical view, calculating, for example, the volume of opioids dispensed in states before and after the adoption of active PDMPs to determine if the presence of the PDMP influences prescribing and dispensing practices.[76] Most decry the underutilization of these programs by prescribers and dispensers of controlled substances.

BRIEF LITERATURE REVIEW OF PDMP EFFECTIVENESS

Reisman et al. in 2009 conducted a retrospective review of prescription opioid shipments to 14 states with PDMPs and 36 states without PDMPs, using data from DEA's ARCOS database for the period 1997 to 2003. The researchers measured "abuse" by using data from the Treatment Episode Data Sets (TEDS).[77] Increasing prescription oxycodone shipments were significantly associated with increasing prescription opioid treatment admission rates ($p < .001$).[77] PDMP states had significantly lower oxycodone shipments than the control group.[77] PDMP states had less increase in prescription opioid treatment admissions per year ($p = .063$).[77] A patient admitted to an inpatient drug abuse rehabilitation program in a PDMP state was less likely to be admitted for prescription opioid drug abuse (odds ratio [OR] = 0.775, 95% confidence interval [CI] 0.764–0.785).[77]

Paulozzi et al. in 2011 measured the relationship of PDMPs to rates of death from drug overdoses and quantities of opioid drugs distributed at the state level. Findings showed that PDMP states consumed significantly greater amounts of Schedule III hydrocodone products (hydrocodone products were rescheduled from Schedule III to Schedule II in October 2014[12]) and nonsignificantly lower amounts of Schedule II opioids.[78] The researchers concluded that PDMPs are potentially important for preventing the nonmedical use of controlled substances, but their impact is not reflected in drug mortality rates.[78]

A four-page letter to the editor of *Pain Medicine* by Green et al. in 2011 criticized this study by Paulozzi et al., stating, for example, that reduction of drug-related mortality was not a goal or purpose of the PDMP program to begin with and therefore should not have been used as a measurement of its effectiveness.[79] Green et al. added that the Paulozzi et al. study took place from 1999 to 2005, when only limited access to PDMP data by healthcare professionals was permitted; hence, the assessment of PDMPs as being something other than a restricted law enforcement tool was questionable.[79]

Wilsey et al. in 2011 examined data from the California PDMP, also known as the Controlled Substance Utilization Review and Evaluation System (CURES), to identify the characteristics of patients who visited two to five prescribers, compared with those visiting only one prescriber.[80] Previously, Parente et al. in 2004[81] had investigated millions of administrative health claims and concluded that a patient who visits six or more prescribers over a 1-year period is potentially exhibiting "aberrant behavior."[80] The Wilsey group reviewed 56.7 million prescriptions collected in the CURES database between 1999 and 2007.[80] Of this number, 2.8 million patients fit the selection criteria of two to five prescriptions for opioids during a 1-year period.[80] The researchers concluded that "the differences were in the opposite direction to those consistent with the assumption that the patients who used more than one provider were manipulating the system."[80] They concluded that using a theoretical number of eight or more prescribers in 1 year was likely a better indicator of probable doctor shopping.[80] This number, they observed, was closer to the six prescribers suggested in the earlier study by Parente et al.[80]

Reifler et al. in 2012 used opioid abuse–related data from poison control centers collected by the Research, Abuse, Diversion and Addiction-Related Surveillance (RADARS®) program and compared them with oxycodone abuse rates per 1,000 unique recipients of a dispensed drug, a specialized metric used by RADARS to measure drug abuse.[82] The study period was from 2003 to mid-2009.[82] Results supported an association between PDMPs and mitigated opioid abuse and misuse trends.[82] Without a PDMP in place, intentional exposures increased, on average, 1.9% per quarter, whereas opioid intentional exposures increased 0.2% ($p = .036$) per quarter with a PDMP in place.[82] Opioid treatment admissions (using the TEDS database) increased 4.9% per quarter, on average, in states without a PDMP versus 2.6% ($p = .058$) in states with a PDMP.[82]

Brady et al. in 2014 used data from DEA's ARCOS program for opioids dispensed in a given quarter of the year for each state and the District of Columbia from 1999 to 2008, and converted them to morphine milligram equivalents (MMEs).[83] These data were compared for states with PDMPs and states without PDMPs.[83] Having a state PDMP was associated with a 3% decrease in MMEs dispensed per capita ($p = .68$).[83] The impact of PDMPs on MMEs dispensed per capita varied markedly by state, from a 66% decrease in Colorado to a 61% increase in Connecticut.[83] The researchers concluded that the implementation of state PDMPs up to 2008 did not show a significant impact on per-capita opioids dispensed.[83]

Gwira Baumblatt et al. in 2014 performed a matched case–control study that analyzed data from the Tennessee PDMP from January 1, 2007, through December 31, 2011, to identify risk factors associated with opioid-related overdose deaths, ascertained from death certificate data.[84] Controls were matched for age and sex and randomly selected among live patients in the PDMP. High-risk factors were identified as four or more prescribers per year and high dosage as a daily mean of more than 100 MMEs per year.[84] In 2011, more than 7.6% of patients in the database used more than four prescribers, 2.5% used more than four pharmacies, and 2.8% had a mean daily opioid dosage greater than 100 MMEs.[84] Increased risk of opioid-related overdose death was associated with having four or more prescribers, four or more pharmacies, and more than 100 MMEs mean daily opioid dose.[84] Persons with one or more of these risk factors accounted for 55% of all drug overdose deaths in the 5-year study period.[84]

Maughan et al. in 2015 investigated the association between PDMP implementation and ED visits involving opioid analgesics for the period 2004 to 2011.[85] Although rates of ED visits increased in all metropolitan areas, the implementation of PDMPs was not associated with a difference in ED visits involving opioid analgesics.[85] The researchers concluded that during 2004 to 2011, PDMP implementation was not associated with a change in opioid-related morbidity, as measured by ED visits involving opioid analgesics.[85]

Ringwalt et al. in 2015 investigated the use of algorithms to survey PDMPs to identify providers with unusual prescribing practices for controlled substances.[86] Using data from a state PDMP, the researchers constructed metrics to use in searching PDMP records for patients who died of a drug overdose within 30 days of their last PDMP record.[86] The strongest concurrent validity with providers identified from the PDMP records related to those who co-prescribed benzodiazepines and high levels of opioid analgesics, as well as those who wrote temporarily overlapping prescriptions.[86]

As this brief review shows, findings that indicate that PDMPs influence prescription drug abuse vary and may even appear to be contradictory from one study to the next. Even so, these studies contribute valuable information about an evolving drug surveillance system whose full potential is yet to be realized. Started decades ago as a law enforcement tool to identify errant prescribers, today's PDMP has evolved to become an active and multifunctional database not only serving its original purpose but also helping to identify patients at risk for substance abuse disorders, including the risk of fatal overdoses.[75]

Despite their reliance on automated systems, PDMPs still have some important limitations.[87] The accidental miscoding of compound surnames, for example, and the use of fraudulent identification by doctor shoppers and prescription forgers, as well as other vulnerabilities common to all online information systems, present limitations in the PDMP data stream.[87] Some of these problems can be addressed successfully by currently available corrective software, while others may have to await further progress in information technology and integrated systems design.[87]

PUBLIC HEALTH OR PUBLIC SAFETY?

Forty of 50 PDMPs (including the PDMP for the District of Columbia) are housed within Health Departments or Boards of Pharmacy; five are managed by state law enforcement agencies; two (Utah and Delaware) are managed by the Department of Professional Licensing; one (Nevada) is managed by both the Board of Pharmacy and the Department of Public Safety; one (Georgia) is managed by the state's Narcotic and Drug Agency at the direction and oversight of the Board of Pharmacy; and one (Connecticut) is managed by the Department of Consumer Affairs.[58]

The expansion of the PDMP from being exclusively a law enforcement tool to a functional healthcare database is reflected in the fact that most states (nearly 80%) in the past decade have assigned these programs to their public health agencies.[58] As discussed in detail below, pilot studies automatically linking PDMP data with electronic health records (EHRs) have proved very beneficial, especially for practitioners in the clinical setting.

UNSOLICITED PDMP REPORTS

Some states provide PDMP users with unsolicited reports of possible diversion.[88] As previously mentioned, algorithms are used to query PDMP systems for likely or probable doctor shoppers based on a patient's pattern of prescriptions obtained from different prescribers in a relatively brief period of time.[89] According to NASMDL, 20 states with PDMPs permit unsolicited reports to be sent to prescribers, pharmacists, law enforcement, and licensing entities.[58] Another 26 states permit unsolicited reports to be sent to one or more of these entities but not all four.[58]

PDMP FUNDING

In 2013, following an investigation by the *Los Angeles Times* that reported half of the state's 3,733 fatal drug overdoses involved prescription drugs, a bill to raise licensing fees and impose a small tax on drug manufacturers to fund California's PDMP (CURES) failed in the legislature.[90] Funding for the PDMP was cut to $400,000 a year.[90] According to media reports, California's PDMP in 2013 was being managed by a single employee.[90] Physicians attempting to access the database reported receiving automated responses advising that no one was available to respond.[90] Despite having the support of the state's attorney general, the California Medical Association, a number of business groups, and the Senate president, the bill to permanently fund California's PDMP failed.[90]

Despite the aforementioned success of its anti-pill mill legislation in 2011, Florida presents a microcosm of the funding problem that affects most PDMPs.[91] The 2011 anti–pill mill statute prohibited state funds from being used to implement the PDMP.[91] This was waived in 2013 when, faced with insolvency, the Florida legislature allocated $500,000 as a one-time expenditure to continue the program.[91] This was repeated by the legislature to fund the PDMP through fiscal year 2015–2016.[91] A bill that would have permanently allocated funds for the PDMP from the Board of Pharmacy Trust Fund was defeated in 2014.[91] To ensure solvency for the program, the Florida attorney general directed a $2 million one-time "contribution" to the PDMP from a settlement award received from CVS/Caremark as a result of unrelated litigation.[92] According to state records, between 2015 and March 31, 2017, federal Rogers grants totaling $1,299,105 have been awarded for Florida's PDMP, along with an additional NASPER grant in the amount of $240,105 from the Substance Abuse and Mental Health Services Administration.[91]

To provide a permanent funding mechanism for the state's PDMP, the Florida legislature authorized the creation of the Florida PDMP Foundation, Inc., a 501c3 nonprofit organization whose sole purpose is to raise funds for the operation of the state's PDMP.[92] The foundation estimates that the PDMP costs between $500,000 and $600,000 per year to manage and operate.[92] Although the foundation has received large donations from several healthcare corporations, including Millennium Laboratories, Automated HealthCare Systems, and AEGIS Science Corporation, and modest contributions from police and sheriff's departments throughout the state, all of these have been one-time donations.[92] The foundation's web page contains an ominous note that because of the legislature's failure to authorize permanent funding for the PDMP, there remains doubt as to whether the PDMP will be able to continue operation.[92]

The Heller School for Social Policy and Management at Brandeis University houses the PDMP Center of Excellence, an expert group of healthcare and policy specialists funded by grants from the US Department of Justice.[93] The Center was founded in 2010 to collaborate with PDMP stakeholders and to use its nationally recognized panel of experts to advise federal and state agencies on best practices in the formation and operation of PDMPs.[93]

Recognizing the importance of funding mechanisms, in 2013 the Center analyzed the current PDMP funding methods employed by states[94] (Table 3.1). As noted, most states use a combination of funding methods to keep their PDMPs operational.[94] This, however, reflects the uncertainty of funding because, with the exception of states that use general revenue funds, many of the other funding sources fluctuate from year to year, depending upon the amount of unscheduled funding received from nonappropriated sources.[94] To address this, the Center has studied alternative ways for states to fund their PDMPs. Each of the suggested funding methods might be used alone or in combination.

TABLE 3.1 PDMP funding methods employed by states (2013)

Types of PDMP Funding	States
Federal Grants	26
Non-federal/Private Grants	4
General Revenue Funds	10
Registration Fees	13
Professional Licensing Fees	3
Regulatory Board Funds	6
Legal Settlements	2
PDMP Licensing Fee	1
Health Insurance Licensing Fee	1
Private Donations (Foundation)	1
Medicaid Fraud Settlements	1

Note: Most states use a combination of funding types.

Source: PDMP Center of Excellence, Brandeis University[93]

ASSESSED FINES

The Center notes that state regulatory boards and state licensing agencies routinely impose fines on entities found to be in violation of state regulations.[94] Fines usually are deposited in the state's general revenue fund.[94] The Center recommends that a percentage of these fines be used to support the state's PDMP program, especially if PDMP data have been used to establish grounds for the fines.[94] The Center notes that the amount of money raised might not be consistent or sufficient to fully fund the PDMP, so other means of support would be needed.[94] The Center believes that establishing this type of funding for PDMPs would likely require legislation.[94]

ASSET FORFEITURE

Law enforcement agencies routinely seize assets acquired as a result, or used during the commission, of certain crimes such as drug trafficking.[94] In states where the PDMP may already be housed within a law enforcement agency, an arrangement that assigns a portion of funds received from liquidating seized drug-related assets could be used to fund the PDMP.[94] This arrangement, the Center notes, might be accomplished through internal administrative means without legislation.[94]

DRUG MANUFACTURERS ASSESSMENT

The Center noted the failure of the California legislative proposal that would have imposed a small tax on drug manufacturers to fund the state's PDMP.[94] The Center believes that this type of legislation would enjoy a more successful outcome if presented to the electorate as a "valuable product stewardship initiative," highlighting drug manufacturers' concern for the public health.[94] The Center estimates that a very small fee, perhaps amounting to as little as one-tenth of one percent of the total revenue from drugs sold in the state, would fully support the funding of a PDMP.[94]

PRESCRIPTION FEES

The Center noted that PDMPs collect data on millions of controlled substances prescriptions each year and that a small fee imposed on each filled prescription could pay for a state's PDMP.[94] For example, if a state PDMP collects data for 10 million prescriptions a year and needs $500,000 to operate its PDMP, the proposed fee would amount to only five cents for each prescription.[94] Although this would shift the cost of the PDMP to the consumer, the Center counters this by saying that a fully operational PDMP lowers the incidence of prescription fraud, thus helping to reduce the overall cost to consumers for healthcare and insurance.[94]

PRIVATE THIRD-PARTY PAYERS OR HEALTH INSURERS

Perhaps the most innovative suggestion from the Center, and the one having the greatest potential for permanently funding PDMPs, is a proposed partnership with state insurance programs in which pilot studies—some of which are described in this chapter—have shown the value of PDMP data to help detect waste, fraud, and abuse in the prescribing and dispensing of controlled substances.[95] To show this potential in just one such program, the Center referenced a 2013 study by the California Workers' Compensation Institute in which multiple opioid prescriptions for claimants were analyzed for potential signals of fraud. According to the study, management controls in the form of denying fraudulent reimbursement claims could have saved the program $57.2 million in just 1 year.[95] The annual operating budget for California's PDMP is estimated at $3.7 million.[94] Thus, it was noted, if the California Division of Workers' Compensation were to fund the state's PDMP and use its information, the return to the state on its investment would be $15.50 for every dollar spent on the PDMP.[94]

SHARING PDMP DATA WITH THIRD-PARTY PAYERS

A promising alternative funding source recommended by the Center would be allowing access to PDMP data for private third-party payers and health insurers.[94] Third-party payers are health insurance providers that reimburse the cost of medical care under insurance or workers' compensation plans.[94] Private insurers like Blue Cross-Blue Shield and

Kaiser Permanente, and public health insurers like Medicare and Medicaid, are considered third-party payers.[94] As of 2013, according to the Center, 31 states were authorized to share PDMP data with Medicaid or Medicare, eight states were authorized to share data with state workers' compensation programs, but only one, Michigan, was authorized to share PDMP data with private third-party payers.[95]

In December 2012, at the request of the Office of National Drug Control Policy (ONDCP) and with a grant from the US Justice Department, the Center held a meeting with more than 75 representatives of third-party payers to explore potential benefits of using PDMP data.[95] One expert at the meeting estimated the cost of fraudulent prescription reimbursements at more than $42 million a year for a medium-sized insurer (≤500,000 lives insured).[95] Another expert, an associate general counsel and director of workers' compensation for the American Insurance Association, warned that opioid abuse was the "most urgent issue facing workers."[95] This expert added that liberal use of long-acting opioids for chronic pain increased the chance of a "catastrophic claim" (>$100,000) by nearly four times, while use of short-acting opioids nearly doubled it.[95]

As previously mentioned, only Michigan allows nongovernment healthcare providers access to PDMP data.[95] Under the Michigan PDMP statute, covered healthcare providers include "a health insurance company, a nonprofit health care corporation, a health maintenance organization, a multiple employer welfare arrangement, a Medicaid contract health plan, or any other person providing a plan of health benefits, coverage, or insurance subject to state insurance regulation."[95]

Although the range of potential savings for third-party insurance payers using PDMP data are in the tens of millions of dollars per year for just medium-sized companies, the aforementioned meeting of insurance company representatives, ONDCP, and the Center exposed a number of issues that must be resolved before private-party access to PDMP data can become a reality.[95] Foremost among these issues is the lack of explicit legislative and regulatory authority in the state PDMP statutes to permit third-party payer access to PDMP data.[95] Noteworthy in this discussion is the model statute for PDMPs authored by NASMDL that contains no language permitting nongovernment third-party access to PDMP data. The pertinent provision in the NASMDL model PDMP statute allows data access *only* for Medicaid or other state-administered payer programs:

> The [designated state agency or entity] may disclose prescription monitoring information to the following persons after such persons have successfully completed the applicable training, education, or instruction regarding the PMP identified in Section 9: (viii) A designated representative of the [state] Medicaid or other state administered health insurance program regarding program recipients, prescribers, or dispensers for the purpose of investigating fraud, waste, or abuse of the [state] Medicaid or other state administered health insurance program.[74]

As evidenced by this provision, the language in the NASMDL model statute does not mention third-party private insurers or federal programs, including Medicare.[74] As of July 2012, it was reported that 23 states permit access to PDMP data by Medicaid officials, and only two states permit access to Medicare officials.[95] The actual extent to which this access is permitted is unknown, as is the format and manner in which outside investigators may access PDMP information.[95] Although critics often cite privacy concerns to oppose sharing PDMP data with private third-party insurance payers, many of these same third-party insurance payers and their respective prescription benefit managers (PBMs) already routinely receive and handle the same data as PDMPs when processing millions of drug reimbursement claims from patients and their providers.[96]

PDMP LIMITATIONS

For more than a decade since the federal grant program brought the modern PDMP to every state and the District of Columbia, policymakers and drug control experts have praised these systems despite little hard evidence that they actually work to reduce problem prescribing, drug diversion, and/or prescription drug abuse.[97,98] As mentioned in the opening paragraphs of this chapter, between 2004 and 2011 (the period when most of today's PDMPs became operational) the number of nonfatal hospital admissions for abuse and/or misuse of opioids more than tripled.[99] During the same period, sales of opioids increased 53.2%, from 4.7 to 7.2 kg per 10,000 persons, and opioid overdose deaths increased 58.8%, from 3.4 to 5.4 per 100,000 persons.[100,101] Thus, by the only measure that matters—reducing prescription drug–related morbidity and mortality—to date PDMPs have failed to deliver except in states where their use is mandated by law, and even then, the evidence of their usefulness is mixed.[75]

On July 9, 2012, the FDA's Safety and Innovation Act became law. It contained several provisions pertaining to PDMPs.[102] The act contained recommendations to improve the interoperability of PDMPs across state lines. The use of open standards—computer language that allows different systems to communicate with each other—and the use of exchange intermediaries, or "hubs," were recommended to promote broader implementation of PDMPs.[102] The act required the Secretary to submit a report assessing the challenges affecting interstate use of PDMPs as well as the integration or interfacing of PDMP data "with other technologies and databases used for detecting and reducing fraud, diversion, and abuse of prescription drugs."[102]

In 2013, the Assistant Secretary for Health submitted the required report to Congress describing in detail a number of problems affecting the PDMP program.[103] The report discussed four major challenges facing PDMPs: legal, technical, fiscal, and privacy/security.[103] Legal questions challenging PDMPs, the report stated, can be solved with amendments to existing statutes or revised administrative regulations.[103] Technical challenges, such as those affecting the interoperability of PDMPs because of different software configurations, can be addressed by establishing compatible standards and including them in upgraded software.[103]

The Assistant Secretary's report referenced the aforementioned study of PDMP funding published in 2013 by the PDMP Center of Excellence at Brandeis University's Heller School for Social Policy and Management.[93] The report included a suggestion by the Assistant Secretary to share PDMP data with public and private third-party payers so that potential savings from reducing fraudulent prescriptions could be used to permanently finance PDMP costs.[93]

PDMP INTEROPERABILITY

On March 26, 2015, the National All Schedules Prescription Electronic Reporting Reauthorization Act of 2015 was introduced in the US House of Representatives.[104] The bill proposed to reauthorize NASPER grants and add provisions to improve the interstate linking of PDMPs and the integration of PDMP data into EHRs and other automated health information systems.[104] The bill cleared the House, was received in the Senate on September 9, 2015. It was placed on the Senate Legislative Calendar under General Orders, where it expired without passage when the 114th Congress ended its second session on January 3, 2017.[105]

While stakeholders and state PDMP agencies had heralded the proposed NASPER reauthorization bill, its contents, according to an accompanying committee report, indirectly revealed key inefficiencies in the current PDMP program that the bill would have addressed.[104] For example, the bill supported the automated incorporation of PDMP data with EHRs. This suggestion had been validated by several pilot studies undertaken by federal authorities and the MITRE Corporation, a private, not-for-profit, consultancy firm.[106] In the MITRE studies, five states (Indiana, Michigan, North Dakota, Ohio, and Washington) were selected to test advanced interoperability experiments.[106] In Indiana, the study team created an automatic interface of PDMP data with a hospital ED's interstate hub for EHRs.[106] In North Dakota, an automated query link was established between the pharmacy system, the existing PBM switch, the interstate hub (for EHR data), and the PDMP.[106] In Ohio, an automated PDMP query was linked to appointment scheduling and patient check-in and configured to display a "patient risk score" in the patient's EHR.[106] In Washington, a direct hyperlink to the state's PDMP was included in the patient's EHR.[106] The results from these pilot studies showed what was described as "immediate improvement" to the patient care process, especially in cases in which heretofore prescribers and dispensers had rarely accessed PDMP data before the experimental links were created.[106] Workflow tasks were streamlined and user satisfaction increased 98% to 100% when systems were designed to automate routine tasks.[106]

Evaluations of these pilot studies showed that 7% of respondents reported an increase in prescriptions written or number of pills dispensed and 58% of prescribers at EDs reported a decrease in prescriptions written or pills dispensed.[106] In the words of one ED physician describing the automated PDMP link to the EHR, "I have to say that this is probably one of the more genius moves of the 21st century . . . having easy access to [PDMP data] without going to a totally different website and have it pop up instantly has taken a lot of time off of decision making for me."[106]

As these pilot studies showed, providing automated PDMP data to hospital emergency departments and other high-risk clinical environments prone to drug diversion can reduce the inefficiencies of the current program, prevent drug diversion, and save lives in the process.

Eligibility for the Rogers grant program that began in 2002 did not include at the outset a requirement for interstate interoperability.[107] Perhaps to avoid the appearance of a federalized program to track prescriptions, states were encouraged to exercise autonomy in the functional design of their individual PDMPs.[107] Upon receiving an initial "feasibility" grant, states were required to enact PDMP laws as a condition for startup and maintenance grants.[107,108] Having the federal government pay the startup costs and early maintenance of PDMPs helped to influence states to accept them.[108] The federal programs, however, were never intended to permanently fund the operation of state PDMPs.

Besides dealing with the challenges presented by policy differences and political considerations, not to mention pressure from industry lobbyists and special interest groups, technical issues continue to plague PDMPs, even in the face of today's advanced information technology.[109] PDMP data structures are based on the National Information Exchange Model, an interagency computer coding initiative that provides the foundation for national-level interoperable data sharing and exchange.[109] The National Information Exchange Model was developed more than a decade ago by the Departments of Justice and Homeland Security to facilitate information sharing among scores of agencies with law enforcement and/or national security responsibilities.[109]

The National Council for Prescription Drug Programs (NCPDP) is an industry organization that develops national standards for electronic healthcare transactions used in prescribing, dispensing, monitoring, managing, and paying for medications and pharmacy services.[110] Its consensus-driven standards and lexicon are used for (1) medication therapy management services; (2) educational purposes in helping pharmacists communicate information to patients about high-risk drugs, as required, for example, by FDA-mandated Risk Evaluation and Mitigation Strategies for opioids; and (3) other pharmacy-related data pertaining to a patient's EHR.[110]

One of the goals of the DHHS is to develop hubs capable of accessing information from various systems, and reformulating it in the electronic language and data structures used to access it.[111] In short, a hub for this purpose would act as a bidirectional translator allowing various parties to share information collected and archived with disparate data structures, coding lexicons, and systems.[111] To assist in meeting this goal, the DHHS Office of National Coordinator for Health Information Technology was tasked to assemble a collaborative community of private- and public-sector representatives to work on the PDMP Initiative, a multiyear effort to identify functional requirements, harmonize core elements, conduct pilot studies (some of which were previously discussed in this chapter), review feedback from pilot studies, and establish industry standards for compatible systems.[111] In October 2016, the group concluded its 2-year effort with a series of findings that expanded the knowledge base and identified key technical areas for additional research and development.[111] As previously mentioned, finding a reliable and permanent source of funding remains a major impediment to pursuing the recommended improvements in the PDMP program.

PRIVATE-SECTOR INITIATIVE

In 2011, the private sector, in the form of the National Association of Boards of Pharmacy (NABP), established PMP InterConnect®, a secure online data-sharing system that permits a participating state PDMP to query PDMPs in other states participating in the NABP program.[112] The NABP is self-funding this program and already has executed participation agreements with 35 states.[112] As of February 2016, the program has been processing more than 3.8 million requests each month.[112]

A typical request originates with a prescriber or dispenser seeking to access PDMP records beyond his or her state.[112–115] If the originating state PDMP and the out-of-state PDMP(s) are participants in PMP InterConnect, special encrypted software will be used to transmit the query to the out-of-state PDMP(s), which will respond accordingly.[112–115] The NABP PMP InterConnect will act as a two-way hub. The number of states participating in this program was expected to reach 40 by the end of 2016.[113] PMP InterConnect was designed to be compatible with national data-sharing standards and architecture adopted by the federal government's Prescription Monitoring Information Exchange.[112–115] PMP InterConnect also is developing an interface with PMP Gateway, a compatible program designed to integrate PDMP data in EHR databanks for delivery to point-of-care authorized users.[112–115]

While the effort of the NABP is commendable, an automated, seamless, user-friendly, interoperable PDMP among the states as currently envisioned by Congress, DHHS, and ONDCP continues to elude the best efforts of federal, state, and private organizations despite a universal consensus that there is a vital need for it.[103] As the pilot studies by DHHS, ONDCP and the MITRE Corporation discovered, the highest PDMP usage levels by prescribers, particularly prescribers assigned to hospital EDs, occurred when systems were fully automated, the user interface required a single sign-on ID/password, software was intuitive, and the PDMP data were integrated in the EHR or directly and immediately accessible via a hypertext link within the EHR record.[106]

Rutkow et al. in 2015 performed a nationwide survey of physicians to identify their awareness of PDMPs. Results showed that 72% of physicians were aware of their state's PDMP and 53% reported using it, although not routinely.[116] Several obstacles were identified, including the time-consuming nature of retrieving PDMP information and the lack of an intuitive interface format for accessing data.[116] The researchers recommended that all states should adopt regulations requiring the use of PDMPs, invest resources in prescriber education and outreach, and improve the PDMP interface format.[116]

A study of 17 emergency medicine providers in Massachusetts compared the physical task of accessing the state's PDMP with performing three other routine online tasks: ordering a computed tomography (CT) scan, preparing a prescription, and searching a medication record in the patient's EHR.[117] Accessing the PDMP took longer than each of the other measured tasks.[117] The PDMP task averaged 4.22 minutes and 50.3 mouse clicks; ordering a CT scan took 1.42 minutes and 24.8 mouse clicks; preparing a prescription took 1.30 minutes and 19.5 mouse clicks; and searching a medication record took 1.45 minutes and 9.5 mouse clicks.[117] The researchers concluded that the complicated processes needed for accessing and navigating the secure PDMP website were barriers preventing more frequent use.[117]

In Florida, a state that has experienced considerable changes in prescription drug regulations in the past 7 years, a survey about the state's PDMP mailed to 5,000 physicians yielded responses from only 390 (7.8%).[118] Of that number, 71.5% (279) agreed or strongly agreed that the PDMP is a useful tool. Sixty-three of 64 physicians (98.4%) conducting 25 or more PDMP searches annually agreed or strongly agreed with its usefulness for monitoring patients' controlled substance histories.[118] Most physicians agreed that use of the PDMP can decrease doctor shopping. Among the 64 most frequent PDMP users, 69.4% agreed or strongly agreed that they have prescribed fewer controlled substances as a result of accessing the PDMP.[118]

In Ohio, where a PDMP has been in operation since 2006, state officials reported 2,482 unintentional drug overdose deaths in 2014.[119] This was an increase of 17.6% over the number of such deaths in 2013.[119] According to state officials, approximately 12,427 prescribers (24% of all prescribers of controlled substances in the state) account for about 84% of Ohio's controlled substances prescriptions.[120,121] On January 1, 2015, PDMP registration became mandatory in Ohio for prescribers of controlled substances.[120,121] The Ohio Board of Pharmacy has reported that the use of the PDMP database has increased each year since 2007, and that the number of doctor shoppers between then and 2014 has been reduced by half.[120,121] The most frequent reason given by doctors who fail to use the PDMP on a regular basis is the amount of time it takes to process a query.[122]

As of December 2014, according to the National Alliance of Model State Drug Laws, all states permit PDMP access by prescribers and dispensers of controlled substances.[58] On January 1, 2017, Nebraska was the 49th state to begin operating its PDMP, and it, too, permits data access by prescribers and pharmacists.[123] On July 17, 2017, Missouri became the 50th state and last state to approve the adoption of a PDMP.[c]

Besides technical and funding issues, PDMPs present other challenges for those who access and use their information. A practitioner, for example, upon reviewing a PDMP report and finding himself or herself confronting a potential doctor shopper needs to know what legal obligation, if any, there is to report the person to the authorities. Principle IV of the American Medical Association's Code of Medical Ethics states that "[a] physician shall safeguard patient confidences and privacy within the constraints of the law."[124] The last phrase, "within the constraints of the law," is important because it controls the issue of patient-privacy, the privileged and confidential relationship that exists between a physician and a patient.

State laws require physicians to alert law enforcement authorities when they encounter patients with violence-related injuries, including knife wounds, gunshot wounds, child, spousal, and elder abuse, etc. Likewise, state laws require that physicians notify state public health officials when they encounter patients with certain specified infectious diseases that may pose a threat to the general public. Many states have "duty to warn" statutes requiring mental health professionals to warn authorities about patients who pose a threat to themselves or others. Physicians who report such patients in good faith to law enforcement authorities generally are statutorily immune from civil liability.[124]

While these breaches of patient privacy and confidentiality, as described, are both lawful and reasonable, the issue becomes far less clear in the case of a physician asked or expected to prescribe controlled substances to someone—that is, to a patient—whose PDMP record suggests is a doctor shopper. Although the federal Controlled Substances Act (CSA) and corresponding state laws provide the prescriber and dispenser with corresponding

c. Office of the Governor of Missouri. (2017) Governor Eric Greitens Announces Statewide Prescription Drug Monitoring Program. Available: https://governor.mo.gov/news/archive/governor-eric-greitens-announces-statewide-prescription-drug-monitoring-program (March 16, 2018).

responsibility and unquestioned discretion to decide when and whether it is proper to issue a patient a prescription for a controlled substance, this largely becomes a subjective determination by the physician and pharmacist as they weigh factors that the law permits and requires. However, the same statutory authority that indemnifies the practitioner who refuses to issue or fill a prescription may not indemnify him or her from civil liability if they go beyond this and report the patient with a suspicious PDMP record to law enforcement authorities, even if done in good faith.

Besides needing official guidance for how to respond to a patient with a questionable PDMP record, practitioners also need to know what officially constitutes a patient's questionable or suspicious PDMP record, and whether it is lawful to prescribe controlled substances for such patients. Practitioners also need to know if current laws in the jurisdictions authorize or oblige them to report that person to the authorities. Because these are practice-related questions, answers are likely to come from individual state medical boards and state regulatory authorities, inasmuch as practices and policies that bear upon these issues differ from state to state.

Discussed in this chapter were several reputable studies of doctor shoppers conducted by experts who differed among themselves in setting baseline criteria for what constitutes doctor shopping behavior. Twenty-seven states and the District of Columbia have statutes conferring immunity from civil liability on practitioners reporting information to their respective PDMP.[125] Most jurisdictions extend this immunity to those receiving, using or relying on, or not using or not relying on information received from their PDMP.[125] As of December 2014, only three states (Indiana, Tennessee, and West Virginia) have added provisions that confer immunity from criminal or civil liability on practitioners who in good faith disclose PDMP information of a suspicious nature to a law enforcement agency.[125] In sum, the legal and ethical uncertainties surrounding the practical use of PDMP information continue in most jurisdictions today and no doubt contribute measurably to the underutilization of these programs.

PREVENTING WASTE, FRAUD, AND ABUSE IN PUBLIC AND PRIVATE HEALTH CARE

PDMPs are not the only programs that can help to reduce prescription fraud by identifying potential doctor shoppers. Two cases discussed at the beginning of this chapter illustrate the usefulness of examining Medicaid reimbursement records to identify waste, fraud, and abuse, including instances of potential doctor shopping.[34,36] Government and private third-party insurers have begun to focus efforts on detecting fraudulent practices identified by excessive reimbursements for certain categories of prescribed drugs.[126] Ironically, according to industry sources, some automated systems in health care that are credited with reducing costs may actually make it easier to commit fraud.[126] An errant pharmacist, for example, may take a 30-day prescription and fraudulently input it into the system as four weekly prescriptions, thus quadrupling his or her Medicaid dispensing fee.[126] Experts note that the digitization of EHRs, required by the Affordable Care Act, has reduced the need for face-to-face information exchanges between parties whose interaction heretofore deterred simple frauds like this.[126]

Whenever a doctor shopper obtains controlled substances by fraud and the cost is reimbursed by a government or private insurance program, besides the drug law violation, there also is a potential charge of insurance fraud for filing, or causing to be filed, a "false" or unsubstantiated claim.[127] The Coalition Against Insurance Fraud, a national alliance of consumer groups, insurance companies, and government agencies, estimates that drug diversion costs health insurers as much as $72.5 billion a year in fraudulent claims for opioid medications (excluding all other classes of controlled substances).[127] More than a third of this cost (>$24.9 billion) is borne by private insurers, with the remainder paid by taxpayers.[127] The Coalition Against Insurance Fraud reports that reimbursements for fraudulent prescriptions may reach $1 billion annually for each of the largest private insurers.[127]

These excessive costs to the insurance industry are but a fraction of the overall economic cost of prescription drug abuse. McAdam-Marx et al. in 2010 studied medical costs of 10,162 Medicaid patients diagnosed with drug abuse or drug-dependent conditions and compared them with the medical costs for a matched control group of 150,486 Medicaid patients during 12 months between 2002 and 2003.[128] After controlling for baseline characteristics, the researchers determined that adjusted costs for abuse/dependent patients averaged $23,556 per patient, versus an average of $8,436 for each patient in the control group ($p < .001$).[128] Not surprisingly, patients diagnosed with drug abuse/dependent conditions were found to have higher rates of costly comorbidities than patients in the control group.[128]

A GAO report in 2014 on Medicare program integrity, among other things, recommended increased use of PDMP data by the Centers for Medicare and Medicaid Services (CMS) to prevent prescription fraud and drug abuse.[129] The report noted that four states (Idaho, Indiana, Massachusetts, and New York) were working with CMS and its primary contractor in pilot programs to make PDMP data available to fraud investigators.[129] Idaho, the report noted, was the only state at the time (2014) that permitted Medicare investigators direct access to PDMP data.[129]

As noted previously, private-sector health insurers annually lose almost $25 billion (circa 2007) as a result of waste, fraud, and abuse, a sizable portion of which involves reimbursements for fraudulent prescriptions for controlled substances.[39] These losses take on added significance because of a provision in the Affordable Care Act that mandates that at least 85% of all premium dollars collected by health insurance companies for large employer plans must be spent on healthcare services and healthcare quality improvement.[130,131] The enormous cost attributed to waste, fraud, and abuse is reflected in higher premiums for enrolees. It also reduces the overall pool of resources that might better be spent by the companies on delivering healthcare services.

THE ROLE OF THE PBM

PBMs are private companies that administer prescription drug plans for more than 266 million Americans with health insurance provided by commercial health plans, self-insured employer plans, union plans, Medicare Part D plans, the Federal Employees Health Benefits Program, state government employee plans, managed Medicaid plans, and others.[132] PBMs' revenues are derived from administrative fees received from insurance companies, transaction fees from pharmacies that use their services, drug pricing rebates from drug companies, other fees received from drug companies, and the markup on drug pricing (difference between what the PBM pays the pharmacy and what the PBM charges its insurance client).[133]

Express Scripts Holding Company is a Fortune 100 company and the nation's largest PBM, with 26,000 employees and a reported annual revenue (2015) of $101.7 billion.[134] The company manages 1.3 billion prescriptions annually for tens of millions of patients.[134] In 2013, Steve Miller, MD, the company's chief medical officer, published a paper on controlled substances in which he noted: "When someone obtains a prescription narcotic using cash, the standard protocols to monitor prescription drugs are bypassed. There is no record that can be cross-checked to ensure that the drugs are not being abused or diverted to the illegal market."[135]

Miller's report indicated that $224 billion is lost annually to healthcare fraud, including $73.5 billion to drug diversion alone.[135] He offered what he called a "simple solution," claiming that the technology already exists, is in place, and just needs a legislative mandate to require pharmacies to report cash transactions involving controlled substances to a transactional PBM (also known as a "cash PBM").[135] Current PBM systems, according to Miller, can be modified to capture these cash payments and a code field already exists in the software template that can be used for this purpose.[135] According to Miller's proposal, pharmacies would be required to process self-paid prescriptions for controlled substances through the transactional PBM, using a universal coding and billing program developed by the National Council for Prescription Drug Programs.[135] If adopted, according to Miller, this system could be used to replace or complement state PDMPs that are "inadequate to address the problem."[135] Miller's proposed system would bring to the table a massive real-time repository of reliable interstate prescription and drug dispensing data, complete with the all-important form-of-payment data.[135]

PBMs have been part of the pharmacy industry for more than four decades, but as a result of mergers and acquisitions, today's PBM sector is dominated by a handful of major players, primarily Express Scripts Holding Company, CVS Health, Catamaran Corp., and OptumRx (UnitedHealth Group Inc.'s pharmacy service).[136,137] In recent years there has been consolidation among pharmacy chains and PBMs.[136,137] Rite Aid Corp., for example, in June 2015, acquired the PBM services of EnvisionRX. The CVS retail pharmacy network of 7,800 stores has had a long and successful business relationship with CVS Caremark, the parent company's PBM and mail service pharmacy.[136,137]

Unlike a PDMP, a PBM is not restricted in its data collection by state boundaries or the control status of the prescribed drug.[138] Chronic pain patients placed on long term opioid therapy often suffer from comorbid conditions requiring non-controlled prescription drugs. A PBM record, therefore, will show the full array of prescribed drugs for a patient and this, in turn, can assist an analyst to determine the appropriateness of a given drug regimen. A doctor shopper may receive prescriptions for controlled and non-controlled drugs, but typically the doctor shopper will forego filling the prescriptions for the non-controlled drugs, especially if paying cash.

PBM systems have their own unique limitations. For example, unlike a PDMP that collects data on all dispensed controlled substances in the state, a PBM system collects data for drugs dispensed by pharmacies only within its network.[132] In addition, while the PDMP has the force of state law behind it, the PBM is a private entity that operates without sovereign immunity ("a judicial doctrine which precludes bringing suit against the government without its consent"[139]).

PBMs like Express Scripts and CVS Caremark and others that, in addition to their prescription processing services, operate central fill pharmacies and/or home-delivery pharmacies are required to register as "pharmacies" with DEA and comply with the provisions of the CSA.[140] Like all registrants, central fill and home-delivery pharmacy services divisions of PBMs by law are required to prevent the theft and diversion of controlled substances.[141] At present, DEA registration is a requirement for only the actual drug-dispensing business activities of the PBM's central fill pharmacy and/or its home delivery service pharmacy.[140] The central fill pharmacy distributes packaged medications, including controlled substances, to pharmacies for pass-through delivery to patients, while the home-delivery pharmacy dispenses and delivers prescribed medications, including controlled substances, directly to patients via postal or courier service.[142] Central fill and home delivery pharmacies operate separately within the PBM structure and are distinct from the PBM employees who service the incoming formulary and reimbursement claims from dispensing pharmacies. In today's busy pharmacy, approval by a PBM that a prescribed drug is covered by the patient's insurer is often a green light for the pharmacist to dispense the drug. The "corresponding responsibility" of the pharmacist (with that of the prescriber) to verify that the drug has been prescribed for a legitimate medical purpose is often overlooked or ignored in the process.

Either through federal legislation or by administrative rulemaking, the prescription processing divisions of PBMs could be added to the list of business activities required by law to register with DEA. This would accomplish at least two important objectives. By imposing upon the PBM's prescription processing division the standard requirement of all DEA registrants to provide effective controls and procedures to guard against the theft and diversion of controlled substances,[141] it would free up enormously rich databases containing billions of prescription records that could be used to identify potential doctor shoppers and corrupt or ineligible prescribers. This, in turn, leads us directly to the second objective: to enable the PBM to perform specific surveillance tasks and report suspicious prescribing patterns to the authorities unencumbered by federal and state privacy laws or the threat of civil litigation for good-faith errors.

In 1970, when the CSA was enacted, there were 10 separate business activities required to register:

1. Manufacturing controlled substances;
2. Distributing controlled substances;
3. Dispensing controlled substances;
4. Conducting research (other than as described in #6);
5. Conducting instructional activities;
6. Conducting research (re: "the development of a narcotic addict rehabilitation program, etc.");

7. Conducting research and instructional activities with controlled substances listed in Schedule I;
8. Conducting chemical analysis;
9. Importing controlled substances; and
10. Exporting controlled substances.[143]

In 2003 and 2005, two additional business activities, "central fill pharmacies" and "reverse distributors," were added to this list by DEA using its rulemaking authority under the CSA and the Administrative Procedure Act.[144,145] These categories did not exist in 1970 when the CSA was enacted, but requiring them to be registered, according to DEA, was important for maintaining the closed system of controlled substances. PBMs and the prescription processing services they provide, like central fill pharmacies and reverse distributors, did not exist in 1970 when the CSA was enacted. The internet that gave rise to businesses like PBMs was in its infancy in 1970 and its limited capabilities were not yet developed sufficiently for this type of commercial use.

PBMs like Express Scripts already perform a broad range of tasks designed to detect and deter waste, fraud, and abuse in their home-delivery and prescription processing services.[146] This includes Drug Utilization Reviews and the use of proprietary algorithms and software to identify atypical prescribing practices. As an industry leader, Express Scripts employs a system that uses "over 290 indicators" to detect potential cases of pharmacy fraud.[146] According to company literature, Express Scripts processes 1.4 billion prescriptions a year from 100 million members of participating benefit programs and its specialized analytics identify the following potential fraud indicators:

1. Number of doctors visited;
2. Distance traveled to physician or pharmacy;
3. Frequency of prescriptions;
4. Geography and patient population; and
5. Mix of drugs dispensed.[146]

In 2013, according to Express Scripts, an estimated $1.49 billion in medical costs was saved by the company's waste, fraud, and abuse program that identified 881 cases of member and physician fraud.[146] Another estimated $14.27 million in savings resulted from identifying 151 cases of pharmacy fraud.[146] While these savings are commendable, they beg the question of why they were not larger in view of data suggesting a relatively high statistical probability of waste, fraud, and abuse in this segment of the industry?

In 2007, an audit of CMS Medicare Part D payments by the Office of Inspector General (OIG) identified 228,000 prescription payment records with invalid prescriber identifications for Schedule II drugs. According to the OIG report, "The prescriber ID field should generally contain one of four types of identification: a Drug Enforcement Administration (DEA) number, a National Provider Identifier (NPI), a Unique Physician Identification Number (UPIN), or a State license number."[147] As a result, OIG investigators reported that they "were unable to identify the top prescribers for oxycodone, Ritalin, and methadone."[147] Overall, according to another OIG report, in 2007, CMS paid $1.2 billion in Medicare Part D prescription drug claims that had invalid prescriber identifiers.[148] These improper payments should have been flagged and denied by the PBM providing prescription processing services for the government's Medicare Part D program.

A 2009 GAO audit of fraud and abuse related to Medicaid payments for controlled substances in several states revealed $2 million in paid prescriptions issued and filled by 65 practitioners and pharmacies barred or excluded from federal health programs for infractions that included illegally selling controlled substances.[149] In addition, investigators identified more than 1,800 beneficiaries who, according to Social Security records, were deceased when their prescriptions for controlled substances were issued and filled.[149]

These and other government audits of irregularities in the Medicare Part D and Medicaid programs suggest that the statistical frequency of fraud involving prescriptions for controlled substances is significantly higher than what present surveillance systems, even one as sophisticated as the Express Scripts program, can address under the current regulatory structure.

Besides helping to reduce prescription fraud and doctor shopping, adding PBM divisions that process prescriptions, including those for controlled substances, to the list of business activities required to register with DEA would provide several benefits for the PBM, including indemnification against civil suits for "good faith" privacy rule violations and other civil law claims that might arise out of the PBM's responsibility as a registrant to provide effective controls and procedures to guard against theft and diversion of controlled substances. DEA registration for PBMs that process prescriptions for controlled substances would help PBMs save millions of dollars a year for pharmacy and insurance clients (including federal and state governments) by taking preventive measures to reduce doctor shopping and prescription fraud. Under the current system, PBMs have limited abilities to address these practices because of bureaucratic and procedural obstacles. Some of these obstacles would be eliminated or significantly reduced by requiring PBMs to register with DEA and comply with the CSA.

In sum, we began this chapter with a description of the scope of the problem of prescription drug abuse, noting that bulk drug distributions of opioids to pharmacies in the United States have declined significantly in the last several years. Based on DEA's ARCOS data, between 2011—the peak year for retail opioid sales in the United States—and 2016, outpatient medical use of oxycodone declined 12.8% (from 60,422 metric tons to 52,051 metric tons); hydrocodone declined by 22.8% (from 45,627 metric tons to 28,616 metric tons); methadone declined 44.4% (from 5,905 metric tons to 3,372 metric tons); and morphine declined 11.7% (from 19,576 metric tons to 17,287 metric tons).[150]

Adding to the refractory nature of the current opioid abuse crisis is the fact that these declines have not been matched with declines in opioid-related overdose deaths. As noted in the beginning of this chapter, researchers at the CDC have written for years about a close linear relationship between retail opioid sales and opioid-related overdose deaths.[8,151] Given this nexus one might expect the converse to be true, that is, that a decline in sales would produce a corresponding decline in overdose deaths. This has not occurred, casting doubt on the CDC's original hypothesis. Several explanations are possible for this and may involve the recent increase in the use of street opioids like heroin and fentanyl analogs.

According to the CDC, heroin-related overdose deaths have more than quadrupled since 2010. In 2015, nearly 13,000 deaths were caused by heroin overdoses—an increase of 20.6% over the previous year. In its report, the CDC noted that Compton et al. in 2016 found that "Past misuse of prescription opioids is the strongest risk factor for starting heroin use—especially among people who become dependent upon or abused prescription opioids in the past year."[4,152]

This dramatic increase in heroin-related deaths is likely driving the overall opioid overdose death rate in the United States. Government databases for tracking nonmedical drug use and related health consequences are obsolete and lack the sensitivity to show which drugs, by chemical name and product formulation, licit or illicit, are responsible for the increasing overdose deaths. The Drug Abuse Warning Network (DAWN) was a unique database that captured drug abuse data directly from hospital EDs throughout the United States. It was begun in the early 1970s in conjunction with the passage of the CSA and for the specific purpose of tracking the health consequences of drug abuse. In 2003, an improved and internet-based version of DAWN was launched by the Substance Abuse and Mental Health Services Administration (SAMHSA) only to be suddenly discontinued in 2011 at the height of the prescription drug abuse epidemic. According to SAMHSA officials at the time, the DAWN program was being transferred to the CDC where its functions would be incorporated into other hospital surveillance programs. A replacement program, SAMHSA officials promised, would be introduced in 2017.[153-155] This, however, did not occur and likely has stymied the government's effort to control a problem it no longer measures.

The government's other drug abuse databases are survey-based and, like DAWN, they trace their origins (and limitations) to the 1970s, when prescription drug abuse was not a significant concern of public health and safety officials. Even today, CDC's reports of opioid-related overdose deaths often do not distinguish between deaths caused by licit opioids (i.e., prescription opioids) and those caused by illicit opioids (i.e., heroin, fentanyl analogs). In purely descriptive terms, an opioid-caused death is one involving an opioid, regardless of whether its origin is licit or illicit. Shaping an effective strategy to reduce the phenomenon, however, requires knowing more about the drugs that are being abused, including their generic or brand name(s) and whether they are prescription or street drugs. The reason for this is obvious. An effective strategy directed against doctor shoppers will have little or no effect against street dealers of heroin and fentanyl analogs, and vice versa. Reporting opioid-related morbidity and mortality without these essential details is like reporting the number of infections in a given population without indicating how many were bacterial and how many were viral. Each, as in the case of addressing the opioid abuse problem, requires its own specific treatment plan for effective control. To control the problem, you first must be able to identify it and its etiology. Since 2011, government systems have been incapable of this.

Meanwhile, the private sector appears to be miles ahead in establishing efficient data systems for monitoring prescription waste, fraud, and abuse even though it lacks the authority to act. Previously mentioned, the private sector does not enjoy sovereign immunity against civil suits, nor is it enabled by statute to acquire and use medical information for law enforcement or public health purposes. Even when practitioners have access to a PDMP, the access is limited to the prescribing records of their own patients.

In this chapter, we discussed some of the benefits and limitations of the PDMPs when used solely as a repository of information. Private and public third-party health insurance payers have been collecting similar data for years. Because of their national presence, private insurers have more expansive databases than any individual state PDMP, yet these private databases are severely limited in how they can be used to identify and block potential doctor shoppers.

If the government cannot or will not collect the information needed to halt the epidemic of prescription drug abuse, it should at least allow the private sector and those other government entities that collect information about patients' prescription records to expand the approved uses of that information to identify, for example, potential doctor shoppers and patients at risk for opioid overdoses.

PDMPs should be integrated with EHRs so that only a single query is needed for a clinician to access sufficient data to decide which drug or therapy is best suited to address the patient's complaint. Pilot studies discussed in this chapter show how improving the efficiencies and ergonomics of integrated information systems can save lives in the clinical setting. Also, the role of the PBM in today's world is far more than that of a clearinghouse for processing reimbursement claims for prescribed drugs. The modern PBM plays a vital and significant role in the process that moves the controlled substance from the pharmacy shelf to the patient's pocket or purse.

Finally, as we described in this chapter, even though a PBM may be authorized to alert clients to overuse or misuse of services, this rarely occurs in day-to-day operations. One obvious reason for this is the lack of indemnification against civil suit if a mistake is made and a patient is denied care in the form of a refused prescription. The cost of litigating such a claim, assuming a PBM would elect to do so, would likely exceed whatever small savings might be had by denying the prescription in the first place. By requiring PBMs to register with DEA, their status would be covered by the CSA and the de facto indemnity it confers on all registrants when, in good faith and with due diligence and compliance with the law, they act to prevent the diversion of controlled substances. It is time to join the best practices of the public and private sectors to address the current opioid crisis.

REFERENCES

1. Centers for Disease Control and Prevention. Understanding the Epidemic: Drug overdose deaths in the United States continue to increase in 2015. 2016. https://www.cdc.gov/drugoverdose/epidemic/. Accessed May 15, 2017.

2. Centers for Disease Control and Prevention. Prescription painkiller overdoses at epidemic levels. 2011. http://www.cdc.gov/media/releases/2011/p1101_flu_pain_killer_overdose.html. Accessed January 23, 2015.

3. Rudd RA, Aleshire N, Zibbell JE, Gladden RM. Increases in drug and opioid overdose deaths—United States, 2000–2014. MMWR Morb Mortal Wkly Rep. 2016;64:1378–1382.

4. Centers for Disease Control and Prevention. Heroin Overdose Data. 2017. https://www.cdc.gov/drugoverdose/data/heroin.html. Accessed May 11, 2017.

5. Centers for Disease Control and Prevention, National Center for Health Statistics. Number and age-adjusted rates of drug-poisoning deaths involving opioid analgesics and heroin: United States, 2000–2014. 2015. http://www.cdc.gov/nchs/data/health_policy/AADR_drug_poisoning_involving_OA_Heroin_US_2000-2014.pdf. Accessed October 4, 2016.

6. US Department of Health and Human Services, Substance Abuse and Mental Health Services Administration, Office of Applied Studies. Drug Abuse Warning Network (DAWN) National &

Metro Tables, 2004–2011 ("All misuse and abuse"). 2013. http://www.samhsa.gov/data/emergency-department-data-dawn/reports?tab=26. Accessed January 21, 2017.

7. Paulozzi LJ, Budnitz DS, Xi Y. Increasing deaths from opioid analgesics in the United States. *Pharmacoepidemiol Drug Safety.* 2006;15(9):618–627.

8. Paulozzi LJ, Weisler RH, Patkar AA. A national epidemic of unintentional prescription opioid overdose deaths: how physicians can help control it. *J Clin Psychiatry.* 2011;72(5):589–592.

9. 21 CFR 1304.33 (Reports to ARCOS). Food and Drugs, Part 1300 to End. 2015. http://www.gpo.gov/fdsys/pkg/CFR-2011-title21-vol9/pdf/CFR-2011-title21-vol9-part1304.pdf. Accessed December 19, 2015.

10. 21 CFR 1305.11-14 (Subpart B, DEA Form 222). Food and Drugs, Part 1300 to End. 2015. http://www.gpo.gov/fdsys/pkg/CFR-2011-title21-vol9/pdf/CFR-2011-title21-vol9-part1301.pdf. Accessed December 19, 2015.

11. Drug Enforcement Administration, Office of Diversion Control. Data from the Automation of Reports and Consolidated Orders System (ARCOS) for average pharmacy distribution of controlled substances in the US from 2007 to 2013. Unpublished data obtained by John J. Coleman from DEA via Freedom of Information Act requests in 2013 and 2014. 2015.

12. Drug Enforcement Administration. Federal Register (79 FR 49661): Schedules of controlled substances: Rescheduling of hydrocodone combination products from Schedule III to Schedule II; Final Rule. 2014. http://www.ncbi.nlm.nih.gov/pubmed/25167591. Accessed May 8, 2017.

13. Jones CM, Lurie PG, Throckmorton DC. Effect of US Drug Enforcement Administration's rescheduling of hydrocodone combination analgesic products on opioid analgesic prescribing. *JAMA Intern Med.* 2016;176(3):399–402.

14. Joranson DE, Ryan KM, Gilson AM, Dahl JL. Trends in medical use and abuse of opioid analgesics. *JAMA.* 2000;283(13):1710–1714.

15. Harris S, Nikulina V, Gelpi-Acosta C, et al. Prescription drug diversion: predictors of illicit acquisition and redistribution in three U.S. metropolitan areas. *AIMS Public Health.* 2015;2(4):762–783.

16. McDonald DC, Carlson KE. Estimating the prevalence of opioid diversion by "doctor shoppers" in the United States. *PLoS One.* 2013;8(7):e69241.

17. Drug Enforcement Administration. National Drug Threat Assessment Summary for 2015 (DEA-DCT-DIR-008-16). 2015. http://www.dea.gov/docs/2015%20NDTA%20Report.pdf. Accessed February 19, 2016.

18. Joranson DE, Gilson AM. Drug crime is a source of abused pain medications in the United States. *J Pain Symptom Manage.* 2005;30(4):299–301.

19. Title 21, Code of Federal Regulations, Sect. 1301.74 (Other security controls for nonpractitioners). Food and Drugs, Part 1300 to End. 2015. http://www.gpo.gov/fdsys/pkg/CFR-2011-title21-vol9/pdf/CFR-2011-title21-vol9-part1301.pdf. Accessed July 11, 2016.

20. Cathy A. Gallagher, U.S. Drug Enforcement Administration, Office of Diversion Control. Drug Theft Prevention. PowerPoint presentation, 2013. http://www.deadiversion.usdoj.gov/mtgs/pharm_awareness/conf_2013/may_2013/gallagher.pdf. Accessed December 20, 2015.

21. Walt Beadling. Cargo Security Alliance: 10 Takeaways from the GPS Cargo Tracking/Monitoring Forum. 2016. https://www.securecargo.org/sites/securecargo.org/files/10_takeaways_from_the_gps_cargo_tracking_forum_rx-360_and_pcsc_0.pdf. Accessed October 6, 2016.

22. Berge KH, Dillon KR, Sikkink KM, Taylor TK, Lanier WL. Diversion of drugs within health care facilities, a multiple-victim crime: patterns of diversion, scope, consequences, detection, and prevention. *Mayo Clin Proc.* 2012;87(7):674–682.

23. Eisler P. Doctors, medical staff on drugs put patients at risk. *USA Today.* April 17, 2014. http://www.usatoday.com/story/news/nation/2014/04/15/doctors-addicted-drugs-health-care-diversion/7588401/. Accessed April 9, 2016.

24. Skinner C. Former New York City hospital executive charged with $5.6 million painkiller theft. Reuters News Service. July 8, 2014. http://www.reuters.com/article/us-drugs-theft-new-york-idUSKBN0FD1XD20140708. Accessed January 23, 2016.

25. Surratt HL, Kurtz SP, Cicero TJ, Dart RC. Street Prices of Prescription Opioids Diverted to the Illicit Market. 2012. http://www.arsh.nova.edu/presentations/forms/street_prices_of_prescription_opioids_diverted_to_the_illicit_market.pdf. Accessed October 1, 2016.

26. Berge KH, Dillon KR, Sikkink KM, Taylor TK, Lanier WL. Diversion of drugs within health care facilities, a multiple-victim crime: patterns of diversion, scope, consequences, detection, and prevention. *Mayo Clin Proc.* 2012;87(7):674–682.

27. Bidgood J. Medical technician is sentenced in hepatitis C outbreak. *New York Times.* December 2, 2013. http://www.nytimes.com/2013/12/03/us/medical-technician-sentenced-in-hepatitis-c-outbreak.html. Accessed January 23, 2016.

28. Walker AK. Patient sues over hepatitis C exposure. *Baltimore Sun.* September 4, 2012. http://articles.baltimoresun.com/2012-09-04/health/bs-hs-hepatitis-c-lawsuit-20120904_1_david-kwiatkowski-hepatitis-c-hays-medical-center. Accessed January 23, 2016.

29. US Department of Justice, Drug Enforcement Administration. National Drug Threat Assessment. 2015. http://www.dea.gov/docs/2015%20NDTA%20Report.pdf. Accessed December 17, 2015.

30. Cai R, Crane E, Poneleit K, Paulozzi L. Emergency department visits involving nonmedical use of selected prescription drugs in the United States, 2004–2008. *J Pain Palliat Care Pharmacother.* 2010;24(3):293–297.

31. Kenan K, Mack K, Paulozzi L. Trends in prescriptions for oxycodone and other commonly used opioids in the United States, 2000–2010. *Open Medicine.* 2012;6(2):e41–47.

32. Food and Drug Administration. FDA Briefing Document: Drug Safety and Risk Management Advisory Committee (DSaRM) Meeting, October 29–30, 2012 (postponed to January 29–30, 2013). 2012. http://www.fda.gov/AdvisoryCommittees/CommitteesMeetingMaterials/Drugs/DrugSafetyandRiskManagementAdvisoryCommittee/ucm334275.htm. Accessed January 9, 2015.

33. Title 21, Code of Federal Regulations, Sect. 1306.07 (Administering or dispensing of narcotic drugs). https://www.gpo.gov/fdsys/pkg/CFR-2014-title21-vol9/pdf/CFR-2014-title21-vol9-chapII.pdf. Accessed December 21, 2015.

34. US Government Accountability Office. Medicaid: Fraud and Abuse Related to Controlled Substances Identified in Selected States. 2009. http://www.gao.gov/assets/300/294710.pdf. Accessed April 3, 2016.

35. Centers for Disease Control and Prevention, Office for State, Tribal, Local and Territorial Support. Doctor Shopping Laws. 2012. http://www.cdc.gov/phlp/docs/menu-shoppinglaws.pdf. Accessed December 21, 2015.

36. Centers for Disease Control and Prevention. Overdose deaths involving prescription opioids among Medicaid enrollees—Washington, 2004–2007. *MMWR Morbid Mortal Wkly Rep.* 2009;58(42):1171–1175. http://www.cdc.gov/mmwr/preview/mmwrhtml/mm5842a1.htm. Accessed December 17, 2015.

37. Jamison RN, Edwards RR. Risk factor assessment for problematic use of opioids for chronic pain. *Clin Neuropsychol.* 2013;27(1):60–80.

38. National Institute on Drug Abuse. The Science of Drug Abuse & Addiction: Trends and Statistics; Cost of Substance Abuse. 2015. http://www.drugabuse.gov/related-topics/trends-statistics. Accessed December 21, 2015.

39. Birnbaum HG, White AG, Schiller M, Waldman T, Cleveland JM, Roland CL. Societal costs of prescription opioid abuse, dependence, and misuse in the United States. *Pain Med.* 2011;12(4):657–667.

40. Coleman JJ. The supply chain of medicinal controlled substances: addressing the Achilles heel of drug diversion. *J Pain Palliat Care Pharmacother.* 2012;26(3):233–250.

41. Florida Legislature. An act (HB 7095) relating to prescription drugs, Chapter 2011-141, amending Florida Statute Sec. 456.072. 2011. http://laws.flrules.org/files/Ch_2011-141.pdf. Accessed December 22, 2015.

42. Washington State Department of Health. Pain Management: Engrossed Substitute House Bill 2876. 2013. http://www.doh.wa.gov/PublicHealthandHealthcareProviders/HealthcareProfessionsandFacilities/PainManagement.aspx. Accessed December 22, 2015.

43. Ohio Legislative Service Commission. Fiscal Note & Local Impact Statement: HB 93 ("The Pill Mill Law"). 2011. http://www.lsc.state.oh.us/fiscal/fiscalnotes/129ga/hb0093in.pdf. Accessed December 22, 2015.

44. Kentucky Board of Medical Licensure. Summary of HB 1: regulation of pain clinics and prescription drug abuse in Kentucky. 2012. http://kbml.ky.gov/hb1/Documents/KBML%20Summary%20of%20HB1.pdf. Accessed December 22, 2015.

45. Florida Department of Law Enforcement. Drugs Identified in Deceased Persons by Florida Medical Examiners 2010 Report. 2011. https://www.fdle.state.fl.us/Content/getdoc/59a8c497-5d9e-4954-b4d7-5dff6bb06e46/2010-Drug-Report.aspx. Accessed December 1, 2015.

46. State of Florida. House Bill 7095: An act relating to prescription drugs; amending s. 456.072. 2011. http://flsenate.gov/Session/Bill/2011/7095. Accessed December 22, 2015.

47. Bondi P. *Florida's Roadmap to End its Prescription Drug Abuse Epidemic.* Testimony by Florida Attorney General Pam Bondi, given before the Subcommittee on Commerce, Manufacturing and Trade, Committee on Energy and Commerce, U.S. House of Representatives, March 1, 2012.

48. Johnson H, Paulozzi L, Porucznik C, et al. Decline in drug overdose deaths after state policy changes—Florida, 2010–2012. *MMWR Morbid Mortal Wkly Rep.* 2014;63(26):569–574.

49. Florida Department of Law Enforcement. Drugs Identified in Deceased Persons by Florida Medical Examiners 2014 Report. 2015. https://www.fdle.state.fl.us/Content/Medical-Examiners-Commission/MEC-Publications-and-Forms/Documents/2014-Annual-Drug-Report-FINAL.aspx. Accessed December 1, 2015.

50. Adams S. Florida's prescription drug crackdown leaves some in need to suffer. *Chicago Tribune.* August 16, 2013.

51. Grant M. Pharmacies denying legitimate prescriptions: pharmacist says patients can be harmed by painkiller restrictions. News broadcast, WESH TV News, Orlando, FL, January 29, 2015. http://www.wesh.com/health/pharmacies-denying-legitimate-prescriptions/30986442. Accessed December 22, 2015.

52. Grant M. Prescription drug denials gaining traction with state leaders: Controlled Substances Standards Committee to address problems. News broadcast, WESH TV News, Orlando, FL, April 22, 2015. http://www.wesh.com/health/prescription-drug-denials-gaining-traction-with-state-leaders/32516338. Accessed December 22, 2015.

53. Resent drug ordinance: say the new one regulating the sale of morphine should be state-wide. *New York Times.* September 25, 1910.

54. Karen Blumenschein, Joseph L. Fink III, Patricia R. Freeman, et al. Review of Prescription Drug Monitoring Programs in the United States. 2010. http://chfs.ky.gov/NR/rdonlyres/85989824-1030-4AA6-91E1-7F9E3EF68827/0/KASPEREvaluationPDMPStatusFinalReport6242010.pdf. Accessed December 23, 2015.

55. Hal Rogers, US Representative. Illegal Drugs: Operation UNITE. 2015. http://halrogers.house.gov/issues/issue/?IssueID=8281. Accessed December 23, 2015.

56. Manchikanti L, Whitfield E, Pallone F. Evolution of the National All Schedules Prescription Electronic Reporting Act (NASPER): a public law for balancing treatment of pain and drug abuse and diversion. *Pain Physician.* 2005;8(4):335–347.

57. Karen Blumenschein, Joseph L. Fink III, Patricia R. Freeman, Kiasha James, Kenneth L. Kirsh, Douglas T. Steinke, Jeffery Talbert. Kentucky All Schedule Prescription Electronic Reporting Program (KASPER). 2010. http://chfs.ky.gov/NR/rdonlyres/85989824-1030-4AA6-91E1-7F9E3EF68827/0/KASPEREvaluationPDMPStatusFinalReport6242010.pdf. Accessed May 15, 2017.

58. National Alliance for Model State Drug Laws. Compilation of Prescription Monitoring Program Maps (Research current through December 2014). 2015. http://www.namsdl.org/library/F2582E26-ECF8-E60A-A2369B383E97812B/. Accessed December 25, 2015.

59. Schwarz A. Missouri alone in resisting prescription drug database. *New York Times.* July 20, 2014.

60. Department of Health and Human Services, Centers for Medicare & Medicaid Services (CMS). Health Insurance Portability and Accountability Act of 1996 (HIPAA). 2005. https://www.cms.gov/Regulations-and-Guidance/HIPAA-Administrative-Simplification/HIPAAGenInfo/downloads/hipaalaw.pdf. Accessed December 25, 2015.

61. National Alliance for Model State Drug Laws. State Prescription Drug Monitoring Programs and HIPAA Privacy Requirements. 2006. http://www.namsdl.org/library/2C1B0E8F-1372-636C-DD624D4C13DB85FF/. Accessed December 26, 2015.

62. Code of Federal Regulations, Title 45 (Public Welfare), Part 160 (General Administrative Requirements), Subpart B (Preemption of State Law), Section 160.203 (General rule and exceptions). http://www.ecfr.gov/cgi-bin/text-idx?SID=6e6fa1320f7ba794f373c91b5ae44345&mc=true&node=se45.1.160_1203&rgn=div8. Accessed December 26, 2015.

63. National Alliance for Model State Drug Laws. History of NASMDL. 2015. http://www.namsdl.org/history.cfm. Accessed December 26, 2015.

64. US General Accounting Office. Prescription Drugs: State Monitoring Programs Provide Useful Tool to Reduce Diversion. 2002. http://www.gao.gov/new.items/d02634.pdf. Accessed December 26, 2015.

65. US Supreme Court. *Whalen v. Roe,* No. 75-839. 1977. http://caselaw.findlaw.com/us-supreme-court/429/589.html. Accessed December 28, 2015.

66. David B. Brushwood, American Pharmacists Association. Unauthorized police access to PDMP data: case of *Brumley v City of Cleveland,* 2013 Tenn. App. LEXIS 274. 2013. https://www.pharmacist.com/unauthorized-police-access-pdmp-data. Accessed December 30, 2015.

67. Ancer L. Haggerty, United States Judge, U.S. District Court for the First District of Oregon, Portland Division. Opinion and Order, Document #60, filed 02/11/14; Case 3:12-cv-02023-HA, *Oregon PDMP v. DEA.* 2014. https://www.techdirt.com/articles/20140212/10133626198/district-court-says-deas-warrantless-access-oregons-prescription-database-is-unconstitutional.shtml. Accessed December 30, 2015.

68. Kyle Simon, Director of Policy and Advocacy, Center for Lawful Access and Abuse Deterrence. Letter to Transportation, Infrastructure, and Public Safety Committee, Missouri Senate, Jefferson City, MO re: PDMP data privacy concerns. 2015. http://claad.org/wp-content/uploads/2015/02/CLAAD-Letter-to-MO-Senate-re-PDMP-Legislation-150206.pdf. Accessed October 7, 2016.

69. Brandeis University, The Heller School for Social Policy and Management, PDMP Training and Technical Assistance Center. History of Prescription Monitoring Programs. PowerPoint slide deck, 2012. http://www.pdmpassist.org/pdf/PPTs/LE2012/1_Giglio_HistoryofPDMPs.pdf. Accessed December 28, 2015.

70. Fox BI, Felkey BG. ComputerTalk for the Pharmacist: The Status of Prescription Drug Monitoring Programs. January/February 2016. http://www.computertalk.com/department-columns/technology-corner-january-february-2016-the-status-of-prescription-drug-monitoring-programs. Accessed May 15, 2017.

71. Drug Enforcement Administration, Office of Diversion Control. Registrant Population by Business Activity: Pharmacy. 2016. http://www.deadiversion.usdoj.gov/drugreg/index.html. Accessed March 5, 2016.

72. Appriss Health. Real-time data for better informed decisions: The national leader in state prescription monitoring program solutions. 2017. https://apprisshealth.com/solutions/pmp-awarxe/. Accessed May 15, 2017.

73. National Association of Model State Drug Laws. History. 2017. http://www.namsdl.org/history.cfm. Accessed May 15, 2017.

74. National Alliance for Model State Drug Laws. Model Prescription Monitoring Program (PMP) Act. 2015. http://www.namsdl.org/library/A72D4573-0D93-65C4-281BD9DB01418276/. Accessed December 28, 2015.

75. Haffajee RL, Jena AB, Weiner SG. Mandatory use of prescription drug monitoring programs. *JAMA*. 2015;313(9):891–892.

76. National Institutes of Health, National Library of Medicine. PubMed Search Engine Query for Prescription Drug Monitoring Program. 2016. http://www.ncbi.nlm.nih.gov/pubmed. Accessed February 12, 2016.

77. Reisman RM, Shenoy PJ, Atherly AJ, Flowers CR. Prescription opioid usage and abuse relationships: an evaluation of state prescription drug monitoring program efficacy. *Subst Abuse*. 2009;3:41–51.

78. Paulozzi LJ, Kilbourne EM, Desai HA. Prescription drug monitoring programs and death rates from drug overdose. *Pain Med*. 2011;12(5):747–754.

79. Green TC, Zaller N, Rich J, Bowman S, Friedmann P. Revisiting Paulozzi et al.'s "Prescription drug monitoring programs and death rates from drug overdose." *Pain Med*. 2011;12(6):982–985.

80. Wilsey BL, Fishman SM, Gilson AM, et al. An analysis of the number of multiple prescribers for opioids utilizing data from the California Prescription Monitoring Program. *Pharmacoepidemiol Drug Safety*. 2011;20(12):1262–1268.

81. Parente ST, Kim SS, Finch MD, et al. Identifying controlled substance patterns of utilization requiring evaluation using administrative claims data. *Am J Manag Care*. 2004;10(11 Pt 1):783–790.

82. Reifler LM, Droz D, Bailey JE, et al. Do prescription monitoring programs impact state trends in opioid abuse/misuse? *Pain Med*. 2012;13(3):434–442.

83. Brady JE, Wunsch H, DiMaggio C, Lang BH, Giglio J, Li G. Prescription drug monitoring and dispensing of prescription opioids. *Public Health Rep*. 2014;129(2):139–147.

84. Gwira Baumblatt JA, Wiedeman C, Dunn JR, Schaffner W, Paulozzi LJ, Jones TF. High-risk use by patients prescribed opioids for pain and its role in overdose deaths. *JAMA Intern Med*. 2014;174(5):796–801.

85. Maughan BC, Bachhuber MA, Mitra N, Starrels JL. Prescription monitoring programs and emergency department visits involving opioids, 2004–2011. *Drug Alcohol Depend*. 2015;156:282–288.

86. Ringwalt C, Schiro S, Shanahan M, et al. The use of a prescription drug monitoring program to develop algorithms to identify providers with unusual prescribing practices for controlled substances. *J Prim Prev*. 2015;36(5):287–299.

87. Department of Health and Human Services, The Office of the National Coordinator for Health Information Technology. Prescription Drug Monitoring Program Interoperability Standards: A Report to Congress. 2013. https://www.healthit.gov/sites/default/files/fdasia1141report_final.pdf. Accessed October 14, 2016.

88. Thomas CP, Kim M, Nikitin RV, Kreiner P, Clark TW, Carrow GM. Prescriber response to unsolicited prescription drug monitoring program reports in Massachusetts. *Pharmacoepidemiol Drug Saf*. 2014;23(9):950–957.

89. Summer Brenwald. Prescription Drug Monitoring Program (PDMP); a study sponsored by the Bureau of Justice Assistance (Contract #GS-10F-0114L). 2013. https://www.bja.gov/Publications/PDMP_PPR_Jan-Dec13.pdf. Accessed May 15, 2017.

90. Girion L, Glover S. Senate rejects bill on prescription monitoring program. *Los Angeles Times*. May 28, 2013.

91. Electronic Florida Online Reporting of Controlled Substances Evaluation (E-FORCE). 2014–2015 Prescription Drug Monitoring Program Annual Report. 2015. http://www.floridahealth.gov/statistics-and-data/e-forcse/news-reports/_documents/2015-pdmp-annual-report.pdf. Accessed February 1, 2016.

92. Florida PDMP Foundation, Inc. Legislature establishes foundation to fund state PDMP database. 2015. http://www.flpdmpfoundation.com/. Accessed January 9, 2016.

93. Brandeis University, The Heller School for Social Policy and Management, The PDMP Center of Excellence, Training and Technical Assistance Center. Technical Assistance Guide No. 04-13, Funding Options for Prescription Drug Monitoring Programs. 2013. http://www.pdmpassist.org/pdf/PDMP_ Funding_Options_TAG.pdf. Accessed January 9, 2016.

94. Thomas Clark, John Eadie, Peter Kreiner, Gail Strickler. Heller School for Social Policy and Management, Brandeis University; Prescription Drug Monitoring Programs: An Assessment of the Evidence for Best Practices. 2012. http://www.pewtrusts.org/~/media/assets/0001/pdmp_update_1312013.pdf. Accessed January 16, 2016.

95. Brandeis University, The Heller School for Social Policy and Management, Prescription Drug Monitoring Program Center of Excellence at Brandeis. PDMPs and Third Party Payers Meeting. 2012. http://www. pdmpexcellence.org/sites/all/pdfs/Brandeis_COE_PDMP_3rd_pty_payer_mtg_rpt.pdf. Accessed January 9, 2016.

96. G. Caleb Alexander, Alex Cahana, Thomas Clark, et al. Prescription Drug Monitoring Programs: Critical elements of effective state legislation (Shatterproof Group). 2016. http://www.aiadc.org/File%20 Library/News/Shatterproof_WP_FINAL.pdf. Accessed May 15, 2017.

97. Griggs CA, Weiner SG, Feldman JA. Prescription drug monitoring programs: examining limitations and future approaches. *West J Emerg Med.* 2015;16(1):67–70.

98. Yarbrough CR. Prescription drug monitoring programs produce a limited impact on painkiller prescribing in Medicare Part D. *Health Serv Res.* 2017 [E-pub ahead of print].

99. US Department of Health and Human Services, Substance Abuse and Mental Health Services Administration, Office of Applied Studies. Drug Abuse Warning Network (DAWN) National & Metro Tables, 2004–2011 ("All misuse and abuse"). 2013. http://www.samhsa.gov/data/emergency-department-data-dawn/reports?tab=26. Accessed September 25, 2016.

100. Grant Baldwin, Centers for Disease Control and Prevention, National Center for Injury Prevention and Control, Division of Unintentional Injury Prevention. Overview of the Public Health Burden of Prescription Drug and Heroin Overdoses. PowerPoint slide program presented November 2, 2015. http://www.nihcm.org/pdf/Baldwin_original.pdf. Accessed January 12, 2016.

101. Personal communication, Len Paulozzi, MD (formerly with Centers for Disease Control and Prevention), via email January 4, 2016, to John J. Coleman. Response Granting Permission to Use Graph: ARCOS data vs Opioid Deaths Slide thru 2013.pptx (with unpublished imbedded Excel data).

102. Department of Health and Human Services, Food and Drug Administration. Regulatory Information: Food and Drug Administration Safety and Innovation Act (FDASIA). 2015. http:// www.fda.gov/RegulatoryInformation/Legislation/SignificantAmendmentstotheFDCAct/FDASIA/ ucm20027187.htm. Accessed October 14, 2016.

103. Department of Health and Human Services, Office of the Assistant Secretary for Health. Prescription Drug Monitoring Program Interoperability Standards: A report to Congress. Submitted to: The Committee on Health, Education, Labor, and Pensions, The Committee on Energy and Commerce (September). 2013. https://www.healthit.gov/sites/default/files/fdasia1141report_final.pdf. Accessed January 12, 2016.

104. US House of Representatives, Committee on Energy and Commerce. Report to accompany H.R. 1725, 114th Congress, 1st Session, Report No. 114-245: National All Schedules Prescription Electronic Reporting Reauthorization Act. 2015. https://www.congress.gov/114/crpt/hrpt245/CRPT-114hrpt245.pdf. Accessed February 8, 2016.

105. Congress.gov. National All Schedules Prescription Electronic Reporting Reauthorization Act of 2015 (all actions). 2017. https://www.congress.gov/search?searchResultViewType=expanded&q={"source":"legi slation","search":"National+All+Schedules+Prescription+Electronic+Reporting+Reauthorization+Act+ of+2015+","congress":"114"}. Accessed May 15, 2017.

106. J. M. Hammer, The MITRE Corporation. Enhancing Access to Prescription Drug Monitoring Programs: A national effort to reduce prescription drug abuse and overdose through technology and policy. PowerPoint

slide format, 2012. http://wiki.siframework.org/file/view/PDMP_Phase1_ResultsOverview.pdf/393951336/PDMP_Phase1_ResultsOverview.pdf. Accessed February 6, 2016.

107. House of Representatives, Subcommittee on Health of the Committee on Energy and Commerce. Hearing: Examining the Federal Government's Response to the Prescription Drug Crisis, June 14, 2013. 2014. https://www.gpo.gov/fdsys/pkg/CHRG-113hhrg85445/html/CHRG-113hhrg85445.htm. Accessed May 15, 2017.

108. Bureau of Justice Assistance. Harold Rogers Prescription Drug Monitoring Program: 19th National Conference on Pharmaceutical and Chemical Diversion. PowerPoint presentation, 2010. https://www.deadiversion.usdoj.gov/mtgs/drug_chemical/2010/rrose.pdf. Accessed May 15, 2017.

109. National Information Exchange Model. NIEM 3.0 Description. 2016. https://release.niem.gov/niem/3.0/. Accessed October 14, 2016.

110. National Council for Prescription Drug Programs. NCPDP Standards. 2016. https://www.ncpdp.org/home.aspx. Accessed October 14, 2016.

111. Department of Health and Human Services, The Office of National Coordinator for Health Information Technology. PDMPConnect: Making Connections with PDMPs. 2016. https://www.healthit.gov/pdmp/PDMPConnect. Accessed October 14, 2016.

112. Danna Droz, National Association of Boards of Pharmacy. Personal communication; telephone discussion between Danna Droz, NABP, and John J. Coleman, on February 19, 2016, pertaining to PMP InterConnect and PMP Gateway.

113. National Association of Boards of Pharmacy. NABP PMP InterConnect: Connecting State Prescription Monitoring Programs Nationwide. 2016. https://www.nabp.net/system/rich/rich_files/rich_files/000/001/264/original/nabpinterconnectflyer022016a.pdf. Accessed February 9, 2016.

114. NABP Continues to Fund PMP InterConnect Participation Supporting States' Momentum in the Fight Against Prescription Drug Abuse: System Facilitates Interstate PMP Data Sharing and Interoperability. PR Newswire-US Newswire. 2015. http://www.prnewswire.com/news-releases/nabp-continues-to-fund-pmp-interconnect-participation-supporting-states-momentum-in-the-fight-against-prescription-drug-abuse-300103465.html. Accessed February 9, 2016.

115. Appriss. PMP Gateway: Access and analyze data from Prescription Monitoring Programs (PMPs) within prescriber and dispenser workflows. 2016. http://www.appriss.com/pmpgateway.html. Accessed February 20, 2016.

116. Rutkow L, Turner L, Lucas E, Hwang C, Alexander GC. Most primary care physicians are aware of prescription drug monitoring programs, but many find the data difficult to access. *Health Affairs*. 2015;34(3):484–492.

117. Poon SJ, Greenwood-Ericksen MB, Gish RE, et al. Usability of the Massachusetts prescription drug monitoring program in the emergency department: a mixed methods study. *Acad Emerg Med*. 2016;23(4):406–414.

118. Gershman JA, Gershman JA, Fass AD, Popovici I. Evaluation of Florida physicians' knowledge and attitudes toward accessing the state prescription drug monitoring program as a prescribing tool. *Pain Med*. 2014;15(12):2013–2019.

119. State of Ohio, Board of Pharmacy. Ohio Automated Rx Reporting System: 2015 Annual Report. 2016. https://www.ohiopmp.gov/portal/documents/2015_OARRS_Report.pdf. Accessed October 14, 2016.

120. Steven W. Schierholt, Esq., Executive Director, State of Ohio Board of Pharmacy. Semiannual report on opioid prescribing in Ohio. 2015. https://www.ohiopmp.gov/portal/documents/OARRS_SemiAnnual_Report_on_Opioid_Prescribing_in_Ohio.pdf. Accessed January 14, 2016.

121. State of Ohio Board of Pharmacy. Mandatory OARRS Registration and Requests. 2015. http://www.pharmacy.ohio.gov/Documents/Pubs/Special/OARRS/H.B.%20341%20-%20Mandatory%20OARRS%20Registration%20and%20Requests.pdf. Accessed January 14, 2016.

122. Ulbrich TR, Dula CA, Green CG, Porter K, Bennett MS. Factors influencing community pharmacists' enrollment in a state prescription monitoring program. *J Am Pharmacists Assoc.* 2010;50(5):588–594.

123. Nebraska Department of Health & Human Services. Prescription Drug Monitoring Program (PDMP) Homepage. 2017. http://dhhs.ne.gov/publichealth/PDMP/Pages/Home.aspx. Accessed May 15, 2017.

124. Schleiter KE. Health law: when patient–physician confidentiality conflicts with the law. *Am Med Assoc J Ethics.* 2009;11(2):146–148.

125. National Alliance for Model State Drug Laws. State PMP Laws that Confer Immunity on Prescribers and/or Dispensers. 2015. http://www.namsdl.org/library/99BC96E9-D3F6-0E64-729A1ED1C3B1668C/. Accessed February 3, 2016.

126. Malida J. Health insurance fraud gets easier; so should stopping it. *Vantagepoint.* 2011;14(6):1–2.

127. Coalition Against Insurance Fraud. Prescription for Peril: How Insurance Fraud Finances Theft and Abuse of Addictive Prescription Drugs. 2007. http://www.insurancefraud.org/downloads/drugDiversion.pdf. Accessed January 6, 2015.

128. McAdam-Marx C, Roland CL, Cleveland J, Oderda GM. Costs of opioid abuse and misuse determined from a Medicaid database. *J Pain Palliat Care Pharmacother.* 2010;24(1):5–18.

129. US Government Accountability Office. Report No. GAO-15-66; Medicare Program Integrity: CMS Pursues Many Practices to Address Prescription Drug Fraud, Waste, and Abuse. 2014. http://www.gao.gov/assets/670/666647.pdf. Accessed January 6, 2016.

130. US House of Representatives, Office of the Legislative Counsel. Compilation of Patient Protection and Affordable Care Act. 2010. http://www.hhs.gov/sites/default/files/ppacacon.pdf. Accessed January 7, 2016.

131. Department of Health and Human Services, HHS.gov. Key Features of the Affordable Care Act by Year. 2015. http://www.hhs.gov/healthcare/facts-and-features/key-features-of-aca-by-year/index.html. Accessed January 7, 2016.

132. Visante. Pharmacy Benefit Managers (PBMs): Generating Savings for Plan Sponsors and Consumers. Prepared for Pharmaceutical Care Management Association, 2016. http://www.pcmanet.org/images/stories/uploads/2016/visante%20pbm%20savings%20study%202016.pdf. Accessed February 25, 2016.

133. Mississippi Independent Pharmacy Association. PBM Model & Facts. 2016. http://mipa.ms/pbm-model-facts/. Accessed February 27, 2016.

134. Express Scripts. Corporate Overview. 2016. http://lab.express-scripts.com/about/. Accessed February 25, 2016.

135. Steve Miller, M.D., Express Scripts. Fighting Rx Abuse and the Cash-Claims Loophole. 2013. http://lab.express-scripts.com/lab/insights/drug-safety-and-abuse/fighting-rx-abuse-and-the-cash-claims-loophole Accessed February 25, 2016.

136. Du J. What is the pharmacy benefit management industry? *Investopedia.* 2015. http://www.investopedia.com/articles/markets/070215/what-pharmacy-benefit-management-industry.asp. Accessed February 28, 2016.

137. EnvisionRX. Rite Aid Acquisition of Leading Independent Pharmacy Benefit Manager EnvisionRx Complete. 2015. https://www.envisionrx.com/LatestNews/pressrelease.aspx. Accessed February 28, 2016.

138. Jo-Ellen Abou Nader, Senior Director of Waste, Fraud & Abuse Services, Express Scripts Holding Company. Curbing Opioid Abuse: A payer perspective. PowerPoint slide deck, 2014. http://www.allhealth.org/briefingmaterials/JANWEBSITE_I3.PDF. Accessed October 9, 2016.

139. Black HC, Nolan JR, Nolan-Haley JM. *Black's Law Dictionary.* 6th ed. St. Paul, MN: West Publishing Co.; 1991.

140. Code of Federal Regulations. Title 21, Section 1301.11 (*Persons required to register, etc.*). *21 C.F.R. 1301.11.* 1970. https://www.gpo.gov/fdsys/pkg/CFR-2016-title21-vol9/pdf/CFR-2016-title21-vol9-part1301.pdf. Accessed May 15, 2017.

141. Code of Federal Regulations. 21 CFR 1301.71(a) ("Security requirements generally"). 2012. http://www.gpo.gov/fdsys/pkg/CFR-2012-title21-vol9/pdf/CFR-2012-title21-vol9-chapII.pdf.   Accessed October 8, 2016.

142. Code of Federal Regulations. 21 CFR 1304, et seq. (Records and Reports of Registrants). 2016. http://www.gpo.gov/fdsys/pkg/CFR-2014-title21-vol9/pdf/CFR-2014-title21-vol9-chapII.pdf. Accessed May 15, 2017.

143. National Archives of the US, Office of the Federal Register. Code of Federal Regulations, Title 21, Food and Drugs, Part 300 to End (Sect. 301.21, "Persons required to register"). 1972. http://loc.heinonline.org/loc/Contents?handle=hein.cfr/cfr1972049. Accessed October 8, 2016.

144. Federal Register, Drug Enforcement Administration: Final Rule. Definition and Registration of Reverse Distributors (70 FR 22591). 2003. https://www.gpo.gov/fdsys/pkg/FR-2005-05-02/pdf/05-8692.pdf. Accessed October 8, 2016.

145. Federal Register, Drug Enforcement Administration Final Rule. Allowing Central Fill Pharmacies and Retail Pharmacies to Fill Prescriptions for Controlled Substances on Behalf of Retail Pharmacies (68 FR 37405). 2003. https://www.gpo.gov/fdsys/pkg/FR-2003-06-24/pdf/03-15912.pdf. Accessed October 8, 2016.

146. Express Scripts Holding Company. Infographic: Prescription Drug Fraud & Abuse: Rx Abuse and Pharmacy Fraud: Deadlier than cocaine and heroin combined. 2014. http://lab.express-scripts.com/lab/insights/drug-safety-and-abuse/infographic-prescription-drug-fraud-and-abuse. Accessed October 9, 2016.

147. Department of Health and Human Services, Office of Inspector General. Oversight of the Prescriber Identifier Field in Prescription Drug Event Data for Schedule II Drugs. 2011. https://oig.hhs.gov/oas/reports/other/140900302.pdf. Accessed October 10, 2016.

148. Department of Health and Human Services, Office of Inspector General. Invalid Prescriber Identifiers on Medicare Part D Drug Claims. 2010. https://oig.hhs.gov/oei/reports/oei-03-09-00140.pdf. Accessed October 10, 2016.

149. U.S. Government Accountability Office. Medicaid: Fraud and Abuse Related to Controlled Substances Identified in Selected States (GAO Report No. GAO-09-957). 2009. http://www.gao.gov/assets/300/294710.pdf. Accessed June 6, 2016.

150. Drug Enforcement Administration, Office of Diversion Control. ARCOS Retail Drug Summary Reports. 2016. https://www.deadiversion.usdoj.gov/arcos/retail_drug_summary/index.html. Accessed May 9, 2017.

151. Paulozzi LJ, Budnitz DS, Youngli Xi. Increasing deaths from opioid analgesics in the United States. *Pharmacoepidemiol Drug Safety.* 2006;15:618–627.

152. Compton WM, Jones CM, Baldwin GT. Relationship between nonmedical prescription-opioid use and heroin use. *N Engl J Med.* 2016;374(2):154–163.

153. Substance Abuse and Mental Health Services Administration, Office of Applied Studies. Drug Abuse Warning Network: Development of a New Design (Methodology Report). DAWN Series M-4, DHHS Publication No. (SMA) 02-3754. Rockville, MD. 2002. http://archive.samhsa.gov/data/dawn/dawninfo/pubs/new-design.pdf. Accessed January 22, 2017.

154. Substance Abuse and Mental Health Services Administration, Drug Abuse Warning Network. New DAWN: Why It Cannot Be Compared with Old DAWN. 2005. http://www.samhsa.gov/data/DAWN/TNDR.htm. Accessed January 23, 2017.

155. Substance Abuse and Mental Health Services Administration. About Emergency Department Data. 2016. https://www.samhsa.gov/data/emergency-department-data-dawn/about. Accessed January 19, 2017.

CHAPTER 4

WHATEVER HAPPENED TO THE *DECADE OF PAIN CONTROL AND RESEARCH?*

John J. Coleman

INTRODUCTION

On October 31, 2000, advocates for improved pain treatment scored a victory when President Bill Clinton signed into law a bill declaring the first decade of the 21st century the *Decade of Pain Control and Research*[1] (Fig. 4.1). This followed on the heels of the Department of Veterans Affairs announcement in 1999 that henceforth pain would be considered a patient's fifth vital sign, to be measured along with pulse, respiration, body temperature, and blood pressure.[2] The prestigious Joint Commission on Accreditation of Healthcare Organizations and the influential American Pain Society joined the Department of Veterans Affairs in supporting this concept.[3]

Although relieving pain has figured prominently in the medical arts since the beginning of recorded history, the management of chronic pain as a subspecialty in medicine is a relatively recent phenomenon.[4] Tompkins et al. attribute the decline in multidisciplinary pain treatment in the 1980s to various regulatory, health system, and provider factors that combined to make opioids the predominant strategy for treating chronic pain.[4]

By the 1990s, opioids had moved from the terminal cancer and end-of-life care setting to the standard of care for treating noncancer chronic pain.[5] To coincide with the growing interest in treating pain, a new opioid product called OxyContin (Purdue Pharma, L.P.) was introduced in 1996.[6] The drug itself—oxycodone—was not new, having been developed some 80 years before by German chemists.[7] What was new, however, was the delivery system.[6] An OxyContin tablet has a biphasic release and absorption profile that provides the user with an immediate release of a portion of the dose; then the remainder of the dose is released and absorbed at a controlled rate over 12 hours.[8]

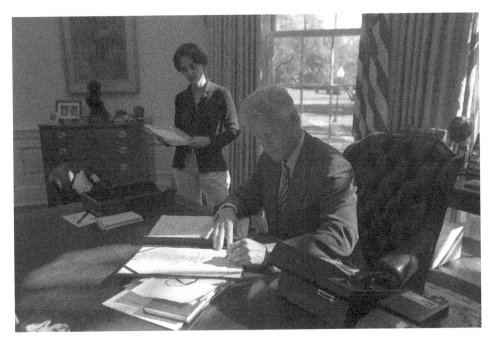

FIGURE 4.1 President Bill Clinton signing into law the *Decade of Pain Control and Research*, October 31, 2000

Courtesy of Clinton Public Library, Little Rock, AR.

For many chronic pain sufferers OxyContin was a godsend. It replaced their immediate-release medications and ended the need to take pain pills every 4 to 6 hours. The drug's sponsor, Purdue, foresaw the commercial potential of its new product and developed an aggressive marketing plan to promote it as a first-line therapy among primary care providers treating chronic malignant and nonmalignant pain, including musculoskeletal and post-operative pain.[9] In its first 5 years on the market OxyContin's annual sales jumped from $48 million to $1.1 billion.[10]

By 2000, however, public health officials were concerned about the increased frequency of abuse reports and overdose deaths involving OxyContin.[11] At first, its abuse appeared centered mostly in the Appalachian states, Maine, and Ohio.[11] Media reports told of opiate addicts crushing the high-dose tablets for oral, inhalation, and injection administration.[9] In 2001, the US Food and Drug Administration (FDA) posted its first public warning about OxyContin abuse.[12]

Hoping to ride, if not push, the wave of excitement was Purdue, the company that introduced the world to extended-release opioids in 1987 with MS Contin, a morphine sulfate drug.[13] The excitement subsided, however, by 2003, when the FDA accused Purdue of violating the law by failing to disclose OxyContin's abuse risks in advertisements placed in the *Journal of the American Medical Association*.[14] By then, there already had been several, sometimes rancorous, congressional hearings into the abuse and misuse of OxyContin.[15–18] The tide was beginning to turn against what some had called a wonder drug.[19]

In 2007, after a lengthy investigation by the FDA, Purdue pled guilty to charges of misbranding OxyContin with the intent to defraud or mislead—a criminal felony under the Food, Drug and Cosmetic Act.[20] The pleading was in response to an Information that, among other things, charged that "[b]eginning on or about December 12, 1995, and continuing until on or about June 30, 2001, certain PURDUE supervisors and employees, with the intent to defraud or mislead, marketed and promoted OxyContin as less addictive, less subject to abuse and diversion, and less likely to cause tolerance and withdrawal than other pain medications."[20] The company's three top executives, including its president, medical director, and general counsel were charged as responsible corporate officials, and pled guilty to criminal misdemeanor charges.[21] The court imposed substantial fines totaling more than $635 million on the company and its three executives.[21]

THE GENESIS OF THE MODERN PAIN-CONTROL ERA

In 1980, a letter by Drs. Herschel Jick and Jane Porter to the editors of the *New England Journal of Medicine* suggested that pain patients receiving treatment with opioids were unlikely to become addicted.[22] The letter reported finding only four cases of drug-seeking behavior among 11,882 hospital patients receiving narcotics for their pain.[22]

In the early days of the *Decade of Pain Control and Research*, the oft-cited Porter and Jick "study" became a rationale for minimizing the risks associated with long-term opioid use.[4] Decades later, Drs. Porter and Jick would reveal that they submitted their information to the journal as a letter to the editor because "the data weren't adequate to be published as a study [and] one couldn't conclude anything about the risks of long-term narcotic use from the figures."[22]

In 1986, Drs. Russell K. Portenoy and Kathleen M. Foley, luminaries in the field of pain and palliative care, conducted a study of 38 pain patients and concluded that "opioid maintenance therapy can be a safe, salutary and more humane alternative to the options of surgery or no treatment in those patients with intractable non-malignant pain and no history of drug abuse."[5] Many in the pharmaceutical industry and the pain-management field would cite this statement to minimize the potential adverse side effects of opioids.[4]

In 2000, *JAMA* published an article by University of Wisconsin researchers comparing medical records of the Drug Abuse Warning Network (DAWN), a public health surveillance system that measures drug abuse, with drug transaction records of the Automation of Reports and Consolidated Orders System (ARCOS), a source of commercial distribution data for controlled substances, for the period of 1990 to 1996.[23] They reported that despite significant increases in the medical use of four of five studied opioids, abuse decreased for all except morphine, which showed a slight increase (3%).[23] They concluded that "The present trend of increasing medical use of opioid analgesics to treat pain does not appear to be contributing to increases in the health consequences of opioid analgesic abuse."[23] The authors of the *JAMA* article were well known in the pain community for their advocacy on behalf of chronic pain patients.[24] Conflict-of-interest disclosures, however, noted that they all were consultants and speakers for various opioid makers.[23]

Despite the pain community's embrace of the *JAMA* article, limitations rendered its findings irrelevant to the growing problem of opioid abuse.[23] Though published in 2000, when concerns about prescription opioid abuse were increasing, the study period was 1990 to 1996, a time that predated the sharp rise in opioid abuse that followed OxyContin's market debut in 1996.[6,23]

Another limitation of the study was its omission of hydrocodone, an opioid prescribed more frequently—and abused more frequently—than all other opioids combined.[25] According to the FDA, in 2011, there were 131 million prescriptions issued for hydrocodone combination products, compared with 57 million for oxycodone-containing products (34.6 million for combination products and 22.3 million for single-entity products), 7.6 million for morphine products, and 2.7 million for hydromorphone products.[25]

The *JAMA* study showed that, collectively, fentanyl, hydromorphone, meperidine, morphine, and oxycodone accounted for a total of 5,573 DAWN abuse mentions in 1996, whereas, for the same year, DAWN abuse mentions for hydrocodone amounted to 11,419—more than double the combined total for all the opioids studied.[26]

In 2004, the authors of the *JAMA* article published a "reassessment" of their original study, noting that in 2002, opioid analgesics accounted for 9.85% of all DAWN drug abuse mentions, up from 5.75% in 1997.[27] As in the original study, the authors omitted hydrocodone and codeine from their reassessment, claiming that they did so because these drugs are not indicated for the treatment of severe pain.[27] Also not included in either study was methadone, which is marketed for the treatment of addiction as well as pain.[27]

GOVERNMENT ACTS TO HALT OPIOID ABUSE

As previously mentioned, between 2001 and 2002, Congress held no fewer than four hearings on OxyContin abuse, two in the House and two in the Senate.[15–18] In 2003, the US Department of Health and Human Services Office of Inspector General (OIG) issued a 56-page document, "Compliance Program Guidance for Pharmaceutical Manufacturers," that warned against certain actions that might violate the federal anti-kickback statute.[28] The federal anti-kickback statute (42 U.S.C. §1320a-7b(b)) is a criminal law that prohibits offering, paying, soliciting, or receiving anything of value to induce or reward referrals or generate federal healthcare program business.[29] Each violation of the statute carries a possible fine of up to $25,000 and a prison sentence of up to 5 years.[29]

The OIG's report zeroed in on some of the industry's most popular and successful promotional activities:

> Manufacturers, providers, and suppliers of health care products and services frequently cultivate relationships with physicians in a position to generate business for them through a variety of practices, including gifts, entertainment, and personal services compensation arrangements. These activities have a high potential for fraud and abuse and, historically, have generated a substantial number of anti-kickback convictions. There is no substantive

difference between remuneration from a pharmaceutical manufacturer or from a durable medical equipment or other supplier—if the remuneration is intended to generate any federal health care business, it potentially violates the anti-kickback statute.[28]

The OIG's report caused pharmaceutical companies to end the practice of providing free educational retreats for top prescribers paid honoraria to listen to sponsored presentations about the companies' products. The industry suffered a more devastating blow in 2007, when, as noted above, Purdue—its putative leader in the opioid sector—and three of its top executives pled guilty to federal criminal charges of unlawfully marketing OxyContin.[30-33] Court documents would show that Purdue used fraudulent marketing practices to mislead physicians about the health and safety risks of OxyContin.[20]

LITIGATING THE *DECADE OF PAIN CONTROL AND RESEARCH*

In 2012, the *Wall Street Journal* published an article in which Dr. Russell Portenoy, a key figure in the pain movement, expressed second thoughts about the use of opioids: "Did I teach about management, specifically about opioid therapy, in a way that reflects misinformation? Well, against the standards of 2012, I guess I did. We didn't know then what we know now."[34,35] Portenoy, however, had acknowledged some concerns about opioids in a 1996 journal article: "The potential for physical dependence and iatrogenic addiction is a major issue in the use of opioid drugs for the management of chronic nonmalignant pain."[36] Portenoy's change of heart came at a time when the White House and Centers for Disease Control and Prevention (CDC) were pondering what to do about the "epidemic," as they called it, of prescription opioid abuse.[37,38]

Portenoy's interview with the *Wall Street Journal* reverberated beyond the medical field and foreshadowed legal action taken against the pharmaceutical industry for alleged wrongdoing in promoting and selling opioids.[39] In 2014, the California counties of Santa Clara and Orange jointly filed suit against Purdue and several other drug makers accusing them of violating the state's false advertising and unfair competition laws, as well as creating a "public nuisance."[40] In a hearing before the Orange County Superior Court, the defendants moved for the case to be dismissed on the grounds that exclusive jurisdiction over the matters in dispute rested with the federal government.[40] The court agreed and dismissed the suit.[40]

Next on the docket was the city of Chicago, which filed a suit charging nine opioid manufacturers with state law violations, including "consumer fraud, misrepresentation, false statements, false claims, insurance fraud, and unjust enrichment."[41] The suit, filed June 2, 2014, in state court, was removed to federal court on July 3, 2014.[41] In its opening brief to the federal court, the city of Chicago asked for a judgment requiring defendants to pay restitution, damages, attorneys' fees, and expenses.[42] On May 8, 2015, on a motion by the defendants, the court dismissed nine of the 11 counts, leaving intact counts one and two (consumer fraud claims) against Purdue.[43] In August 2015, the city of Chicago filed an amended complaint against all the defendants.[43] As of May 16, 2017, the parties have been ordered to confer and agree on written discovery motions by June 7, 2017.[44]

Perhaps the most ambitious case against the drug makers was filed on December 15, 2015, in the Chancery Court of the First Judicial District of Hinds County, Mississippi.[45] In this case, the state of Mississippi charged a number of opioid makers with violations of Mississippi's Medicaid Fraud Control Act, violations of Mississippi's Consumer Protection Act, fraud, negligent misrepresentation, unjust enrichment, and public nuisance.[45] The accusations in the state's 247-page complaint resembled those contained in the California and Chicago cases.[40,43,45]

Unlike the federal case against Purdue, which was based on evidence of false and misleading claims that did not comport with OxyContin's official FDA-approved label, the state cases that have been filed thus far charge a variety of consumer and insurance fraud charges requiring evidence of intent and/or recklessness.[40,43,45] The complaint filed by the city of Chicago, for example, alleged that the defendants "planned to change prescriber habits through the calculated release of false, misleading, and unsupported information."[42] Individually and collectively, the defendants engaged in what the complaint described as a process to "manufacture a body of literature" that would support their interests, using key opinion leaders in the pain movement to author sponsored journal articles "that did nothing more than discuss and cite other studies that came to the same unsupported conclusions."[42]

It also was alleged that the "defendants disseminated false, misleading, imbalanced, and unsupported statements through unbranded marketing materials," described as materials that promoted opioids but omitted using brand names to avoid running afoul of consumer protection laws.[42] This practice, it was alleged, was also intended to avoid having to comply with federal regulations requiring the FDA's approval of promotional materials as consistent with a product's official label.[42]

STATE CASES UNRAVEL HISTORY OF QUESTIONABLE PRACTICES

Among the more inflammatory charges in the Chicago complaint was the alleged creation, support, and direction given by the defendants to "a network of Front Groups to collectively promote the treatment of chronic pain using opioid products over other alternatives."[42] Defendants, it was alleged, engaged a medical publishing firm to produce unbranded pamphlets and DVDs on opioids aimed at the general public.[42] Professional groups, such as the American College of Physicians, were listed as partners, "though the content was drafted by a professional medical writer [and] ... funded by the drug company sponsor."[42]

Prominent names in the pain management field are identified in the Chicago complaint as "key opinion leaders."[42] In return for generous financial compensation, amounting in some cases to millions of dollars, key opinion leaders were alleged to have conducted seminars, given speeches, published journal articles, and performed other promotional activities on behalf of the defendants and their drug products while failing to disclose potential health risks, including the risk of abuse and addiction.[42]

Over time, plaintiffs in these cases amassed voluminous discovery materials to show, among other things, that sales representatives employed by the defendants were trained to misrepresent the risks of addiction associated with opioid products.[45] In the Mississippi complaint, the state charged that sales representatives of one of the defendants were instructed "to promote the misleading concept of 'pseudoaddiction',— i.e., that drug-seeking behavior was not a cause for alarm, but merely a manifestation of undertreated pain."[45]

The concept of pseudoaddiction was defined by Weissman and Haddox (1989) as an "iatrogenic syndrome that mimics the behavioral symptoms of addiction" in patients receiving an inadequate supply of opioids for their pain.[46] The diagnosis was based on a single case involving a 17-year-old patient with acute leukemia who engaged in aberrant behaviors often associated with being addicted.[47] Weissman and Haddox recommended increasing the pseudoaddict's opioid medication to prevent the aberrant drug-seeking behavior.[47] The misinterpretation of this syndrome, according to some pain experts, has been used to justify escalating doses in the face of noncompliance.[48]

IGNORING THE CANARY IN THE MINE

To be sure, there were pain experts who warned their colleagues not to be too cavalier in promoting the use of opioids for long-term chronic nonmalignant pain. In a letter to the *Journal of Pain and Symptom Management* in May 2001, Dr. Steven Passik, a pain psychologist at Memorial Sloan-Kettering Cancer Center, observed that zealous pain specialists relying on faulty information about opioid risks may have contributed to their abuse:

> Unfortunately, the problem of opioid abuse during the course of pain management is an issue over which—I'm afraid—those of us in the pain management community have been somewhat disingenuous. While I certainly believe that the risk of addiction, abuse and poor adherence (aberrant drug-related behavior) in the use of these medications is far less than was once believed to be the case, it is not zero. In our zeal to improve access to opioids and relieve patient suffering, pain specialists have understated the problem, drawing faulty conclusions from very limited data. In effect, we have told primary care doctors and other prescribers that the risk was so low that they essentially could ignore the possibility of addiction. We have also overstated the concept that long-acting drugs have a lower risk of abuse.[49]

In what perhaps was a prescient warning, in 2003 a group of researchers at the Wright State University School of Medicine in Dayton, Ohio, wrote a letter to the editor of the *American Family Physician* in which they reported a small sample study of recent heroin initiates in Ohio.[50] Of 10 subjects surveyed, five reported having abused prescription opioids, "most notably OxyContin," before initiating heroin use.[50] Acknowledging the limitations of their small convenience sample, the researchers concluded that "the abuse of opioid analgesics constitutes a new route to heroin abuse."[50] Poignantly, more than a decade later, the CDC would publish a study of substance abuse trends among heroin users for the period 2002 through 2013, finding, among other things, "the largest percentage increase [of heroin users], 138.2%, occurred among nonmedical users of opioid pain relievers."[51]

THE *DECADE OF PAIN CONTROL AND RESEARCH*

As previously mentioned, a major coup for the advocates of improved pain treatment came in the form of federal legislation enacted in 2000 that officially designated the first decade of the 21st century the *Decade of Pain Control and Research*.[1] The decade lasted from January 1, 2001, to December 31, 2010.[1] During this time, the FDA approved 219 drugs and biologics designated as "new molecular entities."[52] Nine (4.1%) were indicated for acute pain, including three for migraine.[52] Only one (Tapentadol) was indicated for the treatment of moderate to severe *acute* pain.[52] None was indicated for treating chronic pain.[52] On August 26, 2011, Tapentadol extended-release tablets received FDA approval for the management of moderate to severe *chronic* pain.[53] Despite the emphasis on research, not a single new medication to treat chronic pain was approved during the decade.[52] This is somewhat understandable, inasmuch as Congress neglected to provide funding for the *Decade of Pain Control and Research*.[1]

One year after the *Decade of Pain Control and Research* was over, in June 2011, the Institute of Medicine (IOM) published a lengthy report titled *Relieving Pain in America: A Blueprint for Transforming Prevention, Care, Education, and Research*.[54] The IOM was established in 1970 by congressional charter as a division of the National Academy of Sciences, which was founded in 1863 by President Abraham Lincoln as a "body that would operate outside of government to advise the nation 'whenever called upon.'"[55] Its members are elected based on their professional credentials and achievements and they serve without compensation.[55] In 2015, the National Academy of Sciences voted to reorganize the IOM and rename it the National Academy of Medicine.[55] The IOM's pain report was in response to the 2010 Patient Protection and Affordable Care Act, also known as the Affordable Care Act or "Obamacare" that, among other things, required the Department of Health and Human Services to engage the IOM to study pain in America as a public health problem.[54]

The IOM report was not without its critics, who challenged the claim in the report's preface that "Acute and chronic pain affects large numbers of Americans, with approximately 100 million U.S. adults burdened by chronic pain alone."[54] The initial report had stated that 116 million American adults suffered from chronic pain, but this was later revised to 100 million after a math error was discovered and corrected.[56,57] Kennedy et al. (2014) analyzed data from the 2010 Quality of Life Supplement of the National Health Interview Survey and concluded—contrary to the IOM findings—that about 19.0% of adults (approximately 39.4 million persons) in the United States suffer from persistent pain.[58] "Most adults who report conditions such as arthritis, carpal tunnel syndrome, or back or joint pain," the researchers said, "do not describe their pain as 'persistent.'"[58]

If nothing else, the report served the congressional mandate in the Affordable Care Act "to increase the recognition of pain as a significant public health problem in the United States."[59]

MEDIA INVESTIGATIONS STIR CONGRESSIONAL INQUIRIES

In 2011, the *Milwaukee Journal Sentinel*, part of the *USA Today* network, uncovered information linking faculty members of the University of Wisconsin's School of Medicine and Public Health with drug and medical device manufacturers.[60] Reporters noted that a popular pain and policy group housed at the university failed to disclose receiving millions of dollars from opioid makers when, for example, it contested a 2006 report by the CDC linking opioid overdose deaths with a 500% increase in the number of prescriptions written for the drugs.[60]

Using the state's open records law, the *Sentinel* obtained records showing that between 1999 and 2010, the group received about $2.5 million from drug companies, including $1.6 million from Purdue.[61] After these findings were made public, the university reported that it would no longer accept funding from industry sources involved in the marketing of opioids.[61]

In 2012, the *Sentinel* expanded its inquiry to include organizations dedicated to the interests of pain patients and their physicians.[62] Reporters learned that in 1996, the American Pain Foundation (APF) and the American Academy of Pain Medicine—two nonprofit organizations funded in part by the drug industry and representing pain patients and pain physicians, respectively—issued a joint statement endorsing the use of opioids to treat chronic pain and claiming that the risk of addiction was low.[62]

About the same time as the *Sentinel* inquiry, investigative reporters with ProPublica, an independent nonprofit watchdog news agency in New York, were conducting a series of similar inquiries into financial ties between medical specialists and the companies that manufacture and supply devices and drugs used by them in their practice.[63] Pain management was one of several specialties covered by the ProPublica reporters.[63] In December 2011, ProPublica revealed that the APF, self-described as "the nation's largest advocacy group for pain patients," had received almost 90% of its $5 million funding in 2010 from the drug and medical device industry.[64] The report cited examples of how the APF appeared to promote the interests of the industry over those of the pain patients it claimed to represent:

> [The APF] has intervened in court cases in ways that appear to counter its stated mission. In one example, it sided with Purdue Pharma, its longtime funder, to block a 2001 class-action case filed by Ohio patients who had become addicted to or dependent on the company's blockbuster painkiller, OxyContin. And the foundation mobilizes patients to send "outraged" email messages to news organizations that run stories it believes reinforce "stigmas and stereotypes" about the risks of pain medication.[64]

By 2012, the *Sentinel* and ProPublica reports had attracted the attention of Congress.[65] In May, the Chairman and Ranking Member of the Senate Committee on Finance sent letters to Endo Pharmaceuticals, Johnson & Johnson, the American Pain Society, the APF, the Federation of State Medical Boards, Purdue Pharma L.P., the American Academy of Pain Medicine, the Pain & Policy Studies Group, the Center for Practical Bioethics, and the Joint Commission, asking for records showing funds given to, or received from, corporate entities or individuals involved in any way with the manufacture, distribution, or promotion of opioid medications.[65] Addressees were requested to provide records from 1997 to the present (2012) and to comply with the Committee's request "no later than June 8, 2012."[65] (Several requests by this author for additional information, specifically regarding responses to the Committee's request, were sent to Senator Orrin Hatch, current chair of the Senate Committee on Finance. They have not been answered.)

THE ROLE OF THE WHOLESALE DRUG DISTRIBUTOR

Because of its relatively weak pharmacy laws, Florida became a magnet for "pill mills," unlawful enterprises posing as pain management clinics and selling controlled substances to persons posing as legitimate patients.[66,67] As the *Decade of Pain Control and Research* came to an end, it was estimated that more than 900 of these pill mills were operating in Florida, which also served as home to 98 of the top 100 dispensing physicians of oxycodone pills in the United States.[66,67]

In 2005, after several years of investigating pill mills and rogue internet pharmacies, DEA turned its attention to the companies supplying them.[68] Using a provision in the law that heretofore had rarely been enforced, DEA launched an industry-wide special project called the "Distributor Initiative" that focused on registered wholesale distributors that failed to identify and report suspicious orders for controlled substances received from retail customers, including pill mills, rogue internet pharmacies, and registered pharmacies.[69] Between 2006 and 2016, a sizable number of wholesale drug distributors, including the "big three"—McKesson, AmeriSource Bergen, and Cardinal Health—were charged, sometimes more than once, with failing to prevent the diversion of tens of millions of doses of controlled substances, principally oxycodone and hydrocodone (Table 4.1).

Federal law requires DEA-registered manufacturers and distributors of controlled substances to design and operate systems to disclose suspicious orders, which are defined in the law as "orders of unusual size, orders deviating substantially from a normal pattern, and orders of unusual frequency."[70] Orders received for controlled substances fitting any of these criteria must be reported to the nearest DEA field office.[70] Federal law also requires that official order forms (paper or electronic) be used by DEA registrants authorized to purchase controlled substances from registered manufacturers and distributors.[72] Copies of official order forms (paper or electronic) for all classes (C-I to C-V) of controlled substances must be sent to DEA.[71,72] Copies of filled transaction reports (paper or electronic) for C-I and C-II drugs and narcotic substances in C-III must be sent to DEA by the distributor

TABLE 4.1 Major DEA regulatory actions against distributors and other supply-chain entities between 2006 and 2017

Distributor	Date	Drug	Amount (millions of dosage units)	Disposition	DEA Registration(s)
Southwood Pharm.	2006	Hydrocodone	8.7	MOA	1 Restored
Cardinal Health	2007	Hydrocodone	>8	$34 million fine/MOA	3 Restored
AmeriSourceBergen	2007	Hydrocodone	3.8	MOA	1 Restored
McKesson	2008	Hydrocodone	~3	$13.25 million fine/MOA	6 Restored
Masters Pharm.	2009	Hydrocodone	>4	$500,000 fine	1 Restored
Sunrise Wholesale	2010	Oxycodone	NA	n/a	Surrendered
Harvard Medical Grp.	2010	Oxycodone	>13	$8 million fine/MOA	1 Restored
KeySource Medical	2010	Oxycodone	~48	$320,000 fine/MOA	1 Suspended/ Revoked
Omnicare[a]	2012	Various CS	Unknown	$50 million fine	Unaffected
CVS	2012	Various CS	Unknown	$11 million fine	Unaffected
Cardinal Health	2012	Oxycodone	>13	$44 million fine/MOA[e]	1 Suspended, 2 years
Walgreens	2013	Various CS	Unknown	$80 million fine/MOA	7 suspended, 12–16 months
UPS[b]	2013	Various CS	Unknown	$40 million fine	Unaffected
FedEx[c]	2014	Various CS	Unknown	Case dismissed 6/16	n/a
CVS Health	2015	Various CS	Unknown	$22 million fine	2 Revocations
McKesson	2015	Various CS	Unknown	$150 million Fine/MOA[f]	4 Suspended, 1–3 years
Masters Pharm.	2015	Oxycodone	>6.5	DEA Final Order[d]	1 Revocation
Mallinckrodt	2017	Oxycodone	500	$35 million Fine/MOA[g]	Unaffected

[a] Omnicare's fine was for violations of CSA by its pharmacy division.
[b] UPS, for purpose of this case, was considered a common carrier and not a DEA registrant; fine was in return for nonprosecution agreement that stipulated allegations of unlawful profits derived from conducting business with illegal internet pharmacies.
[c] The FedEx case was dismissed by the court on a motion by the government on June 17, 2016.
[d] Masters Pharmaceutical, Inc's petition for review was denied by the US Court of Appeals for the District of Columbia (Case No. 15-1335) on June 30, 2017.
[e] Imposed December 2016.
[f] Imposed January 2017.
[g] Settlement agreed April 2017.
CS = controlled substances; MOA = memorandum of agreement.

Adapted and updated with permission of the author, John J. Coleman.[68] Public Sources: US District & Appeals Court files (PACER), DEA/DOJ press releases, company statements, Securities & Exchange Commission filings, media news and information reports, etc.

when orders are filled.[71,72] Tens of millions of these reports, now mostly filed electronically through a secure internet portal, are received by DEA annually and archived in the ARCOS database.[71]

Analyzing ARCOS records enables DEA to identify suspicious orders for controlled substances that were not reported by drug distributors to DEA as the law requires.[73] Upon identifying the unreported suspicious orders, the agency may take action against the distributors (and their customers) for failing to report the suspicious orders and thereby failing to prevent the diversion of controlled substances.[68] The regulations permit DEA to issue an "Order to Show Cause" why a registration should not be suspended or revoked for failing to comply with the law.[74]

In passing the Controlled Substances Act, Congress created what it called a "closed system" of distribution for controlled substances.[68] Only certain classes of registrants may distribute bulk supplies of controlled substances to other classes of registrants authorized to purchase them.[75] Registered wholesale distributors purchase drugs from manufacturers and in turn distribute them to customers (e.g., hospitals, pharmacies, buying groups, health maintenance organizations) that have purchase agreements with the manufacturer.[68] Given these relationships and the ARCOS transaction records that must be supplied to DEA, an irregularity discovered at any juncture in the supply chain will cause investigators to search for corresponding irregularities elsewhere in the closed system.[68]

In February 2012, DEA issued an immediate suspension order against the registration of Cardinal Health's Lakeland, Florida, distribution facility for law violations involving suspicious orders that were filled and not reported to DEA.[76] In a court filing, DEA provided ARCOS data showing that between 2008 and 2011, the Cardinal facility sold 12,913,100 dosage units of oxycodone to four retail pharmacies in Florida.[76] The records showed that in 2011 alone, Cardinal distributed over 3 million dosage units of oxycodone to two CVS pharmacies in Sanford, Florida, a town with a population of 53,570 and 14 other pharmacies with DEA registrations.[76] The orders received and filled by Cardinal were clearly suspicious, annually increasing in volume by several hundred percent, and, although subpoenaed records would show that the company identified them as suspicious, they were not reported to DEA and, instead, were filled in violation of the law.[76] On November 13, 2012, after a "show cause" hearing before a DEA administrative law judge, the DEA registrations for the two CVS pharmacies in question were permanently revoked.[77] In 2015, CVS Health, parent company of the two CVS pharmacies in Sanford, agreed to pay $22 million to the government to resolve claims connected with the DEA charges.[78] Cardinal Health had its DEA registration at its Lakeland facility suspended for 2 years and was fined $44 million to resolve outstanding claims involving Cardinal's operations in Florida, Maryland, Washington, and New York.[79]

GENERIC DRUG GIANT TURNS A BLIND EYE TO SUSPICIOUS ORDERS

On August 23, 2011, DEA headquarters officials met with representatives of Mallinckrodt plc, a British-owned company with its US offices in St. Louis, Missouri.[80] Mallinckrodt is registered by DEA as an importer and manufacturer of controlled substances in the United States.[80] Cardinal at the time was one of 43 wholesale drug distributors having marketing agreements for controlled substances with Mallinckrodt.[81]

According to the Securities and Exchange Commission, in calendar year 2015, Mallinckrodt had an estimated 25% of the DEA's total annual quota for controlled substances that it manufactured.[82] Industry estimates for the same period show that Mallinckrodt had a 23% market share of DEA Schedules II and III opioid and oral solid-dose medications sold in the United States.[82] For fiscal 2016, Mallinckrodt posted $3.4 billion in revenue and $489 million in profit.[83]

Less than a month after the meeting between Mallinckrodt and DEA, a senior manager in charge of Mallinckrodt's Controlled Substance Compliance unit sent a letter to the company's wholesale drug distributors reminding them of the need to have suspicious order monitoring programs.[81] The letter advised that "effective immediately," Mallinckrodt would no longer process "charge backs" submitted by distributors for sales of Mallinckrodt's controlled substances to a list of pharmacies identified in an attachment.[81] (A charge back is a payment made by a drug manufacturer to a distributor to reimburse it for the difference between the full price the distributor paid for the manufacturer's drug and the discounted price the distributor received for it when it was sold to the manufacturer's customers.[68] In the pharmaceutical industry, charge backs are a major source of revenue for distributors.)[68]

Among the 43 wholesale drug distributors receiving the Mallinckrodt letter were AmerisourceBergen Progenerics, Cardinal Healthcare, Masters Pharmaceuticals, Harvard Drug, KeySource Medical, Inc., and McKesson.[81] A year or more before receiving the Mallinckrodt letter in September 2011, each of these distributors had been charged by DEA with failing to report suspicious orders to the agency[68] (see Table 4.1). Cardinal Health and AmerisourceBergen had been charged by DEA in 2007, McKesson in 2008, Masters Pharmaceuticals in 2009, and Harvard Medical Group and KeySource Medical in 2010.[68] They were charged with failing to prevent the diversion of tens of millions of dosage units of hydrocodone and oxycodone.[68] Some paid modest fines in return for an out-of-court settlement and the restoration of one or more suspended DEA registrations.[68] All signed agreements stipulating to the facts in the DEA charges and pledging to comply with the law.[68] McKesson and Cardinal Health, however, violated their pledges by reengaging in similar offenses.[68] Cardinal Health settled its second DEA case in 2012 and McKesson in 2015.[68,84–87]

Despite the actions of Mallinckrodt's Controlled Substance Compliance Unit, the damage had already been done by at least six of Mallinckrodt's distributors between 2007 and 2010.[68] As previously mentioned, the regulation requiring distributors of controlled substances to design and implement systems to identify and report suspicious orders of controlled substances to DEA applies equally to manufacturers in their sales of controlled substances to their authorized distributors.[88]

Wholesale distributors purchase controlled substances from manufacturers at full price and agree to sell them to customers that have negotiated discounted pricing with the manufacturer.[68] A distributor is not just delivering drugs on behalf of a manufacturer but actually takes title to the drugs when purchased from the manufacturer.[68] This, then, makes the distributor a "customer" of the manufacturer who, in turn, has an obligation under the law to report suspicious orders received from its customers.[68]

On April 2, 2017, the *Washington Post*, citing confidential sources, published a lengthy report describing DEA's investigation of Mallinckrodt as the "largest prescription-drug case" ever pursued by the agency:

> Ultimately, the DEA and federal prosecutors would contend that the company ignored its responsibility to report suspicious orders as 500 million of its pills ended up in Florida between 2008 and 2012—66 percent of all oxycodone sold in the state. Government investigators alleged in internal documents that the company's lack of due diligence could have resulted in nearly 44,000 federal violations and exposed it to $2.3 billion in fines, according to confidential government records and emails obtained by the *Washington Post*.[83]

The *Post* described a 6-year effort on the part of prosecutors and DEA officials to hold Mallinckrodt responsible for failing to prevent the diversion of hundreds of millions of dosage units of oxycodone, a good portion of which included Mallinckrodt's blue 30-milligram oxycodone tablet that among drug users and dealers had "acquired a street name—'M's', for the company's distinctive block-letter logo."[83] In 2015, according to the *Post*, government lawyers prepared draft charges of civil conspiracy against Mallinckrodt but backed away from this charge following discussions with Mallinckrodt's legal team, which included a former federal prosecutor and a former associate chief counsel for DEA's diversion division—who, ironically, was one of the original architects of the agency's crackdown on the pharmaceutical industry.[83]

In July 2015, according to the *Post*, the US Attorney's Office in Detroit sent a proposed settlement offer to Mallinckrodt: "Prosecutors said they could fine the company as much as $2.3 billion because 222,107 orders to Florida were 'excessive' and should have been reported as suspicious. Or they could fine the company up to $1.3 billion based on an analysis of the 217,022,834 Mallinckrodt 30 mg oxycodone tablets that were sold for cash in Florida in 2009 and 2010."[83] Mallinckrodt, according to the *Post*, was willing to accept responsibility for failing to report suspicious orders received from distributors but not for suspicious orders that were not reported by Mallinckrodt's distributors.[83] If true, this was contrary to a position expressed in Mallinckrodt's September 2011 letter to 43 of its distributors stating that "Effective immediately, Mallinckrodt will no longer process charge backs from distributor sales of Mallinckrodt's products to the pharmacies identified on Attachment 1 hereto."[81] In that letter, Mallinckrodt clearly accepted responsibility for monitoring sales of its products facilitated by its distributors.[81]

Despite the billion-dollar fines being threatened, the *Post* article stated that federal prosecutors proposed settling the case for $70 million.[83] Reasons for proposing such a modest settlement, according to the *Post*, included uncertainties in the government's claim that Mallinckrodt had a legal responsibility to monitor the sales of its products by its distributors.[83] On more than one occasion in discussions with Mallinckrodt, according to the *Post*, even DEA investigators expressed uncertain views about this.[83]

On April 5, 2017, three days after the *Post* article was published and possibly in response to it, Mallinckrodt issued a press release stating:

> Mallinckrodt plc has reached an agreement in principle with the U.S. Drug Enforcement Administration (DEA) and the U.S. Attorneys' Offices (USAOs) for the Eastern District of

Michigan and the Northern District of New York, respectively, to settle previously disclosed investigations relating to the company's monitoring program, reporting, record keeping and security measures related to manufacturing and distribution of controlled substances. As part of the agreement, the company will pay $35 million to resolve all potential claims. The agreement in principle is subject to additional review and approval by the Department of Justice and DEA.[89]

CONGRESS BEFRIENDS THE INDUSTRY

Mallinckrodt and most of the accused distributors eventually agreed to settle their cases with the government.[68] In most cases, to avoid further litigation, the accused registrant companies agreed to pay relatively modest fines and implement measures to ensure future compliance with the law.[68]

Behind the scenes, however, things were different. The distributors and their powerful lobbying arm, the Healthcare Distribution Alliance—previously known until June 2016 as the Healthcare Distribution Management Association—were lobbying for legislation that would weaken DEA's authority to issue Immediate Suspension Orders (ISOs) and Orders for Show Cause Hearings to registrants accused of failing to maintain effective controls against the diversion of controlled substances.[90] The Ensuring Patient Access and Effective Drug Enforcement Act of 2016 was enacted on April 19, 2016, and included a new definition of "imminent danger" in the context of an ISO: "there is a substantial likelihood of an immediate threat that death, serious bodily harm, or abuse of a controlled substance will occur in the absence of an immediate suspension of the registration."[91]

The new law was consistent with arguments made by defendants in cases listed in Table 4.1.[92,93] Before litigating the merits of some of the cases, defendants challenged the "imminent danger" provision of the regulation under which the ISO was issued by DEA immediately suspending the plaintiffs' registrations and halting transactions involving controlled substances.[92,93] One distributor argued that its alleged unlawful actions had been halted long *before* DEA issued its ISO, and, consequently, the agency's decision to issue an ISO did not meet the legal standard of "imminent danger."[93] The Court disagreed and denied this distributor's motion for a preliminary injunction.[94] With the prodding of industry lobbyists, though, Congress sided with the industry and amended the statute to narrow the definition of "imminent danger."[90]

In addition, the Ensuring Patient Access and Effective Drug Enforcement Act of 2016 requires that a DEA Order to Show Cause henceforth must "notify the applicant or registrant of the opportunity to submit a corrective action plan on or before the date of appearance."[91] This notice effectively enjoins enforcement action until the registrant's corrective plan is reviewed: "Upon review of any corrective action plan submitted by an applicant or registrant . . . the Attorney General [i.e., DEA] shall determine whether denial, revocation, or suspension proceedings should be discontinued, or deferred for the purposes of modification, amendment, or clarification to such plan."[91]

In October 2016, the *Guardian* published a lengthy article that quoted Joseph Rannazzisi, a licensed pharmacist, attorney, and the recently retired head of DEA's Office of Diversion Control, as saying that the 2016 Act

> doesn't ensure patient access and it doesn't help drug enforcement at all. . . . What this bill does has nothing to do with the medical process. . . . What this bill does is take away DEA's ability to go after a pharmacist, a wholesaler, manufacturer or distributor. . . . This was a gift. A gift to the industry. . . . As long as the industry has this stranglehold through lobbyists, nothing's going to change. The bill passed because "Big Pharma: wanted it to pass.[90]

According to the *Guardian*, the bill was backed by the Healthcare Distribution Management Association, which claimed that DEA was misusing its powers to go after pharmacists and drug distributors for minor mistakes.[90] The *Guardian*'s report went on to describe how lobbyists for the industry have changed public policy:

> Industry groups have spent hundreds of millions of dollars in lobbying to stave off measures to reduce prescriptions and therefore sales of opioid painkillers. Among the most influential drug industry groups is the Pain Care Forum, co-founded by a top executive of Purdue Pharma— the manufacturer of the opioid which unleashed the addiction epidemic, OxyContin—and largely funded by pharmaceutical companies. It spent $740m lobbying Congress and state legislatures over the past decade according to the Center for Public Integrity.[90]

TROUBLE INSIDE DEA

In October 2016, the *Washington Post* began a series of articles that focused on trouble inside DEA.[95] The *Post* interviewed former employees of the agency, including Rannazzisi, who advised that efforts to go after wholesale distributors often were thwarted by higher-ups in the agency and their counterparts and superiors at the Department of Justice.[95] Rannazzisi told the *Post* about an "unusual meeting" with the deputy attorney general that he was ordered to attend in 2012: " 'That meeting was to chastise me for going after industry, and that's all that meeting was about,' " recalled Rannazzisi, who ran the diversion office for a decade before he was removed from his position and retired in 2015."[95]

Rannazzisi told the *Post* that on February 1, 2012, he was preparing to sign ISOs against Cardinal Health and CVS when he received a call from James H. Dinan, Chief of the Organized Crime Drug Enforcement Task Forces program at the Department of Justice.[95] Dinan, who worked for Deputy Attorney General James M. Cole, the second-in-charge at the Department, told Rannazzisi, "We're getting calls from attorneys, former Justice people, that are saying you guys are doing some enforcement action."[95] At the time, the *Post* article noted, Cardinal already had been served by DEA with administrative search warrants and records had been seized.[95] The *Post* article noted that among the attorneys representing Cardinal at the time were two former deputy attorneys general, Jamie S. Gorelick and Craig S. Morford.[95] In 2008, Morford left the Department of Justice to become Chief Legal and Compliance Officer for Cardinal Health. Both, it would turn out, had already been in contact with DEA.[95,96] Morford, formerly the then-DEA administrator's immediate supervisor, had sent the administrator a handwritten personal note on behalf of Cardinal Health asking for an "opportunity to meet with you and your team to address these issues in a non-adversarial way."[96]

When contacted by *Post* reporters, both Gorelick and Morford declined to comment and instead referred questions to D. Linden Barber, a former associate chief counsel for DEA, who was then in private practice with Quarles & Brady, a law firm that represents Cardinal and other clients in the pharmaceutical industry.[95] In 2017, Barber left Quarles & Brady to become Senior Vice-President and Chief Regulatory Counsel for Cardinal Health. As previously mentioned, Barber had been a member of the Mallinckrodt legal team that negotiated a $35 million settlement with the Department of Justice and DEA to settle pending investigations and claims that Mallinckrodt failed to identify and report suspicious orders received from distributors for controlled substances.[83]

IF YOU CAN'T BEAT THEM, HIRE THEM

In December 2016, the *Post* continued its investigation of DEA and the pharmaceutical industry with the publication of a lengthy article reporting that "Pharmaceutical companies that manufacture or distribute highly addictive pain pills have hired dozens of officials from top levels of the Drug Enforcement Administration during the past decade."[97] The *Post* investigation found that pharmaceutical companies and law firms that represent them have hired at least 42 officials from DEA, including 31 of them directly from the Office of Diversion Control, the division that regulates the industry.[97]

At least five of the 31 DEA employees were hired by McKesson, the nation's largest drug distributor and fifth-largest corporation, according to *Fortune* magazine.[97,98] McKesson was fined $13.25 million by DEA in 2008 after being charged with selling approximately 3 million dosage units of hydrocodone products to a rogue internet pharmacy.[68] It was alleged that six of McKesson's distribution centers failed to file suspicious order reports and one failed to report the theft and loss of controlled substances, as required by law.[68] In 2015, McKesson was again the subject of a DEA investigation.[86] A preliminary settlement in April resulted in the suspension for periods ranging from 1 to 3 years of four registrations held by McKesson facilities in Colorado, Michigan, Ohio, and Florida.[86] In January 2017, McKesson entered into an Administrative Memorandum of Agreement with the Department of Justice and DEA to settle allegations of wrongdoing against a dozen McKesson distribution facilities located throughout the United States.[86] In return for releasing McKesson from any and all administrative claims within DEA's authority under the Controlled Substances Act, McKesson agreed to pay $150 million and to implement improvements and changes to ensure compliance with the law.[68,86,87,97]

THE REVOLVING DOOR

The *Post's* investigation found that DEA's associate chief counsel from 2006 to 2010, D. Linden Barber, played a key role in shaping most of the early cases against wholesale distributors, including the 2008 case against Cardinal.[97] Barber, according to the Post, was "deeply involved in crafting a memorandum of agreement to settle the allegations against Cardinal."[97] In September 2011, noted the Post, Barber left DEA and joined the law firm Quarles & Brady.[97] Larry Cote, Barber's subordinate at DEA, took over the job as DEA's associate chief counsel.[97] A month later, on October 26, 2011, DEA executed an administrative inspection warrant on Cardinal's Lakeland facility to "determine whether Cardinal Health has failed to report suspicious orders to DEA."[99] According to the Post, "Seven months later, in May 2012, Cote, who helped to coordinate the second Cardinal case while at the DEA, joined Barber at Quarles & Brady, becoming the co-director of compliance and litigation. Cote had appeared in court on behalf of the DEA in the case against Cardinal three months earlier, records show."[97]

Contacted by the Post, Barber claimed to have sought advice from Roberto D. DiBella, the DEA's ethics lawyer, before and after leaving the agency, and to have complied fully with the law.[97] The DEA, however, provided the Post with a copy of DiBella's ethics opinion indicating that Barber asked for guidance on his representation of Cardinal and that "DiBella told him that he was banned for life from representing Cardinal on any issues connected to the 2008 memorandum of agreement (MOA)."[97] DiBella, according to the Post, told Barber, "Your representation of Cardinal to address an alleged violation of the MOA would on its face appear that you switched sides on a matter that you participated in as a DEA employee."[97] In July 2017, Barber was hired by Cardinal Health as the company's Chief Regulatory Counsel and Senior Vice President.

The Post reported that Cote also sought DiBella's advice and that DEA records show that Cote had participated "personally and substantially" in specific matters relating to at least 10 drug companies while he was at DEA.[97] Cote, too, is banned for life from communicating with or appearing before DEA or any other federal agency on behalf of certain companies, including McKesson, AmerisourceBergen, CVS, Walgreens, Rite Aid, and Walmart.[97] Cote told the Post that he has followed DiBella's advice that included his work for the DEA on the Cardinal case. Although his and Barber's employer, Quarles & Brady, represents Cardinal, Cote told the Post that he has been "walled off" from the firm's representation of Cardinal.[97] The descriptions of DiBella's opinions mirror the language of the relevant statute at 18 U.S.C. §207 calling for a permanent ban on former government officers and employees appearing before any agency, department, or court of the United States in connection with a particular matter in which the person participated personally and substantially such as an officer, an employee, or so forth.[100]

DEA's Office of Diversion Control is relatively small considering the enormous task of keeping track of 1.7 million registrants (as of April 2017), as well as regulating the controlled substances sector of the pharmaceutical industry.[101] In 2016 the diversion control office had 1,497 permanent positions, about a third of which are diversion investigators assigned to DEA field offices.[102] Diversion investigators represent a separate item and employment series in DEA's budget, which includes 5,174 special agents (as of 2016).[102] According to a June 2014 quarterly report mentioned in the Post's investigative series and obtained from DEA under the Freedom of Information Act, DEA's Chief Administrative Law Judge John J. Mulrooney II is quoted as saying, "There can be little doubt that the level of administrative Diversion enforcement remains stunningly low for a national program."[95]

The Post found that in fiscal 2011 there had been 131 civil cases filed by DEA against distributors, manufacturers, pharmacies, and doctors; by 2014, the number of such cases had dropped to 40.[95] The number of ISOs issued by DEA in the same period dropped from 65 to nine.[95] The slowdown in cases began in 2013, according to former DEA supervisors interviewed by the *Post*, "after DEA lawyers started requiring a higher standard of proof before cases could move forward."[95]

While DEA officials, including Judge Mulrooney, Administrator Chuck Rosenberg, Chief Counsel Wendy H. Goggin, and Rannazzisi's replacement, Louis J. Milione, declined to be interviewed for the *Post*'s investigative series, the Department of Justice issued a statement explaining that "the drop in diversion cases reflects a shift from crackdowns on 'ubiquitous pill mills' toward a 'small group' of doctors, pharmacists and companies that continues to violate the law."[95]

A spokesperson for the Department of Justice told the *Post* reporters that "diversion investigators are also increasingly using criminal procedures to force targets to surrender their licenses without administrative hearings."[95] This, however, was not borne out by the department's own statistics, which, according to information obtained by the *Post*, showed a 34% drop (from 924 to 610) in the number of surrendered registrations between fiscal year 2011 and fiscal year 2016.[95] In addition, several former DEA officials interviewed by the *Post* disputed the department's claim and blamed the drop in cases and surrendered registrations on the DEA's chief counsel's office, which, they said, simply refused to move forward on cases submitted by field investigators.[95]

THE UNINTENDED CONSEQUENCE: REAL OR IMAGINARY?

By law, DEA is required to establish annual manufacturing and production quotas for controlled substances in Schedule I and Schedule II.[103] Since 2011, the Government Accountability Office (GAO) has conducted several inquiries into reported shortages of medications, including controlled substances.[104–106] An exhaustive inquiry by the GAO concluded in 2015:

> While we cannot establish a causal relationship between shortages of drugs containing controlled substances and DEA's management of the quota setting process, the shortcomings we have identified prevent DEA from having reasonable assurance that it is prepared to help ensure an adequate and uninterrupted supply of these drugs for legitimate medical need.[104]

The "shortcomings" found by the GAO audit pertained to workflow issues inside the DEA on processing applications for quotas and supplemental applications for increases, as well as coordination with FDA on estimating the annual quotas needed by the medical and scientific communities.[104]

Despite GAO's findings, ARCOS data for opioids dispensed to patients for medical use by pharmacies in the United States between 2001 and 2016 show sizable increases: 184.7% for oxycodone, 338.9% for hydromorphone, 94.4% for hydrocodone, 103.1% for methadone,

150.1% for morphine, and 127.8% for fentanyl. Codeine was the only major opioid to show a decrease (minus 19.9%) over this 16-year period.[107] The US population during this same period increased only 13.4% (from 284,968,955 to 323,127,513 persons).[108]

Adding to the complexity of the purported drug shortage issue, in 2016 the CDC issued a highly detailed study and list of guidelines for the prescribing of opioids for chronic pain.[109] The CDC's main finding surprised the pain community: "In summary, evidence on long-term opioid therapy for chronic pain outside of end-of-life care remains limited, with insufficient evidence to determine long-term benefits versus no opioid therapy, though evidence suggests risk for serious harms that appears to be dose-dependent."[109] Patient advocacy groups like the U.S. Pain Foundation, a nonprofit funded in part by the pharmaceutical industry, warned that the guidelines would lead to "further restrictions on access to opioids for people with unremitting pain."[110] The American Cancer Society's Cancer Action Network, an advocacy group with drug company sponsorship, asked the CDC to withdraw the guidelines because they were based on "low quality" evidence and the process used to formulate them lacked transparency.[111] To be fair, the CDC's guidelines had their fans as well as their critics: one of the early supporters was the *Washington Post*, which published an editorial supporting the CDC's plan.[112]

TAKING THE *DECADE OF PAIN CONTROL AND RESEARCH* ABROAD

In 2016, the *Los Angeles Times* conducted an award-winning investigative inquiry of Purdue and OxyContin.[113,114] Using what the *Times* claimed were "internal" reports and sources, reporters learned that Purdue's labeling claim that OxyContin worked for 12 hours was false, and that the company knew this before the drug was marketed in 1996. The FDA-approved package insert (PI) for OxyContin describes the drug's pharmacokinetics and metabolism, in part, as follows: "OxyContin Tablets are designed to provide controlled delivery of oxycodone over 12 hours."[115] The clinical significance of this claim, the *Times* noted, was that "More than half of long-term OxyContin users are taking doses that public health officials consider dangerously high, according to an analysis of nationwide prescription data conducted for the *Times*."[113,114]

Internal documents uncovered by the *Times* showed that Purdue officials responded to the "12-hour problem" by instructing hundreds of sales representatives to tell doctors "to prescribe stronger doses, not more frequent ones."[114] Theodore J. Cicero, a neuropharmacologist at the Washington University School of Medicine and a leading authority on how opioids affect the brain, told the *Times* that OxyContin could be "the perfect recipe for addiction" because patients in whom the drug's effect was less than 12 hours could experience a return of their underlying pain and "the beginning stages of acute withdrawal."[114] "That," Cicero warned, "becomes a very powerful motivator for people to take more drugs."[114]

In response to the *Times*' article, Purdue issued a formal statement on its website defending OxyContin's 12-hour dosing and criticizing the *Times* for "its attempt to resurrect a long-discredited theory."[116] In a follow-up article published by the *Times* on May 6, 2016, Purdue's responses were refuted.[117]

Besides exposing OxyContin's "12-hour problem," the *Times* reported that Purdue was planning to "globalize" its sales campaign for OxyContin, using some of the same marketing tactics that, according to the *Times*, caused the company legal problems in the United States.[118]

In the third installment of its series, the *Times* led off its report with this first sentence: "OxyContin is a dying business in America."[118] Reporters noted that due to the fallout from years of controversy and being in the "grip of an opioid epidemic that has claimed more than 200,000 lives, the U.S. medical establishment is turning away from painkillers."[118] They noted that since 2010, prescriptions for OxyContin had fallen nearly 40%—"meaning billions in lost revenue for . . . Purdue Pharma."[118]

The response, according to the *Times*, was that Purdue's owner, the Sackler family, was using its family-owned network of international companies to market the drug in Latin America, Asia, the Middle East, Africa, and other parts of the world, places that the *Times* labeled "ill-prepared to deal with the ravages of opioid abuse and addiction."[118] In 2016, *Forbes* described the Sackler family as follows: "The family fortune began in 1952 when three doctors—Arthur (d. 1987), Mortimer (d. 2010) and Raymond Sackler—purchased Purdue, then a small and struggling New York drug manufacturer.[119] The company spent decades selling products like earwax remover and laxatives before moving into pain medications by the late 1980s."[119]

Operating as Purdue's wholly owned subsidiary, Mundipharma International maintains a worldwide presence in 51 countries, including 23 countries in Europe, where it was founded in 1967 in Frankfurt, Germany, by Drs. Raymond Sackler and Mortimer Sackler.[118,120,121] According to the *Times*, Mundipharma companies are conducting training seminars in Brazil, China, and other countries in which "doctors are urged to overcome 'opiophobia' and prescribe painkillers."[119] In addition, the Mundipharma companies, according to the *Times*, are sponsoring public awareness campaigns that encourage people to seek medical treatment for chronic pain and "are even offering patient discounts to make prescription opioids more affordable."[119]

The *Times* series pointed out that many of the nations where Mundipharma has a presence have national healthcare systems in which prescription drugs are centrally regulated.[118] The *Times* speculated that practices that are common in the United States, such as doctor shopping and paying cash for medical services and drugs, may be less common in single-payer countries where controlled substances are dispensed in most cases upon presentation of one's government-issued national healthcare identification card.[122–124]

MEANWHILE . . . BACK HOME THINGS HAVE NOT IMPROVED

The government's crackdown on drug companies and others in the pharmaceutical industry has had a negligible effect on reducing the morbidity and mortality resulting from the abuse of opioids. Data compiled by the CDC's National Center on Health Statistics

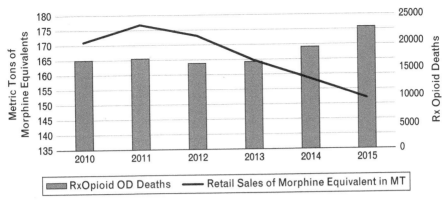

FIGURE 4.2 As prescription opioid deaths increase, retail sales of prescription opioids decrease

Sources: DEA-ARCOS[107] and National Center on Health Statistics[125]

from death certificates show that the total number of overdose deaths from select prescription drugs and illicit drugs increased 211% between 1999 and 2015 (from 16,849 to 52,404).[125] It is likely that mortality figures associated with the misuse of prescription opioids are undercounts since, according to the CDC, almost one in four death certificates received in 2014 and 2015 that listed "drug overdose" as the cause of death failed to specify the drugs involved.[126]

Beginning in 2011, as Figure 4.2 shows, retail sales of prescription opioids began to decline. Prescription opioid deaths, however, after a brief and modest decline lasting 2 years (2012 and 2013), began to increase rapidly and inversely to the decline in sales. Between 2011 and 2015, retail sales of prescription opioids decreased 14.1%, while overdose deaths increased 33.6%.[107,125,127]

Research indicates that a high proportion of users of heroin report problematic prescription opioid use before initiating heroin use.[128] Some have theorized that regulatory crackdowns that have reduced the volume of diverted drugs and increased their street price, as well as the development of abuse-deterrent opioids, have caused some prescription opioid addicts to switch to heroin, which is cheap and readily available on the street.[129]

Statistics showing total drug abuse, prescription drug abuse, opioid abuse, and heroin abuse are all trending upward in a close linear relationship.[125] The data show that prescription opioid deaths and heroin deaths are increasing concurrently.[125] This suggests that we may be observing multiple epidemics at the same time (or, perhaps, a series of mini-epidemics) and that crossovers from one to the other, based on the limited research we have, are unpredictable and opportunistic, largely depending upon what is available to the opiate addict at any given time[125] (Fig. 4.3).

CONCLUSION

Despite the problems discussed in this chapter, during the *Decade of Pain Control and Research*, the essential point of those advocating for chronic pain patients was made: chronic

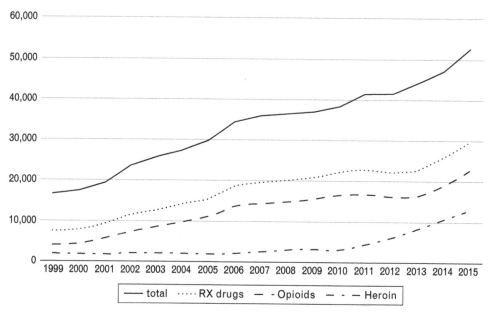

FIGURE 4.3 National overdose deaths from select prescription and illicit drugs
Source: CDC, National Center on Health Statistics[125]

pain indeed is a national public health problem that deserves more attention than it has been afforded. Arguably, more government funding is needed. In fiscal year 2017, funding by the National Institutes of Health for pain research was budgeted at $481 million. This is about 0.3% of the $164 billion budgeted for 265 research/disease areas funded by the National Institutes of Health for 2017.[130] This, however, does not include funding spent on pain research by the private sector. In addition, it does not include research funded for diseases, such as cancer and diabetes, that cause or contribute to chronic pain.

Clifford J. Woolf, a professor of neurology and neurobiology at Harvard Medical School and director of the F.M. Kirby Neurobiology Center at Children's Hospital Boston, notes that pharmaceutical companies have departed the field of pain medicine because they failed to develop new and more effective medications.[131] Woolf suggests that what is needed is a paradigm shift in thinking about how pain should be treated.[131] The industry's search for the "magic bullet," the single drug to relieve all forms of pain, he says, was a costly mistake because pain has no common etiology and is therefore unlikely to respond to a common remedy.[131]

If something positive at this late date can be said about the accomplishments of the *Decade of Pain Control and Research*, perhaps it is the emergence of thinkers like Woolf who brings to the table fresh ideas. For example, in 2013, Woolf reported on the structural biology of proteins at the mu-opioid receptor that appear to mediate analgesia, euphoria, and respiratory depression produced by opium.[132] Understanding these structures, Woolf says, someday may enable scientists "to use the receptor structure to design drugs that retain therapeutic actions of opioids but not their unwanted side-effects."[132] The development of nonaddictive opioids, he claims, is now potentially achievable.[132] Should this come to pass, it may very well be the lasting legacy of the *Decade of Pain Control and Research*.

In closing, we note that Reid Hunt, a Harvard University pharmacologist, wrote to the National Research Council in 1922 citing "the urgent need of non-habit-forming opiates."[133] Such a discovery, he said, would reduce the medical need for abusable drugs and return hundreds of thousands of ordinary people who had become opiate addicts to healthy and productive lives.[133] For several decades the National Research Council searched unsuccessfully for Hunt's non-habit-forming opiate and in the process developed several new opiates, some of which still are used for treating pain.[133] National Research Council scientists and pharmacologist Hunt had the foresight to envision what was needed but lacked the technical tools needed to achieve it. In the coming years, if Dr. Woolf and others are successful in their work, it could bring us to the cusp of an entirely new generation of drugs, including opiates, with improved efficacy and fewer or no adverse side effects. It could finally fulfill Hunt's "urgent need" for a non-habit-forming opiate, which was voiced for the first time almost a century ago but is needed now more than ever. If this comes to pass, the "second" *Decade of Pain Control and Research* will be more fruitful than the first.

REFERENCES

1. Victims of Trafficking and Violence Protection Act of 2000, Title VI, Sec. 1603: *Decade of pain control and research*; H.R. 3244 (Public Law No: 106-386). 2000. http://www.gpo.gov/fdsys/pkg/BILLS-106hr3244enr/pdf/BILLS-106hr3244enr.pdf. Accessed February 16, 2017.

2. Mularski RA, White-Chu F, Overbay D, Miller L, Asch SM, Ganzini L. Measuring pain as the 5th vital sign does not improve quality of pain management. *J Gen Intern Med*. 2006;21(6):607–612.

3. Lanser P, Gesell S. Pain management: the fifth vital sign. *Healthcare Benchmarks*. 2001;8(6):68–70, 62.

4. Tompkins DA, Hobelmann JG, Compton P. Providing chronic pain management in the "Fifth Vital Sign" Era: historical and treatment perspectives on a modern-day medical dilemma. *Drug Alcohol Depend*. 2017;173(Suppl 1):S11–S21.

5. Portenoy RK, Foley KM. Chronic use of opioid analgesics in non-malignant pain: report of 38 cases. *Pain*. 1986;25(2):171–186.

6. Anjelina Pokrovnichka, MD, Medical Officer, Division of Anesthesia, Analgesia, and Rheumatology Products, Office of Drug Evaluation II, Food and Drug Administration. History of OxyContin: Labeling and Risk Management Program. PowerPoint presentation given to a joint meeting of the Anesthetic and Life Support Drugs Committee and the Drug Safety and Risk Management Advisory Committee on November 13 and 14, 2008. http://www.fda.gov/ucm/groups/fdagov-public/@fdagov-afda-adcom/documents/document/ucm248776.pdf. Accessed May 16, 2017.

7. Sneader W. *Drug Discovery: A History*. 1st ed. Hoboken, NJ: John Wiley and Sons; 2005.

8. Purdue Pharma, L.P., Stamford, CT 06901-3431. FDA-approved label for OxyContin (NDA #OT00367K/300514-OH). 2007. http://www.accessdata.fda.gov/drugsatfda_docs/label/2008/020553s059lbl.pdf. Accessed October 31, 2016.

9. Anjelina Pokrovnichka, MD, Medical Officer, Division of Anesthesia, Analgesia, and Rheumatology Products, Office of Drug Evaluation II, Food and Drug Administration. History of OxyContin: Labeling and Risk Management Program. PowerPoint presentation given to a joint meeting of the Anesthetic and Life Support Drugs Committee and the Drug Safety and Risk Management Advisory Committee on November 13 and 14, 2008. http://www.fda.gov/ucm/groups/fdagov-public/@fdagov-afda-adcom/documents/document/ucm248776.pdf. Accessed November 7, 2016.

10. Van Zee A. The promotion and marketing of OxyContin: commercial triumph, public health tragedy. *Am J Public Health*. 2009;99(2):221–227.

11. National Drug Intelligence Center. OxyContin Diversion and Abuse. 2001. https://www.justice.gov/archive/ndic/pubs/651/abuse.htm. Accessed May 16, 2017.

12. Addressing OxyContin abuse. *FDA Consum*. 2001;35(4):3.

13. Purdue Pharma L.P. MS Contin (morphine sulfate extended-release tablets). 2017. http://www.purduepharma.com/healthcare-professionals/products/ms-contin/. Accessed May 16, 2017.

14. Thomas W. Abrams, Director, Division of Drug Marketing, Advertising, and Communications, Food and Drug Administration. FDA Warning Letter, dated January 17, 2003, issued to Michael Friedman, Executive Vice President and Chief Operating Officer, Purdue Pharma L.P.; Re: *NDA 20-553, OxyContin*. 2003. https://www.fda.gov/downloads/Drugs/GuidanceComplianceRegulatoryInformation/EnforcementActivitiesbyFDA/WarningLettersandNoticeofViolationLetterstoPharmaceuticalCompanies/UCM168946.pdf. Accessed March 10, 2017.

15. US House, Subcommittee on Commerce, Justice, State and Judiciary. Hearing: On OxyContin. September 13, 2001. https://www.congress.gov/congressional-record/2001/9/6/daily-digest/article/d873-1?q=%7B%22search%22%3A%5B%22Oxycodone+OR+OxyContin%22%5D%7D&r=8. Accessed April 8, 2017.

16. US Senate, Committee on Health, Education, Labor, and Pensions. Hearing: To hold hearings to examine the effects of the drug OxyContin. September 20, 2002. https://www.congress.gov/congressional-record/2001/9/14/daily-digest/article/d900-2?q=%7B%22search%22%3A%5B%22Oxycodone+OR+OxyContin%22%5D%7D&r=5. Accessed April 8, 2017.

17. US Senate, Committee on Health, Education, Labor, and Pensions. Hearing: To examine the effects of the painkiller OxyContin, focusing on risks and benefits. February 12, 2002. https://www.congress.gov/congressional-record/2002/2/11/daily-digest/article/d82-4?q=%7B%22search%22%3A%5B%22Oxycodone+OR+OxyContin%22%5D%7D&r=2. Accessed April 8, 2017.

18. US House, Subcommittee on Commerce, Justice, State and Judiciary. Hearing: Painkiller OxyContin abuse. December 11, 2001. https://www.congress.gov/congressional-record/2001/12/11/daily-digest/article/d1237-1?q=%7B%22search%22%3A%5B%22Oxycodone+OR+OxyContin%22%5D%7D&r=1. Accessed April 8, 2017.

19. Meier B. *Pain Killer: A "Wonder" Drug's Trail of Addiction and Death*. Emmaus, PA: Rodale; 2003.

20. James P. Jones, US District Judge, US District Court, Western District of Virginia, Abingdon Division. Opinion & Order in case No. 1:07CR00029 (JPJ), *US v. The Purdue Frederick Company, Inc.*, et al., *Defendants* (Document No. 77, filed July 23, 2007). http://www.vawd.uscourts.gov/OPINIONS/JONES/107CR00029.PDF. Accessed December 17, 2016.

21. James P. Jones, US District Judge, US District Court, Western District of Virginia, Abingdon Division. Opinion by James P. Jones, US District Judge, issued in Case No. 1:07CR00029, *US v. The Purdue Frederick Company, Inc.* (Document No. 141, filed August 5, 2013). Accessed November 16, 2016 (Via PACER).

22. Porter J, Jick H. Letter to the editor: addiction rare in patients treated with narcotics. *N Engl J Med*. 1980;10(302-2):123.

23. Joranson DE, Ryan KM, Gilson AM, Dahl JL. Trends in medical use and abuse of opioid analgesics. *JAMA*. 2000;283(13):1710–1714.

24. University of Wisconsin: Pain & Policy Studies Group. About PPSG. 2017. http://www.painpolicy.wisc.edu/about-ppsg. Accessed May 16, 2017.

25. Food and Drug Administration. FDA Briefing Document: Drug Safety and Risk Management Advisory Committee (DSaRM) Meeting, October 29–30, 2012 (postponed to January 29–30, 2013). 2012. http://www.fda.gov/AdvisoryCommittees/CommitteesMeetingMaterials/Drugs/DrugSafetyandRiskManagementAdvisoryCommittee/ucm334275.htm. Accessed January 9, 2015.

26. Substance Abuse and Mental Health Services Administration. *Emergency Department Trends From the Drug Abuse Warning Network, Final Estimates 1995–2002, DAWN Series: D-24, DHHS Publication No. (SMA) 03-3780*. Rockville, MD; 2003.

27. Gilson AM, Ryan KM, Joranson DE, Dahl JL. A reassessment of trends in the medical use and abuse of opioid analgesics and implications for diversion control: 1997–2002. *J Pain Symptom Manage*. 2004;28(2):176–188.

28. Department of Health and Human Services, Office of Inspector General. Compliance Program Guidance for Pharmaceutical Manufacturers. 2003. https://oig.hhs.gov/fraud/docs/complianceguidance/042803pharmacymfgnonfr.pdf. Accessed March 4, 2017.

29. Department of Health and Human Services, Office of Inspector General. Comparison of the anti-kickback statute and Stark Law. 2011. https://oig.hhs.gov/compliance/provider-compliance-training/files/StarkandAKSChartHandout508.pdf. Accessed March 3, 2017.

30. James P. Jones, US District Judge, US District Court, Western District of Virginia, Abingdon Division. Judgment in a criminal case No. DVAW107CR000029-001, *US v. The Purdue Frederick Company, Inc.* (Document No. 79, filed July 25, 2007). Obtained via PACER (restricted). Accessed December 17, 2016.

31. James P. Jones, US District Judge, US District Court, Western District of Virginia, Abingdon Division. Judgment in a criminal case No. DVAW107CR000029-002, *US v. Michael Friedman* (Document No. 81, filed July 25, 2007). Obtained via PACER (restricted). Accessed December 17, 2016.

32. James P. Jones, US District Judge, US District Court, Western District of Virginia, Abingdon Division. Judgment in a criminal case No. DVAW107CR000029-003, *US v. Howard R. Udell* (Document No. 83, filed July 25, 2007). Obtained via PACER (restricted). Accessed December 17, 2016.

33. James P. Jones, US District Judge, US District Court, Western District of Virginia, Abingdon Division. Judgment in a criminal case No. DVAW107CR000029-004, *US v. Paul D. Goldenheim* (Document No. 85, filed July 25, 2007). Obtained via PACER (restricted). Accessed December 17, 2016.

34. Frakt A. Painkiller abuse, a cyclical challenge. *New York Times*. December 22, 2014. http://www.nytimes.com/2014/12/23/upshot/painkiller-abuse-a-cyclical-challenge.html. Accessed November 18, 2016.

35. Catan T, Perez E. A pain-drug champion has second thoughts. *Wall Street Journal*. December 17, 2012. http://www.wsj.com/articles/SB10001424127887324478304578173342657044604. Accessed March 31, 2016.

36. Portenoy RK. Opioid therapy for chronic nonmalignant pain: a review of the critical issues. *J Pain Symptom Manage*. 1996;11(4):203–217.

37. Executive Office of the President, Office of National Drug Control Policy. Epidemic: Responding to America's Prescription Drug Abuse Crisis. 2011. http://www.whitehouse.gov/sites/default/files/ondcp/policy-and-research/rx_abuse_plan.pdf. Accessed January 21, 2015.

38. Centers for Disease Control and Prevention. Prescription painkiller overdoses at epidemic levels. 2011. http://www.cdc.gov/media/releases/2011/p1101_flu_pain_killer_overdose.html. Accessed January 23, 2015.

39. *City of Chicago, Plaintiff v. Purdue Pharma, L.P.,* et al., *Defendants*. US Court for the Northern District of Illinois (Eastern Division); Case No. 1:14-cv-04361 (Judge Jorge L. Alonso). 2014. Accessed Via PACER, November 20, 2016.

40. Giron L. Judge halts counties' lawsuit against 5 narcotic drug manufacturers. *Los Angeles Times*. August 28, 2015. http://www.latimes.com/local/california/la-me-pharma-20150828-story.html. Accessed November 21, 2016.

41. Clerk of the Circuit Court, Cook County, Illinois. Case Information Summary for Case Number 2014-L-005854, *City of Chicago v. Janssen Pharmaceuticals*, et al. 2014. https://w3.courtlink.lexisnexis.com/cookcounty/Finddock.asp?DocketKey=CABE0L0AAFIFE0LD. Accessed November 20, 2016.

42. Stephen R. Patton, Corporation Counsel of the City of Chicago. First Amended Complaint, *City of Chicago v. Purdue Pharma, L.P.,* et al. Case No. 14-cv-04361 (Hon. Elaine E. Bucklo), US District Court for the Northern District of Illinois (Eastern Division). 2014. Accessed Via PACER, November 21, 2016.

43. *City of Chicago, Plaintiff v. Purdue Pharma, L.P.,* et al., *Defendants.* US Court for the Northern District of Illinois (Eastern Division); Case No. 1:14-cv-04361 (Judge Jorge L. Alonso), document no. 552, filed April 14, 2017. Accessed via PACER, April 19, 2017.

44. Young B. Kim, US Magistrate Judge, US District Court for the Northern District of IL Eastern Division. Minute Entry in *City of Chicago v. Purdue Pharma L.P.,* et al., Case No. 14 CV 4361, regarding discovery by parties to be discussed and resolved by June 7, 2017. 2017. https://ecf.ilnd.uscourts.gov/doc1/067119109569. Accessed via PACER restricted data source, May 16, 2017.

45. Jim Hood, Attorney General, State of Mississippi. Complaint filed 12/15/2015 in The Chancery Court of the First Judicial District of Hinds County, Mississippi, titled: *State of Mississippi v. Purdue Pharma, L.P.,* et al.; Case No. 25CH1:15-cv-001814, Doc. #2. 2015. Accessed via Public Access to Mississippi Electronic Courts (PAMEC), November 21, 2016.

46. Weissman DE, Haddox JD. Opioid pseudoaddiction—an iatrogenic syndrome. *Pain.* 1989;36(3):363–366.

47. Greene MS, Chambers RA. Pseudoaddiction: fact or fiction? An investigation of the medical literature. *Curr Addict Rep.* 2015;2(4):310–317.

48. Passik SD, Kirsh KL, Webster L. Pseudoaddiction revisited: a commentary on clinical and historical considerations. *Pain Manage.* 2011;1(3):239–248.

49. Passik SD. Responding rationally to recent report of abuse/diversion of OxyContin. *J Pain Symptom Manage.* 2001;21(5):359.

50. Siegal HA, Carlson RG, Kenne DR, Swora MG. Probable relationship between opioid abuse and heroin use. *Am Fam Physician.* 2003;67(5):942, 945.

51. Jones CM, Logan J, Gladden RM, Bohm MK. Vital signs: demographic and substance use trends among heroin users—United States, 2002-2013. *MMWR Morb Mortal Wkly Rep.* 2015;64(26):719–725.

52. Food and Drug Administration. New Molecular Entity (NME) Drug and New Biologic Approvals. 2016. http://www.fda.gov/Drugs/DevelopmentApprovalProcess/HowDrugsareDevelopedandAppr oved/DrugandBiologicApprovalReports/NDAandBLAApprovalReports/ucm373420.htm. Accessed December 9, 2016.

53. Johnson & Johnson. NUCYNTA® ER (Tapentadol extended-release tablets) receives FDA approval for the management of moderate to severe chronic pain. 2011. https://www.jnj.com/media-center/press-releases/nucynta-er-tapentadol-extended-release-tablets-receives-fda-approval-for-the-management-of-moderate-to-severe-chronic-pain. Accessed February 7, 2017.

54. National Academies of Sciences, Engineering, and Medicine. *Relieving Pain in America: A Blueprint for Transforming Prevention, Care, Education, and Research.* 2011. http://www.nationalacademies.org/hmd/Reports/2011/Relieving-Pain-in-America-A-Blueprint-for-Transforming-Prevention-Care-Education-Research.aspx. Accessed November 25, 2016.

55. National Academies of Sciences, Engineering, and Medicine. Press release: Institute of Medicine to Become National Academy of Medicine. 2015. http://www.nationalacademies.org/hmd/Global/News%20Announcements/IOM-to-become-NAM-Press-Release.aspx. Accessed November 25, 2016.

56. Steglitz J, Buscemi J, Ferguson MJ. The future of pain research, education, and treatment: a summary of the IOM report "Relieving Pain in America: A Blueprint for Transforming Prevention, Care, Education, and Research." *Transl Behav Med.* 2012;2(1):6–8.

57. Mackey S. National Pain Strategy Task Force: the strategic plan for the IOM Pain Report. *Pain Med.* 2014;15(7):1070–1071.

58. Kennedy J, Roll JM, Schraudner T, Murphy S, McPherson S. Prevalence of persistent pain in the U.S. adult population: new data from the 2010 National Health Interview Survey. *J Pain.* 2014;15(10):979–984.

59. Institute of Medicine Committee on Advancing Pain Research C, Education. The National Academies Collection: Reports funded by National Institutes of Health. *Relieving Pain in America: A Blueprint for Transforming Prevention, Care, Education, and Research.* Washington, DC: National Academies Press, National Academy of Sciences; 2011.

60. Fauber J. UW a force in pain drug growth: Research group receiving millions from pharmaceutical firms helped liberalize use of opioids. *Milwaukee Journal Sentinel.* April 3, 2011. http://nl.newsbank.com/sites/mwsb/. Accessed November 26, 2016.

61. Fauber J. UW group ends drug firm funds: more than $2.5 million was accepted from companies. *Milwaukee Journal Sentinel,* April 21, 2011. http://nl.newsbank.com/sites/mwsb/. Accessed November 26, 2016.

62. Fauber J. Networking fuels painkiller boom: doctors, researchers with financial ties to drug-makers set stage for surge in prescriptions. *Milwaukee Journal Sentinel.* February 19, 2012. http://nl.newsbank.com/sites/mwsb/. Accessed November 26, 2016.

63. Ornstein C, Weber T, Nguyen D. Dollars for docs: how industry dollars reach your doctors. ProPublica. 2016. https://www.propublica.org/article/about-our-pharma-data. Accessed November 27, 2016.

64. Ornstein C, Weber T. The champion of painkillers. ProPublica. 2011. https://www.propublica.org/article/the-champion-of-painkillers. Accessed November 27, 2016.

65. Charles E. Grassley, Max Baucus, Senators, US Senate Committee on Finance. Various letters sent on May 8, 2012 to pharmaceutical company presidents and heads of pain organizations seeking information. 2012. http://www.finance.senate.gov/search/?q=Opioids&start=15&as_sitesearch=www%2Efinance%2Esenate%2Egov%2Fdownload&page=2. Accessed November 25, 2016.

66. Pam Bondi, Attorney General, Florida Office of Attorney General. Pill Mill Initiative. 2011. http://myfloridalegal.com/pages.nsf/Main/AA7AAF5CAA22638D8525791B006A30C8. Accessed April 10, 2016.

67. Bondi P. *Florida's Roadmap to End Its Prescription Drug Abuse Epidemic.* Testimony by Florida Attorney General Pam Bondi, given before the Subcommittee on Commerce, Manufacturing and Trade, Committee on Energy and Commerce, US House of Representatives, March 1, 2012.

68. Coleman JJ. The supply chain of medicinal controlled substances: addressing the Achilles heel of drug diversion. *J Pain Palliat Care Pharmacother.* 2012;26(3):233–250.

69. Drug Enforcement Administration. DEA Congressional Testimony: Written Statement of Joseph T. Rannazzisi, Deputy Assistant Administrator, Office of Diversion Control, Drug Enforcement Administration, in testimony given May 16, 2007, before US Senate Judiciary Committee. http://www.dea.gov/divisions/hq/2007/ct051607p.html. Accessed May 2, 2016.

70. Code of Federal Regulations. 21 CFR 1301.74(b) Other security controls for non-practitioners, etc. 2016. https://www.gpo.gov/fdsys/pkg/CFR-2016-title21-vol9/xml/CFR-2016-title21-vol9-chapII.xml. Accessed December 19, 2016.

71. Drug Enforcement Administration. Automation of Reports and Consolidated Orders System (ARCOS). 2012. http://www.deadiversion.usdoj.gov/arcos/index.html. Accessed March 28, 2017.

72. Drug Enforcement Administration, Office of Diversion Control. Controlled Substances Ordering System (CSOS). 2017. https://www.deaecom.gov/overview.pdf. Accessed March 28, 2017.

73. *Cardinal Health Inc. v. Eric Holder, Jr., Attorney General,* et al. US District Court, District of Columbia, Case 1:12-cv-00185-RBW; Document No. 14, filed February 10, 2012; Page 39 of 49.

74. Code of Federal Regulations. 21 CFR 1316.31 (Authority for enforcement proceedings). 2016. http://www.gpo.gov/fdsys/pkg/CFR-2014-title21-vol9/pdf/CFR-2014-title21-vol9-chapII.pdf. Accessed May 16, 2017.

75. Code of Federal Regulations. 21 CFR Part 1300 to end. 2016. http://www.gpo.gov/fdsys/pkg/CFR-2014-title21-vol9/pdf/CFR-2014-title21-vol9-chapII.pdf. Accessed May 16, 2017.

76. *Cardinal Health Inc. v. Eric Holder, Jr., Attorney General,* et al. US District Court, District of Columbia, Case 1:12-cv-00185-RBW; Document No. 14, filed February 10, 2012.

77. Federal Register. Drug Enforcement Administration [Docket Nos. 12–37 and 12–38], Holiday CVS, L.L.C., d/b/a CVS Pharmacy Nos. 219 and 5195; Decision and Order (FR Vol. 77, No. 198, Friday,

October 12, 2012, Notices). https://www.gpo.gov/fdsys/pkg/FR-2012-10-12/pdf/2012-25047.pdf. Accessed April 26, 2017.

78. Department of Justice, US Attorney's Office, Middle District of Florida. Press release: United States Reaches $22 Million Settlement Agreement with CVS for Unlawful Distribution of Controlled Substances. 2015. https://www.justice.gov/usao-mdfl/pr/united-states-reaches-22-million-settlement-agreement-cvs-unlawful-distribution. Accessed April 26, 2017.

79. Department of Justice, US Attorney's Office, District of Maryland. Press release: Cardinal Health Agrees to $44 Million Settlement for Alleged Violations of Controlled Substances Act; Settlement resolves multiple investigations against Cardinal in Maryland, Florida, New York and Washington. 2016. https://www.justice.gov/usao-md/pr/cardinal-health-agrees-44-million-settlement-alleged-violations-controlled-substances-act. Accessed April 26, 2017.

80. *Holiday CVS, L.L.C., d/b/a CVS Pharmacy Nos. 5195/219 v. Michelle Leonhart, In her official capacity as Administrator of the Drug Enforcement Administration,* et al. US District Court, District of Columbia, Case 1:12-cv-00191-RBW; Document No. 5, filed February 7, 2012 at pp. 12–13.

81. Harper K. Mallinckrodt LLC ("A Covidien Company") letter of September 16 and 19 sent to 43 distributors. Filed February 10, 2012, as document no. 14-16 in *Cardinal Health Inc. v. Eric Holder, Jr., Attorney General,* et al., Civil Action No. 1:12-cv-00185-RBW, US District Court, District of Columbia, 2011.

82. US Securities and Exchange Commission. Form 10-K for the fiscal year ended September 30, 2016, for Mallinckrodt plc. 2016. http://www.mallinckrodt.com/investors/annual-reports. Accessed April 5, 2017.

83. Bernstein L, Higham S. The government's struggle to hold opioid manufacturers accountable: sixty-six percent of all oxycodone sold in Florida came from this company. But the DEA's case against it faltered. *Washington Post.* April 2, 2017. https://www.washingtonpost.com/graphics/investigations/dea-mallinckrodt/?utm_term=.ab20bdfc4364. Accessed April 6, 2017.

84. R. Kerry Clark, John J. Carney, Jodi L. Avergun, et al. Settlement Agreement signed o/a October 2, 2008, between Cardinal Health, Inc., and six United States Attorneys. Document No. 14-15 (Appendix F), filed February 10, 2012, in case: *Cardinal Health, Inc., v. Holder;* No. 1:12-cv-0185-RBW, US District Court for the District of Columbia. 2012. Obtained via PACER (restricted), December 26, 2016.

85. Lacy R. Harwell, Jr., Katherine M. Ho, Jeffrey T. Walsh, et al. Settlement Agreement, dated December 16, 2016, between Cardinal Health, Inc., and United States Department of Justice, Drug Enforcement Administration, US Attorney's Offices for the Middle District of Florida, District of Maryland, and Western District of Washington. http://www.bizjournals.com/tampabay/news/2016/12/23/cardinal-health-agrees-to-44m-settlement-in.html. Accessed December 24, 2016.

86. Mark Walchirk, President, McKesson Corporation; Chuck Rosenberg, Acting Administrator, DEA; Louis J. Milone, Assistant Administrator, Diversion Control Division, DEA. Administrative Memorandum of Agreement between McKesson and DEA. 2017. https://www.justice.gov/opa/press-release/file/928476/download. Accessed March 14, 2017.

87. US Securities and Exchange Commission. Form 8-K, Current Report Pursuant to Section 13 or 15(d) of the Securities Exchange Act of 1934, filed April 30, 2015, by McKesson Corporation. https://www.sec.gov/Archives/edgar/data/927653/000119312515161747/d919028d8k.htm. Accessed January 3, 2017.

88. Code of Federal Regulations. 21 CFR 1301.74(b) Other security controls for non-practitioners, etc. 2016. https://www.gpo.gov/fdsys/pkg/CFR-2016-title21-vol9/xml/CFR-2016-title21-vol9-chapII.xml. Accessed March 14, 2017.

89. Mallinckrodt plc. News releases: Mallinckrodt Statement on DEA and USAOs Agreement in Principle. 2017. https://www.mallinckrodt.com/about/news-and-media/2259303. Accessed April 5, 2017.

90. McGreal C. Opioid epidemic: ex-DEA official says Congress is protecting drug makers. *The Guardian.* October 31, 2016. https://www.theguardian.com/us-news/2016/oct/31/opioid-epidemic-dea-official-congress-big-pharma. Accessed January 3, 2017.

91. US Congress. Ensuring Patient Access and Effective Drug Enforcement Act of 2016; enacted and signed into law on April 19, 2016 as Public Law 114-145 (130 STAT. 354). https://www.congress.gov/114/plaws/publ145/PLAW-114publ145.pdf. Accessed December 29, 2016.

92. *Holiday CVS, L.L.C. d/b/a CVS Pharmacy #5195 and #219 vs. Eric H. Holder, Jr.,* et al. US District Court, District of Columbia, Case 1:12-cv-00191-RBW, Document No. 4-1, filed February 6, 2012, Plaintiff's Statement of Points and Authorities in Support of Motion for Temporary Restraining Order. https://ecf.dcd.uscourts.gov/doc1/04513733360 (PACER restricted database). Accessed May 17, 2017.

93. *Cardinal Health, Inc., v. Eric Holder, Jr., Attorney General,* et al. US District Court, District of Columbia, Case 1:12-cv-00185-RBW, Document No. 1 (Complaint), filed February 3, 2012. Obtained via PACER (Restricted). Accessed January 3, 2017.

94. *Cardinal Health, Inc., v. Eric Holder, Jr., Attorney General,* et al. US District Court, District of Columbia, Case 1:12-cv-00185-RBW, Document No. 32, filed March 7, 2012. Obtained via PACER (Restricted). Accessed December 31, 2016.

95. Bernstein L, Higham S. Investigation: the DEA slowed enforcement while the opioid epidemic grew out of control. *Washington Post.* October 22, 2016. https://www.washingtonpost.com/investigations/the-dea-slowed-enforcement-while-the-opioid-epidemic-grew-out-of-control/2016/10/22/aea2bf8e-7f71-11e6-8d13-d7c704ef9fd9_story.html?tid=a_inl&utm_term=.e865ae6fb62c. Accessed January 3, 2016.

96. Craig Morford, Chief Legal and Compliance Officer, Cardinal Health, Inc. Handwritten note to "Michele" from "Craig," requesting meeting. Obtained from DEA by John J. Coleman on September 16, 2014, pursuant to Freedom of Information Act request in: Case No. 13-00090-F, "Information Pertaining to Cardinal Health, Inc., Etc." 2012.

97. Higham S, Bernstein L, Rich S, Crites A. Drug industry hired dozens of officials from the DEA as the agency tried to curb opioid abuse. *Washington Post.* December 22, 2016. https://www.washingtonpost.com/investigations/key-officials-switch-sides-from-dea-to-pharmaceutical-industry/2016/12/22/55d2e938-c07b-11e6-b527-949c5893595e_story.html?utm_term=.c64b7bb3da92. Accessed January 3, 2016.

98. Fortune 500 Rankings of Companies for 2016. Fortune.com. 2017. http://beta.fortune.com/fortune500/list. Accessed February 8, 2017.

99. *Cardinal Health Inc. v. Eric Holder, Jr., Attorney General,* et al. US District Court, District of Columbia, Case 1:12-cv-00185-RBW; Document No. 14, filed February 20, 2012 at p. 10 of 49. 2012. Obtained via PACER (Restricted). Accessed January 3, 2017.

100. 18 U.S.C. § 207—Restrictions on former officers, employees, and elected officials of the executive and legislative branches. 1982. http://uscode.house.gov/. Accessed January 3, 2017.

101. Drug Enforcement Administration, Office of Diversion Control. Registrant Population—Summary. 2017. https://apps.deadiversion.usdoj.gov/webforms/odrRegSummaryReport.do;jsessionid=3767AFE068A901D4DFF5B8DC54C81520. Accessed May 19, 2017.

102. Drug Enforcement Administration. FY 2016 Budget Request at a Glance. 2016. https://www.justice.gov/sites/default/files/jmd/pages/attachments/2015/01/30/28_bs_section_ii_chapter_-_dea.pdf. Accessed May 19, 2017.

103. 21 CFR Part 1303, *Quotas* (Sec. 306 of Title 21, U.S.C., Sect. 826). 2016. http://www.gpo.gov/fdsys/pkg/CFR-2014-title21-vol9/pdf/CFR-2014-title21-vol9-chapII.pdf. Accessed May 19, 2017.

104. General Accountability Office. Drug Shortages: Better Management of the Quota Process for Controlled Substances Needed; Coordination between DEA and FDA Should Be Improved. Report#GAO-15-202 to Congressional Requesters, February 2015. http://www.gao.gov/assets/670/668252.pdf. Accessed May 19, 2017.

105. General Accountability Office. Drug Shortages: FDA's Ability to Respond Should Be Strengthened. Report #GAO-12-116 to Congressional Requesters; November 2011. http://www.gao.gov/assets/590/587000.pdf. Accessed May 19, 2017.

106. General Accountability Office. Drug Shortages: Public Health Threat Continues, Despite Efforts to Help Ensure Product Availability. Report#GAO-14-194 to Congressional Requesters; February 2014. http://www.gao.gov/assets/670/660785.pdf. Accessed May 19, 2017.

107. Drug Enforcement Administration, Office of Diversion Control. ARCOS Retail Drug Summary Reports. 2016. https://www.deadiversion.usdoj.gov/arcos/retail_drug_summary/index.html. Accessed January 11, 2017.

108. US Census Bureau. US Population Growth by Region. 2017. https://www.census.gov/popclock/data_tables.php?component=growth. Accessed March 29, 2017.

109. Dowell D, Haegerich TM, Chou R. CDC guideline for prescribing opioids for chronic pain—United States, 2016. *JAMA*. 2016;315(15):1624–1645.

110. US Pain Foundation. Transparency (IRS 990 Tax Return for 2014). 2016. https://www.uspainfoundation.org/transparency/. Accessed January 7, 2017.

111. Foreman J. Analysis: controversy over CDC's proposed opioid prescribing guidelines. WBUR. January 9, 2016. http://www.wbur.org/commonhealth/2016/01/09/analysis-controversy-over-cdcs-proposed-opioidprescribing-guidelines. Accessed January 7, 2017.

112. The CDC's promising plan to curb America's opioid dependence [editorial]. *Washington Post*. October 20, 2015. https://www.washingtonpost.com/opinions/guidelines-that-could-save-lives/2015/10/20/9fd65dba-775e-11e5-a958-d889faf561dc_story.html?utm_term=.1fb26cc4789b. Accessed January 7, 2017.

113. Ryan H, Girion L, Glover S. *LA Times* OxyContin report receives investigative journalism honors. October 4, 2016. http://www.latimes.com/local/readers-rep/la-rr-times-oxycontin-barlett-steele-awards-20161004-snap-htmlstory.html. Accessed January 9, 2017.

114. Ryan H, Girion L, Glover S. A *Times* investigation: "You want a description of hell?"—OxyContin's 12-hour problem. *Los Angeles Times*. May 5, 2016. http://www.latimes.com/projects/oxycontin-part1/. Accessed January 9, 2017.

115. Purdue Pharma, L.P., Stamford, CT 06901-3431. Package Insert: OxyContin. 2007. http://www.accessdata.fda.gov/drugsatfda_docs/label/2009/020553s060lbl.pdf. Accessed January 9, 2017.

116. Purdue Pharma L.P. Setting the record straight on OxyContin's FDA-approved label. 2016. http://www.purduepharma.com/news-media/get-the-facts/setting-the-record-straight-on-oxycontins-fda-approved-label/. Accessed January 9, 2017.

117. Ryan H. Purdue Pharma issues statement on OxyContin report; *L.A. Times* responds. 2016. http://www.latimes.com/projects/purdue-response/. Accessed January 9, 2017.

118. Ryan H, Girion L, Glover S. A *Times* investigation: OxyContin goes global—"We're only just getting started." *Los Angeles Times*. December 18, 2016. http://www.latimes.com/projects/la-me-oxycontin-part3/?utm_campaign=Rx+Summit&utm_source=hs_email&utm_medium=email&utm_content=40127701&_hsenc=p2ANqtz-8-A_di00xr0B7qt7mflionRcGgXHYp4D0vFEKQfWRRkhpHbuIsmau1 1xDWM5SwpebtrO160SgNWIq4NL41pYQVe7a04A&_hsmi=40127 701#nt=oft12aH-1gp2. Accessed January 5, 2017.

119. Peterson-Withorn C. Fortune of family behind OxyContin drops amid declining prescriptions. *Forbes*. June 29, 2016. http://www.forbes.com/sites/chasewithorn/2016/06/29/fortune-of-family-behind-oxycontin-drops-amid-declining-prescriptions/#21bd8e267535. Accessed December 17, 2016.

120. Mundipharma International. Overview of Mundipharma: From 1967 to 2015. 2017. https://translate.google.com/translate?hl=en&sl=de&u=https://de.wikipedia.org/wiki/Mundipharma&prev=search. Accessed January 9, 2017.

121. Mundipharma International. About us: The Mundipharma network of independent associated companies. 2014. http://www.mundipharma.com/AboutUs. Accessed January 9, 2017.

122. Rossow I, Bramness JG. The total sale of prescription drugs with an abuse potential predicts the number of excessive users: a national prescription database study. *BMC Public Health.* 2015;15:288.

123. Lapeyre-Mestre M, Gony M, Carvajal A, et al. A European community pharmacy-based survey to investigate patterns of prescription fraud through identification of falsified prescriptions. *Eur Addict Res.* 2014;20(4):174–182.

124. Birke H, Kurita GP, Sjogren P, et al. Chronic non-cancer pain and the epidemic prescription of opioids in the Danish population: trends from 2000 to 2013. *Acta Anaesthesiol Scand.* 2016;60(5):623–633.

125. National Institute on Drug Abuse, National Center on Health Statistics, CDC Wonder. National Overdose Deaths from Select Prescription and Illicit Drugs (All underlying causes of death as coded in the International Classification of Diseases, 10th Revision). 2017. https://www.drugabuse.gov/related-topics/trends-statistics/overdose-death-rates. Accessed January 7, 2017.

126. Warner M, Trinidad JP, Bastian BA, Minino AM, Hedegaard H. Drugs most frequently involved in drug overdose deaths: United States, 2010–2014. *Natl Vital Stat Rep.* 2016;65(10):1–15.

127. Centers for Medicare & Medicaid Services (CMS). Opioid Morphine Equivalent Conversion Factors. 2015. https://www.cms.gov/Medicare/Prescription-Drug-Coverage/PrescriptionDrugCovContra/Downloads/Opioid-Morphine-EQ-Conversion-Factors-March-2015.pdf. Accessed January 11, 2017.

128. Pollini RA, Banta-Green CJ, Cuevas-Mota J, Metzner M, Teshale E, Garfein RS. Problematic use of prescription-type opioids prior to heroin use among young heroin injectors. *Subst Abuse Rehabil.* 2011;2(1):173–180.

129. Cicero TJ, Ellis MS, Surratt HL. Effect of abuse-deterrent formulation of OxyContin. *N Engl J Med.* 2012;367(2):187–189.

130. National Institutes of Health. Estimates of Funding for Various Research, Condition, and Disease Categories (RCDC). 2016. https://report.nih.gov/categorical_spending.aspx. Accessed March 26, 2017.

131. Woolf CJ. Overcoming obstacles to developing new analgesics. *Nat Med.* 2010;16(11):1241–1247.

132. Woolf CJ. Pain: morphine, metabolites, mambas, and mutations. *Lancet Neurol.* 2013;12(1):18–20.

133. Acker CJ. Addiction and the laboratory: the work of the National Research Council's Committee on Drug Addiction, 1928-1939. *Isis (University of Chicago).* 1995;86(2):167–193.

CHAPTER 5

EVALUATION AND TREATMENT OF THE CHRONIC PAIN PATIENT

Practice and Complexity

John F. Peppin, Pravardhan Birthi, Bill H. McCarberg, and Yvonne D'Arcy

INTRODUCTION

Few issues in medicine have generated as much fiery and impassioned debate as the use of opioid medications in the treatment of chronic pain of noncancer origin. (The term "chronic pain of noncancer origin" is used in a conscientious effort to disabuse the pain community from the philosophically charged terms "chronic noncancer pain" and "cancer pain." A discussion of this topic is beyond the scope and goal of this chapter.[1]) Concepts in this chapter can be applied to pain of both noncancer and cancer origin, although the patient with chronic pain of noncancer origin will be the current focus. In the appropriately selected patient, these medications can provide relief of significant suffering, which is the goal of medicine.[2,3] Patients with chronic pain of noncancer origin are routinely marginalized and their care has changed little over the past 20 years.[4,5]

The recent Institute of Medicine (IOM) report "Relieving Pain in America: A Blueprint for Transforming Prevention, Care, Education, and Research" estimated that 100 million people in the United States suffer from chronic and undertreated pain.[6] Further, the economic cost of chronic pain is staggering: the estimated annual cost of chronic pain in the United States is $560 billion to over $600 billion, including both healthcare costs ($261–300 billion) and lost productivity ($297–336 billion).[6] The IOM report emphasized that effective pain management is a "moral imperative" and added that pain should be considered a disease with a distinct pathology that requires an interdisciplinary, multimodal treatment approach (Multi-disciplinary, multi-modal treatment programs are described further in Chapter . . .).[6] Ferrell has described the status of chronic pain treatment as "the moral outrage of unrelieved pain."[7]

Much of the problem with the treatment of chronic pain rests in a lack of knowledge about pain; its physiology, progression, and treatment; and its profound impact on an individual patient and society. The importance and knowledge of how to assess these patients is not taught in medical school (or other professional schools), nor in residencies.[8] These patients are extremely complex, similar to those with other chronic diseases, in their presentations and their diagnoses.[9] At a pain medicine board review course a few years ago, one of the lecturers stated, "To treat pain you have to know everything about medicine."[10] Although tongue and cheek, there is truth to this statement. Every single specialty in medicine deals with pain, either acute or chronic. Every physician, nurse practitioner, and physician assistant is presented with patients in pain. The pain clinician will need a working knowledge of many disciplines and treatment modalities, physiology, and pathophysiology, and will need close relationships with a multitude of other specialists to appropriately treat these patients—in other words, they need to "know everything."

The term "pain clinician" will be used throughout this chapter to indicate practitioners who provide full assessment and treatment for chronic pain patients. They would not focus exclusively on one modality, but would embrace the multimodal, multidisciplinary approach to chronic pain treatment. Further, the pain clinical would be aware of the complexities of treating these patients as well. They would also be knowledgeable concerning medical management, including opoids. This would include physicians, nurse practitioners, and physician assistants, although we realize that in some states nurse practitioners and physician assistants may not be able to prescribe scheduled medications.[11-13]

There are obvious benefits to the appropriate treatment of pain, and this appropriate treatment requires appropriate evaluation. Intuitively, it makes sense that appropriate treatment would reduce costs, improve outcomes, and reduce the potential for medication abuse, misuse, and diversion. Treating acute pain aggressively, which requires appropriate acute evaluation and assessment, may prevent progression to a more severe chronic pain state.[14]

For the nonmedical person who is professionally involved in opioid use, abuse, misuse, diversion, and overdose deaths, an understanding that single and simplistic approaches to the treatment of chronic pain of noncancer origin will undoubtedly fail is critical. Further, if the evaluation and diagnoses tend to be "boilerplate," one should be suspect. Having said this, it is the rare clinician who is willing to take on this challenge. It is easier to refer a patient, or give a prescription or an injection, rather than go through the long, laborious process of a thorough evaluation, treatment, and reevaluation of patients in chronic pain.

The chronic pain patient is one of the most challenging and complicated of those seen in clinical medicine. As stated, single approaches or therapies will routinely fail, since, such an approach does not take into account the complexities involved in these patients. Linear approaches will inherently be failures as well when dealing with these patients.[9] What is needed is a new paradigm, not a restructuring of the old. However, until that new paradigm appears, we must work with the current one, imperfect though it may be. We hope that we have sufficiently defined the goals of this chapter.

EVALUATION OF THE CHRONIC PAIN PATIENT

Multiple problems and issues can affect a patient's pain level and ability to function. These include motivational, educational, psychiatric and behavioral, social, and medical variables. The IOM report on pain noted, "We believe pain arises in the nervous system but represents a complex and evolving interplay of biological, behavioral, environmental, and societal factors."[6] A comprehensive biopsychosocial, multidisciplinary, multimodal approach to evaluation and treatment decision-making seems intuitive in dealing with a complex pain patient but is rarely utilized.

The evaluation of these patients begins with a full history.[14] A patient's chronic pain does not exist in a vacuum but rather is affected by multiple aspects and issues in a patient's life. Intuitively, it makes sense that there would be a strong negative correlation between comorbidities, insomnia, pain, and other symptoms, but little has been written about this intuition. In addition, patients with chronic pain commonly present with multiple psychiatric comorbidities, especially depression and anxiety, the "depression–anxiety spectrum of disorders."[15] In patients with depression, 75% to 80% have persistent pain, such as headaches or low back pain.[16] In patients with fibromyalgia or persistent spinal pain, the incidence of persistent pain is 20% to 40%.[16,17] The effect of pain and mood states on central nervous system dysregulation is profound.[18,19]

Multiple medical comorbidities are common in patients with chronic pain. For example, in a study from the Netherlands on patients with hip and knee osteoarthritis, 98.6% had one or more coexistent diseases; of this group, 84.4% had one or more moderate or severe coexistent diseases, with cardiac disease being the most prevalent.[20]

Patients with chronic pain in both Europe and the United States frequently have more than one pain complaint.[21,22] It seems obvious that the more pain complaints, the more difficult it will be to evaluate and treat a give pain patient. The notion that a focused evaluation of a single chief complaint will be enough to treat a patient with chronic pain is clearly misguided.[23] If a patient presents for a "focused" evaluation for back pain yet also has migraines, chronic generalized myofascial pain syndrome, and knee pain, it seems unlikely that a single intervention (e.g., spinal surgery, injection) focusing on a single pain complaint will be successful.

There has been a growing understanding of the development of chronic pain states and past surgeries. A thorough evaluation of past surgeries should be undertaken at the first visit. The true nature of the relationship between tobacco use and chronic pain is not clear, but tobacco use has been correlated with chronic pain.[24,25] Therefore, an evaluation of the use of tobacco products needs to be part of a full evaluation for the chronic pain patient.

A dramatically underdiagnosed problem is traumatic brain injury (TBI).[26] TBI predisposes patients to substance abuse, depression, and other psychiatric disabilities.[27,28] Traumatic migraines are well described, but other pain states may be common in the presence of TBI.[29] In one article, although many of the studies reviewed had limitations, the authors concluded, "Chronic pain is a common complication of TBI and contributes to morbidity and potentially poor recovery after brain injury."[30]

Obesity is another issue in patients with chronic pain that needs to be evaluated and addressed.[31,32] For example, obesity and osteoarthritis are correlated.[33] Further bariatric surgery has been shown to reduce lower back pain.[34]

The interaction of sleep and chronic pain is complex. A majority of patients with chronic pain describe disrupted sleep, and it has been shown that lack of sleep can exacerbate chronic pain.[35,36] A full history of sleep patterns, use of soporifics, and timing of sleep is important in the evaluation of these patients. Patients without appropriate goals have pain that is more difficult to treat. Unrealistic goals may never be met, and the ensuing frustration and hopelessness in patients will translate into poor adherence to prescribed therapies and treatment failure. Goals should be set with the patient during the initial assessment phase of patient care. They should be realistic and well defined and should be reassessed at subsequent visits. "Pain-free" is often not an option for patients with chronic pain. Asking the patient what pain intensity would be needed to perform a daily task, such as a daily walk, will provide better information. In one study, the endpoint of which was the goal of returning to work, the single most predictive factor in the patient returning to work was that specific goal.[37] At each visit the pain clinician should chart progress toward the established goals to ensure that opioid therapy, or any therapy, is providing the desired outcome.

Educational level, pain coping skills, and social support can all affect a patient's ability to cope with pain, the patient's functionality, and the pain specialist's ability to treat.[38–40] Polypharmacy is the rule rather than the exception in the treatment of all chronic illnesses, and chronic pain is no different.[41] Medication errors and adverse drug reactions can occur if a thorough medication history is not taken and if that history is not reevaluated at every visit.[42] The patient's level of exercise is a critical historical component. Participating in aerobic exercise for only 2 minutes a day will reduce pain levels.[43] In obese patients, participating in resistance exercise can produce a sense of positive well-being and reduce pain as well.[44] However, lack of exercise increases the risk for treatment failure and increased pain. A short study looking at physical therapy evaluation of patients with chronic pain in a pain clinic over 6 to 9 months using the 6 minute walk as a primary outcome, found that the patients, regardless of treatment, showed statistical improvement.[45] Unfortunately, these patients (average age of 40–50 years), even after this improvement, did not reach the lower limit of functioning for normal 65-year-olds. Pain patients tend to fear movement (kinesiophobia), which can lead to further deconditioning and more pain.[46]

Even obtaining a history of immunizations is important. Did the patient have the herpes zoster vaccine? What is the patient's risk for hepatitis C and HIV? All of these factors, and more, are needed for a thorough and high-quality evaluation of chronic paint patients. Most of the history collection can be done at the initial visit, but continued reevaluation is crucial. No clinician would prescribe a dose of insulin and never obtain another blood sugar measurement, so why would that same clinician prescribe an opioid and never do a reassessment to see if the therapy continues to be effective?

Because of the rise in the prevalence of opioid abuse and overdose deaths, pain clinicians must evaluate every patient's potential for abuse, misuse, abuse, substance use disorder, and diversion. Further, given that the rate of substance dependency (i.e., use disorders, see the American Psychiatric Association, Diagnostic and Statistical Maual of mental disorders (DSM-5), American Psychiatric Publications, 2013. "Substance-Related and Addictive

Disorders", 481-490) in the United States is more than 12%, assessments for potential abuse of illicit substances, alcohol, or prescription medications should be part of the evaluation of every patient, regardless of the presence of pain. Screening tools to evaluate the risk of misuse, abuse, and diversion of opioids include the Screener and Opioid Assessment for Patients with Pain (SOAPP-R); Opioid Risk Tool (ORT); Diagnosis, Intractability, Risk and Efficacy Score (DIRE); and Current Opioid Misuse Measure (COMM).[47,48] A complete patient history should include a thorough family history as well. This can point to genetic disorders as well as the potential for substance use disorder.

The pain level is purposefully left to the end of such evaluations since other complexities are frankly more important in the evaluation. A myopic focus on reducing a number is an inappropriate approach to the outcomes in these patients. If pain levels do not change but function increases, mood improves, and the patient sleeps better and has an improved quality of life, pain level numbers are a non sequitur.

A thorough physical examination should be performed. Areas of pain should be examined, palpated, and documented. Evaluating the skin, nails, heart, and so forth can give clues to other diagnoses that may hinder or complicate treatment. It is almost routine to find areas of pain other than the "primary complaint" (see earlier). The goal is not to add therapies but to consider the patient as a whole: each comorbidity may be contributing to the overall picture.

Part of the evaluation might include laboratory studies or radiologic imaging, but there is no need to reproduce recent testing. Many if not most patients have been evaluated in the past. Old records are a valuable source of information, both diagnostic and therapeutic. They should be sent for, not brought in by the patient, and reviewed in detail.

TREATMENT OF THE CHRONIC PAIN PATIENT

Treatment of the chronic pain patient depends, as just discussed, on an appropriate and in-depth evaluation. As mentioned above, most chronic pain patients will have more than one pain complaint. Since multiple pain generators will probably be present, it is crucial that all of these be evaluated and an overall treatment plan be implemented that takes into consideration these generators, comorbidities, and other issues.

Treatment should be a combination of pharmacologic therapies, interventions (e.g., injections, radiofrequency ablation, spinal cord stimulation), physical therapy, cognitive-behavioral therapy, and/or integrative/complementary therapies. The spectrum of pharmacologic therapies should be broad and include "adjuvants" such as antiepileptic agents, muscle relaxants, serotonin and norepinephrine reuptake inhibitors (SNRIs), selective serotonin reuptake inhibitors (SSRIs), tricyclic antidepressants (TCAs), and other medications. Opioids are one option and should be used within the confines of the risks and complexity stratifications described. There should never be a "cookie cutter" approach to the chronic pain patient but rather an attempt to use all the modalities and therapies available in a logical way.

Not every patient who complains of pain needs an opioid or is a candidate for opioid therapy. Opioids should be prescribed only when the benefit outweighs the risks. Functional improvement should be a primary goal, along with improved sleep and mood, regardless of the therapy used. Focusing only on pain levels misses the complexities involved in the evaluation and treatment of chronic pain and will hinder treatment success.

Universal Precautions provide a standardized approach to the use of opioids in chronic pain treatment.[49] Using these precautions along with prescribing agreements, accessing the state prescription monitoring program and urine drug monitoring, should reduce the risk of abuse, misuse, and diversion.[50] Using a prescribing agreement can also define the opioid prescribing process and help patients better understand the "rules" for their opioid management as well as educating them about risks and benefits.

Once the assessment process is completed, and an opioid has been selected, a trial period should be used to determine if the opioid fits the patient's pain management needs. In the first step of the current treatment approach, a single agent or therapy is tried. If this is successful, the clinician stops. If not, the clinician moves on to option #2, and so on, until a successful therapy is found. During this trial period the patient will need frequent reevaluation and should be seen more frequently, with follow-up discussions about pain relief, functionality, and adverse effects.

Pain that is unrelieved should elicit reevaluation. Perhaps the diagnosis was in error, or some other issue has taken precedence or was missed. Clinicians should always bear in mind that opioids are *not* a panacea for chronic pain, and they may be ineffective, cause significant and unrelieved side effects, or contribute to inappropriate drug-taking behaviors.

Aging changes the way medications are utilized and excreted in several ways. Muscle-to-fat ratios and body fat composition change. Poor nutrition may decrease drug-binding ability. Changes in protein-binding mechanisms may cause medications to compete for binding sites. The physiologic mechanisms of metabolism, absorption, medication clearance, slowed gastrointestinal motility, decreased cardiac output, and decreased glomerular filtration rates can all affect medication utilization. Drug excretion and elimination are reduced by 10% for each decade after age 40 because of decreased renal function.[51–53] For the older patient, doses may need to be decreased and careful monitoring is necessary.

OPIOID SIDE EFFECTS AND TREATMENT OPTIONS

All opioids, like all pharmaceuticals, can cause side effects. All patients should have their medications, including over-the-counter medications, vitamins, or supplements reviewed at each visit. Medicinal as well as recreational marijuana is legal in many states. Patients may be hesitant to disclose their use of marijuana. Despite legalization and more societal acceptance of marijuana, clinicians should specifically ask patients about this compound. Ideally, patients should bring all these items to their appointments. Polypharmacy, as discussed above, is the norm rather than the exception in these patients. Making sure that medications not needed have been discontinued, that interactions have been reviewed, and that medications are being taken as indicated is a critical part of such regular reevaluations.

Pharmacogenomics is a rapidly developing field and can provide some guidance in directing pharmacotherapy: drug dosing can be reduced, drug–drug interactions can be anticipated, and patients who are "poor metabolizers" can be identified.[54] As this field develops it will have a dramatic effect on medicine as a whole, and pain medicine in particular.

Nausea has been reported in 25% of patients on chronic opioid therapy (COT), while vomiting is less common.[55] Nausea and vomiting are usually transient, lasting 2 to 3 days, although much of this information was obtained in the postoperative setting rather than in patients on COT.[56] The pathophysiologic mechanisms of nausea includes direct stimulation of the chemoreceptor trigger zone (CTZ) in the brain, reduced gastrointestinal motility (gastroparesis), and enhanced vestibular sensitivity.[57] Understanding the pathophysiology can reduce redundant medications and increase the use of combination therapy directed at different mechanisms, which can reduce the total drug burden and dose.[58,59] Antiemetics are beneficial and may have secondary benefits such as antipruritic, anxiolytic, sedative, or pro-motility activity. Antipsychotics such as haloperidol and prochlorperazine are inexpensive and will block dopamine receptors in the CTZ. However, these treatments also have side effects, such as dystonic reaction, akathisia, and hypotension.[60] Metoclopramide also blocks dopamine receptors in the CTZ and promotes peristalsis through acetylcholine release.[61] Serotonin antagonists, such as ondansetron, block serotonin release mainly in the gastrointestinal tract but also centrally. These agents are mainly used in postoperative ileus and nausea related to chemotherapy and radiation.[62] Patients experiencing nausea with ambulation, due to opioid-induced vestibular sensitivity, may get benefit from antihistaminic and anticholinergic agents like diphenhydramine and meclizine.[59] Although corticosteroids have an unclear mechanism of action for treating nausea, they are routinely used in chemotherapy-related nausea and vomiting.[63] Further, there is little data on their use in opioid-induced nausea, and long-term use is problematic.[64] Other options to treat opioid-induced nausea and vomiting include decreasing the opioid dose to a minimally acceptable level for adequate analgesia, or opioid rotation.[65] Once a patient has been started on COT and has improved, the clinician should consider carefully reducing the dose to achieve the minimal opioid level for the maximal amount of analgesic benefit.

Dental caries have been related to the use of opioids that contain sugars as part of their delivery systems.[66] However, opioids can cause xerostomia, and the combination of xerostomia and sugar may have a greater impact on dental caries than xerostomia alone.[67] The mechanism here is thought to be due to induced xerostomia.[68] Perhaps the best-studied relationship between xerostomia and opioids is with methadone.[69] Fentanyl, especially in the submucosal formulations, has also been linked to xerostomia and dental caries.[70] Xerostomia has been shown with the use of buprenorphine submucosal film as well.[71,72] As part of any assessment of any patient on COT, an oral examination should be performed. A dry oral cavity should be treated with patient education, appropriate hydration, elimination of tobacco products, and even artificial saliva as necessary.

There have been recent suggestions that dysphagia is more common in the chronic pain population, regardless of the addition of exogenous opioids.[73] A recent telephone survey of physicians suggested that the incidence of dysphagia in chronic pain was 20%, regardless of the medication used.[74] Gastroesophageal reflux disease is common in patients who take opioids. A 2008 Canadian study demonstrated that patients who were given laxatives for opioid-induced constipation also received proton-pump inhibitors or histamine-2 blockers.[75] Other factors associated with opioid-induced gastrointestinal adverse effects, specifically constipation and reflux, escalated with increasing age and duration of opioid use. The distribution of opioid receptors in the esophagus is poorly understood; however, opioid use is associated with esophageal dysmotility.[76] A study in 2010 showed a statistically significant degree of esophageal dysmotility in the 15 patients studied.[76] The reduction in gastric and intestinal motility can have far-reaching effects. Patients can become intolerant of intragastric tube feedings, and absorption of other medications may be inhibited.[77]

Constipation is a common side effect of opioid use to which the patient may not become tolerant. Stool softeners such as Colace can be used to ease bowel movements. Stimulant laxatives and osmotic laxatives can be used prophylactically to help keep the bowels regular. In 2017 the ROME group developed a standard definition of Opioid Induced Constipation which was included in the updated ROME 4 text.[77a] Studies on traditional approaches, e.g., increased hydration, exercise, bisacodyl, lack research support and tend to be based more on tradition than science. For example, bulk agents are routinely avoided in patients taking opioids since, these agents could worsen constipation.[78] However, actual research to support this claim is lacking. The treatments suggested above may not be enough, and an injectable or oral opioid antagonist (e.g., methylnaltrexone or naloxagol) may be needed.[79]

Sedation is another potential side effect of opioid therapy. It occurs with the initiation of opioids but can be a chronic problem. It can also occur with dosage changes or the addition of other types of medications that are also sedating, such as benzodiazepines, antihistamines, and antiemetics. Sedation should be taken seriously since it is a more consistent sign for the potential of respiratory failure and should be actively queried.[80,81] Combining opioids with other centrally sedating drugs is strongly discouraged by many treatment guidelines and state medical boards. Patients should be educated about the risks of combining medications and should be instructed to take their medications according to the prescribed doses and time intervals. However, "despite the frequency of opioid-induced sedation, there are no universally accepted guidelines to direct effective and safe assessment and monitoring practices for patients receiving opioid analgesia."[82] Unfortunately the problem of sedation is probably much more common than currently believed. For example, Saunders in 2012 found a high level of use of other central nervous system depressants, including alcohol, in patients taking opioids, regardless of their substance use disorder prevalence.[83] To counteract sedation, stimulants such as caffeine, dextroamphetamine, methylphenidate, or modafinil have been recommended in the past but are seldom used today except in terminal cancer and palliative care patients. As with many side effects, opioid rotation and dose reduction are other approaches.[65]

The incidence of pruritus with the use of opioids is 2% to 10%.[84] Although the mu receptor clearly seems to be involved, the mechanism is poorly understood.[85] Antihistamines have been used in the treatment of pruritus, and for hospitalized patients with intravenous access low-dose nalbuphine or naloxone can be used.[86]

The incidence of delirium associated with the use of opioids (in patients at risk for delirium) has been estimated to be up to 50%.[87] However, one study found "no association between the use of any postoperative opioid and incident delirium in both demented and cognitively intact patients after hip fracture repair."[88p2260] The presence of confusion and delirium, when opioids are being used, should always trigger a thorough evaluation and review.

There are many causes of delirium, including medications (benzodiazepines), infections, lack of sleep, and other causes. The pain clinician should never automatically believe that opioids are the cause of mental status changes.[4] Rather, evaluation without such bias should be the appropriate response and frequently will indicate other etiologies.[4] Opioid rotation and the use of analgesic adjuvants are both potential approaches to the treatment of delirium and mental status changes.[65]

Myoclonus, tremor, rigidity, catalepsy, and akathisia are closely related symptoms that are occasionally reported in patients treated with opioids. The incidence of myoclonus has been reported to be 2.7% to 11% in cancer patients on COT.[89] The pathophysiology of these disorders is obscure, In patients on morphine, a metabolite of morphine, morphine-3-glucuronide, may be partially responsible.[89] Others have suggested neurotoxicity, specifically related to hydrocodone.[90,91] Treatment of myoclonus is hampered by lack of clinical data, few studies, and studies with small numbers and low power. Clonidine and dantrolene have been studied and shown to be effective in small studies.[89] In the palliative medicine population caffeine, dexamphetamine, and ketamine have also been used.[92,93] Opioids are not the only cause of iatrogenic movement disorders, so other etiologies should be considered.[94]

Patients with chronic pain frequently have sleep disorders, with rates ranging from 30% to 87%.[95,96] Sleep disorders are frequently associated with movement disorders. The discussion of movement disorders and opioids is complicated by the complexity involved in these disorders. For example, in patients with restless leg syndrome and periodic limb movement disorder, opioids have been used successfully to treat these disorders.[97] In this 2012 study, the chronic pain group spent more time in bed with the lights off, and sleep efficiency was lower than for the control group (81.2% vs. 89.49%). Other studies have found similar results.[98]

Opioids are known to have respiratory complications, particularly in patients who are opioid-naïve or who have overdosed. Increased susceptibility can be seen in obese, elderly, and neonatal patients as well as patients with comorbid cardiopulmonary conditions. Also, the addition of other central nervous system depressants, specifically benzodiazepines (or nonmedications, such as ETOH) places these patients at much higher risk for serious respiratory issues.[99] The mechanism of opioid-induced respiratory depression is obscure but thought to be related to stimulation of mu and delta receptors.[100] These opioid receptors have been identified in the respiratory center of the brain, the pons and medulla, which provides respiratory drive.[101] The incidence of opioid-induced respiratory depression varies from 0.2% to 1.0%. A meta-analysis by Cashman et al. showed that the incidence of respiratory depression determined by respiratory rate was less than 1%; the analysis included patients who were taking intramuscular, epidural, and intravascular opioids.[102] Although the risk of respiratory depression in the outpatient setting appears to be minimal, pain clinicians using opioids should have a low index of suspicion and should use screening, such as the Epworth Sleepiness Scale, in their repeated evaluations in patients on COT.[103]

The respiratory effects of opioids, in the acute setting, have traditionally been measured using changes in breathing frequency and/or by oxygen saturation (SpO_2).[104] Wheatley et al. defined postoperative hypoxemia related to epidural opioid administration as SpO_2 < 94% (for >6 minutes for 1 hour) and moderate and severe hypoxemia as SpO_2 < 85%.[105] Respiratory depression is frequently regarded as a breathing rate of less than 8 to 10 breaths per minute.[106] However, the SpO_2 and breathing frequency give limited information on ventilator drive. Inspired minute ventilation and arterial carbon dioxide concentration are a direct measure of ventilatory drive, but they are difficult to assess on a continual basis in the outpatient pain clinic.[104] The extrapolation of the use of SpO_2 and breathing rate as simple measures of respiratory depression in COT lacks a firm foundation in research. However, one study found that the Epworth Excessive Sleepiness Scale, a simple and easy screen, was much more sensitive correlation to morphine equivalent dose than other measures, such as the respiratory rate.[107]

Opioids can reduce dyspnea; this effect can be used for comfort in terminally ill patients and in palliative care patients with chronic lung disease. A systemic review by Jennings et al. showed the usefulness of opioids in reducing dyspnea in these patients.[108] Further, in patients with advanced chronic obstructive pulmonary disease, dyspnea can be difficult to control. Increasingly, data show that opioids can be effective in relieving the feeling of dyspnea. However, as a Canadian study has shown, the reluctance of physicians to prescribe opioids has hindered the use of this effective therapy in patients with severe chronic obstructive pulmonary disease.[109]

Sleep apnea, especially central sleep apnea (CSA), can be seen with opioid use. Wang et al. examined 50 former heroin and polysubstance abusers who were on methadone maintenance therapy.[110] The study showed a high incidence of CSA, and obstructive sleep apnea was no more prevalent than in the control group. The researchers also found that in patients taking methadone, "blood concentrations are the most significant predictor of the severity of CSA."[110p1354] Walker et al., in a 2007 study, looked at the development of CSA and ataxic breathing and opioid serum levels.[111] They concluded that "chronic opioid use is a dose-related and independent risk factor for the development of irregular breathing with central apneas and chronic use of opioid medication (i.e., longer than 6 months), predisposing patients to the development of an irregular breathing pattern with central apneas during sleep."[111p458] However, this study did not differentiate between opioid class and used morphine equivalence for comparisons. Walker et al. further suggested that patients receiving COT of greater than a 200-mg morphine equivalent should be objectively evaluated with polysomnography for sleep-disordered breathing.[111] The rare ventilatory patterns of Biot's respiration and ataxic breathing are not usually seen in the general population but are seen in patients on COT.[112] One of the initial studies to look at sleep-disordered breathing and opioids found this to be a common issue in patients on COT.[113] Patients on long-term methadone maintenance therapy have a much higher incidence of CSA and disordered sleep breathing, although only six patients were included in the study.[114] In a single 2014 case study, CSA was reversed with the discontinuation of COT; this was the first such reported case of opioid discontinuation with reversal of CSA.[115]

The current literature on opioids and CSA should give all pain clinicians great concern. Patients should continually be evaluated for the presence of obstructive sleep apnea and potential risk factors using screening and pertinent questioning. Further, once placed on COT, patients should be reevaluated regularly for the development of CSA. The benefit must exceed the risk, so pain levels, activity, etc . . . should have increased to balance the risk of effects on respiratory function.

The cardiac side effects of opioids are fortunately very uncommon. Early studies suggested that noncardiogenic pulmonary edema was seen with use of many opioids, including morphine, methadone, heroin, and codeine.[116,117] Osler first described a case of noncardiogenic pulmonary edema in a patient with morphine overdose.[118] However, clinicians should remember that opioid-induced noncardiac pulmonary edema is rare. Other cardiac effects are more specific to distinct opioids, such as methadone.

Methadone has been linked to electrocardiographic (ECG) changes, specifically QT-interval prolongation with resultant torsades de pointes. Methadone in the United States comes as a racemic mixture and QTc prolongation is thought to be related to the (R)-enantiomer.[119] Methadone is increasingly used in pain medicine, and many insurance plans consider methadone to be on the first tier for COT, based solely on price rather than patient safety.[120] Kornick, in a study of 190 cancer patients taking intravenous methadone for pain, found that there was a dose–response increase in the QTc interval.[121] However, there was no specific dose below which the QTc was not prolonged. Interestingly, the only commercial formulation of parenteral methadone available in the United States contains the preservative chlorobutanol, which may also induce QT prolongation and torsades.[122] Cruciani et al., in 104 addicted patients who were taking more than 200 mg of daily oral methadone, found that 33% had QTc prolongations, although none had prolongation greater than 500 ms.[123] They stated in their conclusions that "methadone does not increase the risk of torsades." Some data suggest that one of the more important periods of risk is when the dose is being titrated upward.[124] Ower et al., in their case report, suggest that ECG monitoring "should be conducted regularly to rule out prolonged QTc in patients on long-term methadone, as a single ECG is not sufficient to dismiss this risk."[125p76] Gil et al. recommend measuring the QT interval before starting methadone treatment and monitoring the QT interval, "especially in cases of an increase in the dosage of methadone."[126p997] Methadone is not the only potential cause for a prolonged QT interval. Hypokalemia and other electrolyte abnormalities, cocaine usage, and especially medications that might change the methadone serum levels through their influence on the cytochrome P 450 enzyme system, particularly CYP3A4 and CYP2D6 inhibitors, should be considered.[127] Also, many patients have multiple comorbid diseases (e.g., cardiac disease) and may be taking cardiac medications that can cause or contribute to QT prolongation. And there is also the potential of congenital prolonged QT syndrome. In a study of critically ill postoperative patients, up to 42% had prolonged QT intervals, which is obviously a high rate.[128] However, in a screening study of neonates, 1 in 2,534 apparently healthy live births had a QTc of more than 450 ms.[129] The actual incidence in populations seen by pain clinicians is not known, but it seems very prudent, inexpensive, and simple to check the ECG before prescribing a medication that may prolong the QT interval (e.g., methadone, TCAs).

The data on QT prolongation due to methadone to date consist mostly of retrospective case studies. There is no clear relationship on dosage, time of use of methadone, dose threshold for QT prolongation, duration of dosing before QTc prolongation, increased incidence of prolongation with dosage change, or whether dosage route makes a difference. Until there is a clear prospective study that correlates methadone dose with prevalence of QT prolongation it is difficult to specify a clinical course of action, but evaluation and consistent reevaluation are critical.

However, since the result of torsades due to QT prolongation can be swiftly fatal, ECG evaluation of a patient who may be a candidate for COT with methadone is warranted. Once placed on methadone, continued ECG monitoring should be standard. Krantz

TABLE 5.1 Krantz recommendations for the evaluation of torsades risk

Recommendation 1 (Disclosure)	Clinicians should inform patients of arrhythmia risk when they prescribe methadone.
Recommendation 2 (Clinical History)	Clinicians should ask patients about any history of structural heart disease, arrhythmia, and syncope.
Recommendation 3 (Screening)	Obtain a pretreatment electrocardiogram for all patients to measure the QTc interval and a follow-up electrocardiogram within 30 days and annually. Additional electrocardiography is recommended if the methadone dosage exceeds 100 mg/d or if patients have unexplained syncope or seizures.
Recommendation 4 (Risk Stratification)	If the QTc interval is greater than 450 ms but less than 500 ms, discuss the potential risks and benefits with patients and monitor them more frequently. If the QTc interval exceeds 500 ms, consider discontinuing or reducing the methadone dose; eliminating contributing factors, such as drugs that promote hypokalemia; or using an alternative therapy.
Recommendation 5 (Drug Interactions)	Clinicians should be aware of interactions between methadone and other drugs that possess QT interval prolonging properties or slow the elimination of methadone.

From reference 130.

in 2009 published recommendations for the evaluation of torsades risk in the *Annals of Internal Medicine*; until better data are available, they seem prudent (Table 5.1).[130] Even though the Krantz recommendations have been criticized, in the absence of better data, they provide a working set of recommendations for the clinician when considering the use of methadone.[131]

It is not unusual to find a pregnant patient who is on COT for chronic pain, so pain clinicians will be involved in the treatment of these patients. Pregnant patients taking licit or illicit opioids present their unborn fetus with continuous opioids during pregnancy. Opioids cross the placenta and are taken up into the fetal tissues. When the neonate is born the abrupt cessation of this opioid milieu can result in withdrawal, which has been termed the "neonatal abstinence syndrome" (NAS has been expanded to include abstinence from serotonin, alcohol, and other drugs as well[132]). NAS can occur anytime during the pregnancy when maternal opioids are stopped abruptly. It is associated with significant morbidity and can result in prolonged hospital stays, especially if not recognized and treated early. Neonates who have NAS have an increased risk of fetal distress and death, impaired fetal growth, and an increased risk of sudden infant death syndrome.[133] Few studies have examined the impact of dosage on the incidence of NAS, although a recent study found a correlation between maternal methadone dose and rate of NAS.[134] This study included 388 neonates over a 10-year period and was retrospective in design. Interestingly, it seems that heavy smokers have neonates with more severe NAS of longer duration and preterm infants seem to have less severe NAS than those born at term.[135]

NAS can occur in any pregnant patient who is taking chronic opioids for pain. Pain clinicians should assume that pregnant patients on COT will have neonates with some degree of NAS. Further, they should be familiar with the presentation of this syndrome (e.g., recent guidelines that elaborate management of NAS).[136,137] Therefore, a pregnant patient who is being treated in a pain clinic should be referred to an obstetrician and neonatologist familiar with NAS and should be followed closely throughout her pregnancy.

Opioid-induced hyperalgesia (OIH) has been defined by Chu as "a state of nociceptive sensitization caused by exposure to opioids."[138] Much of the research on OIH in humans is anecdotal or involves small studies with poor power. However, there is a plethora of animal studies—as Chu states, "more than 90 publications"—suggesting OIH in a variety of animal models.[138] Regardless, discussion of OIH in humans is plagued by (1) inability to diagnostically determine the difference between OIH and tolerance, (2) a lack of universally accepted definitions of OIH, (3) lack of universally accepted diagnostic criteria for OIH, (4) lack of quality prospective randomized trials evaluating for the presence of OIH, (5) lack of a clear understanding of the physiology of this problem, (6) lack of understanding of opioid differentiation in regard to OIH (i.e., which opioids have higher or lower potential for OIH), (7) lack of a universally accepted and appropriate treatment of OIH, (8) a lack of understanding of the plastic central nervous system changes that may occur in addiction, which may be different from chronic pain, (9) inability to appreciate the role depression, other psychiatric disturbances, and disrupted sleep play in reducing pain thresholds (the previous studies on OIH did not evaluate these variables as potential confounders), and (10) lack of understanding of how sleep apnea (potentially induced or exacerbated by opioids and shown to reduce pain thresholds), either central or obstructive, influences the presentation of OIH.

In one of the most thorough reviews of OIH currently extant, Fishbain et al. in 2010 reviewed 504 articles with reference to OIH and found that only 48 articles met inclusion and exclusion criteria.[139] Their conclusion was that "There is not sufficient evidence to support or refute the existence of OIH in humans except in the case of normal volunteers receiving opioid infusions."[139p837]

OIH may occur in selected patients and, anecdotally, some patients do seem to respond to an opioid taper or rotation to another opioid class. However, claims that OIH is a *common* clinical entity are not consistent with current reviews and evidence. The clinical relevance of OIH has yet to be established. This does not mean that OIH does not occur, or that pain clinicians should ignore this as a possibility when pain seems to worsen in patients on COT. However, many other etiologies should be ruled out before one leaps to a diagnosis of OIH (e.g., worsening disease state, new disease etiology).[140]

Endocrinopathy is becoming a more recognized issue in patients on COT. The majority of studies have focused on androgens, although other endocrinopathies have been described. Testosterone (both free and total), estrogen, luteinizing hormone (LH), gonadotropin-releasing hormone (GnRH), corticotrophin-releasing hormone (CRH), dehydroepiandrosterone (DHEA), adrenocorticotropin (ACTH), dehydroepiandrosterone sulfate (DHEAS), thyroid-stimulating hormone (TSH), and cortisol have all been shown to decrease in COT.[141,142] When testosterone is affected due to COT, a condition called "opioid-induced androgen deficiency" results.[143] When this condition occurs pain worsens, depression is common, and efforts to treat the pain become complicated.[144] These opioid endocrine effects have been documented in men and women who are taking oral, intravenous, transdermal, and intrathecal opioids.[145] In women these effects are more complicated and less studied. Opioid endocrinopathy results in hypogonadism due to central suppression of hypothalamic secretion of GnRH.

One of the first reports to discuss the effect of opioids on sexual function was by Abs et al.[146] They studied 73 patients taking intrathecal opioids, either morphine or hydromorphone, and a variety of endocrine parameters were evaluated. In this study, a majority of both men and women developed hypogonadotropic hypogonadism, while 15% developed central hypocorticism and about 15% developed growth hormone deficiency. Daniell, in three studies (two in men and one in women), found reductions in sex hormones. In the first study, patients were found to have dose-dependent reductions in sex hormone levels.[147] A second study found dose-dependent reductions in DHEA levels for both oral and transdermal opioids, and the third study found that there was "profound inhibition of ovarian sex hormone and adrenal androgen production among women chronically consuming sustained-action opioids."[148,149p34] Patients with these endocrinopathies can present with altered menstrual flow, reduced fertility, opioid-associated depression, and osteoporosis. The relationship between cancer, cancer treatment, and the use of opioids seems to suggest that the addition of opioids may lead to an increased risk of hypogonadism in these patients, but the relationships are complex.[150] In this review there was a suggestion that type of opioid and dosage may be important in determining the impact of opioids on endocrine function in these patients. A recent review of testosterone suppression in patients on COT suggests that the reduction in testosterone appears to be a class effect of opioids.[151] This review also suggested that men much more than women are affected by these endocrine changes. However, to date, there have been no head-to-head comparison studies on the effects of individual opioids on testosterone suppression, much less in other endocrine disorders. Thus it is not clear at all if opioids generally have the potential to cause endocrinopathies, or whether there are differences between classes of opioids. In support of potential differences between classes of opioids, Bliesener found that patients with a history of heroin addiction who were taking buprenorphine had significantly higher testosterone levels than patients on chronic methadone maintenance alone.[152]

Nonetheless, these correlations are not necessarily straightforward. For example, statistically significant associations has been found between hypogonadism and hypertension, tobacco abuse, work-related stress, depression, and especially sleep apnea.[153] This illustrates the common theme of this chapter: evaluation and reevaluation, without biases, is the appropriate approach to these patients. Opioids may be a cause, but endocrine abnormalities seen in patients on COT may be due to a nonpharmacologic etiology or a combination of a number of factors.

There has been increased concern that chronic use of opioids can lead to reduced bone density, the etiology of which is still unclear.[154] When combined with the increased incidence of falls in elderly patients taking opioids, this places patients, especially elderly ones, at a much higher risk for fracture.[155] One study found that 44% of men with chronic pain who were taking opioids had bone mass densities in the osteopenic or osteoporotic range.[156]

The changes in thyroid function brought about by opioids have been equivocal.[157] However, it is recommended that thyroid function tests be part of an endocrine evaluation in all patients with chronic pain, regardless of the use of opioids.[158] Whether or not other endocrine studies should be performed in patients on COT is still not clear. Pain clinicians should use their judgment and clinical suspicion to guide further endocrine studies and testing.

As emphasized throughout this chapter, evaluation and reassessment is key in treating any side effect of opioids. As should be obvious, patients are reluctant to discuss issues and problems related to sexual dysfunction. Since it is unclear how quickly endocrinopathy develops or how these abnormalities will progress over time, obtaining a general endocrine panel in patients who are to be placed on COT, when symptoms occur, or once a year seems to be a reasonable approach.[158] Further, it seems prudent to perform a bone density evaluation in patients who are to be placed on COT, and routinely as they age. Obviously, a working relationship with an endocrinologist is a necessity.

There are six general approaches to treating side effects in COT:

1. Stop the opioid completely.
2. Reduce the opioid dose.
3. Rotate to a different opioid class.[65]
4. Assess to see if the patient could get the same analgesia on a lower dose of opioid.
5. Add analgesic adjuvants to help lower the total amount of opioid being delivered per day.
6. Treat the side effect per se, leaving other therapies consistent.[159]

NONOPIOID MEDICATIONS

Since physiologic generation of chronic pain has a multitude of potential mechanisms, applying different approaches to treatment to engage those mechanisms makes intuitive sense. There are few well-designed studies evaluating the treatment of patients with a chronic pain diagnosis, with most of the medications commonly used over long periods of time (i.e., greater than 4–6 months). A recent review of adverse events and cost in the treatment of low back pain found that the short-term use of most drugs produced symptomatic relief, but long-term benefits, regardless of drug, have yet to be determined.[160] Nonopioid therapies are both pharmacologic and nonpharmacologic. The following is not meant to be an exhaustive list of potential nonopioid therapies, but rather an overview of some other potential therapies for the patient with chronic pain.

There are a number of potential medications in the class of antiepileptic drugs that can be additive to a pharmacologic regimen for chronic pain. However, the exact mechanisms for these medications have not been clearly established and they can have significant side effects. The goal is to add a medication whose benefits are synergistic, thereby reducing doses of other medications (e.g., opioids) and increasing analgesia. Unfortunately, even though prima facie the use of medications that affect multiple mechanisms makes physiologic sense, there are few data in support of this approach and only a few studies have been published. In one pilot study, the combination of gabapentin and morphine was found to be synergistic.[161] In another recent study on postoperative pain, gabapentin and morphine were also found to be synergistic in their level of analgesia.[162] However, a 2015 study found that the benefit was small and side effects increased with the combination of gabapentin and morphine.[163] The study had only 16 patients, however.

The gabapentinoids are a class of medications used extensively for neuropathic pain and have a fairly robust set of published data. Gabapentin, pregabalin, and microgabalin are the three currently on the market, with others in the pipeline. This class of medications is said to work through modulation of the alpha-2 delta subunit of a sodium channel.[164]

Nonsteroidal anti-inflammatories (NSAIDs) are ubiquitous drugs that can provide significant relief for acute pain. The benefit for long-term use in chronic pain is hindered by the significant side effects of this class of medications and lack of evidence that inflammation is a pain generator when acute pain transitions to chronic pain. Peptic ulcer disease, cardiac effects, coagulation effects, and kidney and liver failure are all potential issues when these medications are used.[165–167] One of the risk factors for these side effects is total dose and length of time dosed. Although NSAIDs can be helpful for acute exacerbations, their use in the long term, in standard doses, is hard to rationalize, especially considering the type of patients with chronic pain. Many of these patients have relative and absolute contraindications to the use of NSAIDs.

The mechanism of acetaminophen, or paracetamol, (APAP) is still unknown. Further, there has been significant concern from political entities that the use of APAP is a significant public health threat.[168] In the United States recently, combination APAP products were mandated to contain no more than 325 mg APAP.[169] Since APAP contributes to 50% of the cases of acute liver failure and since liver transplantation is the primary treatment, with concomitant significant costs, this concern is reasonable.[170] Although APAP remains the initial treatment recommended by the American Rheumatological Association, recent reviews suggest that this drug produces minimal benefits.[171] For example, Chou in a recent review suggested that APAP did not alleviate lower back pain and helped only a "small amount" in hip and knee osteoarthritis.[172] Further, a 2015 review of APAP and NSAIDs in osteoarthritis found that ibuprofen was "usually superior" to APAP.[173] This review questioned "the practice of routinely using paracetamol as a first line analgesia."[173p1213] However, APAP can be beneficial in some situations. For example, studies in demented patients show that the use of scheduled APAP can lead to improved interactions and fewer behavioral problems.[174]

The term "muscle relaxants" is very broad and includes a variety of drug classes. Of interest, a recent review found that the use of "muscle relaxants" increased the risk for both emergency department visits and hospital admissions in elderly patients.[175] These data reinforced the recommendations by professional organizations that "muscle relaxants" should be used with caution and are considered "high risk" in the elderly.[176] In a Cochrane review of "muscle relaxants" in the treatment of rheumatoid arthritis pain, few studies were identified and most used benzodiazepines (BZDs). This review found weak evidence for no or little benefit from BZDs, especially overuse of NSAIDs in the treatment of rheumatoid arthritis pain.[177] Long-term BZD use is common,[178] even though they are problematic when used chronically or for treating chronic pain patients. "BZDs are used in a variety of psychiatric and nonpsychiatric disorders. In most cases, such a wide use is not supported by scientific evidence but is mostly empirical."[179p11] This 2013 review suggests that "the risk/benefit ratio is positive in short-term use but debatable once treatment exceeds the recommended duration."[179p12] A very recent study in US Veterans Gressler, et. al., found that the concomitant use of opioids and benzodiazepines resulted in a significant increase in adverse outcomes (Gressler LE, Martin BC, Hudson TJ, painter JT. Relationship between concomitant benzodiazepine-opioid use and adverse outcomes among US veterans. pain. 2018;159:451-459.) Regardless, long-term use for chronic pain has poor scientific support and should be discouraged and avoided, especially if opioids are being added to the regimen.[99]

The International Association for the Study of Pain's definition of pain begins by stating that "pain is an unpleasant sensory and emotional experience."[180] There is a connection between pain and depression, with both having shared neurobiology.[181] Clearly the emotional component of chronic pain must be addressed if chronic pain is to be treated successfully. Antidepressants are routinely used by the pain clinician and have become commonly prescribed in primary care as well. The mechanisms here are diverse, but they mainly reduce pain by strengthening the inhibitory signal of descending pathways from the brain. The greatest amount of evidence for the use of antidepressants in chronic pain is for neuropathic pain, specifically diabetic neuropathic pain and postherpetic neuralgia pain. TCAs have been used for decades for neuropathic pain and are considered the "gold standard" in the use of antidepressants for chronic pain.[182] There is level 1 evidence for the use of amitriptyline in diabetic neuropathy and level 2 evidence for the use of TCAs in neuropathic pain generally.[183] SSRIs are inferior to TCAs and to SNRIs. They have been found to be superior to placebo in a number of studies, but the difference is minimal (though statistically significant). SNRIs have been investigated extensively. Venlafaxine, duloxetine, and milnacipran have all been shown to improve analgesia in neuropathic pain. In acute pain, Wong, in a 2014 review of current data on antidepressants and postoperative pain, suggested that "there is currently insufficient evidence to support the clinical use of antidepressants . . . for treatment of acute, or prevention of chronic, postoperative pain."[184]

Cannabinoids have shown some benefit when given in preparations of specific metabolites (specifically, cannabidiol). The use of smoked cannabis for analgesia is at best questionable, and many feel the data are plagued by poor study design and poor consistency of experimental drug and steeped in sociopolitics.[185] As stated in a recent publication, "Owing to rising THC concentrations of products, 'medical' marijuana is rarely good medicine."[186]

Physical therapy, chiropractic, and other nonpharmacologic approaches should always be considered in the chronic pain patient. Improving function, as previously mentioned, should be a primary goal. Further, nonpharmacologic approaches get patients more involved in their own therapy. Complementary or integrative therapies are becoming commonly used by patients with chronic pain. One of the major issues facing the clinician is how to integrate such therapies with completely different philosophical foundations into some kind of combined therapeutic approach (e.g., acupuncture and Western medicine). Further, high-quality studies on many of these approaches are lacking. For example, a recent review of integrative therapies for pain made the following judgment: "Only a small number of [randomized controlled trials and controlled clinical trials] with a limited number of patients and lack of adequate control groups assessing integrative health care research are available. These studies provide limited evidence of effective integrative health care on some modalities. However, integrative health care regimen appears to be generally safe."[187p1]

CONCLUSION

This chapter gave an overview of the evaluation and therapeutic approach to the chronic pain patient. Chronic pain is complex.[9] Its diagnosis and treatment are also complex and are not limited to the pain *per se*. A single therapeutic modality will usually not be successful in treating the chronic pain patient. A multidisciplinary, multimodal approach appears to be the best approach for these patients, and clinicians who do not have access to all these resources will need to be creative. This chapter is not meant to suggest that the approaches discussed here constitute some kind of legal standard of care, nor is this chapter meant to be a clinical guide. We are suggesting that clinicians prescribing opioids should also consider many other issues, diagnoses, and approaches for chronic pain patients. In addition, these patients need a "wholistic" approach, taking into consideration co-morbidities and other diagnoses that need to be treated concomitantly with the treatment of their chronic pain. As emphasized, these patients much more complex and requires an approach including thorough evaluation, diagnosis, and treatment.

REFERENCES

1. Peppin J, Schatman M. Commentary: terminology of chronic pain: the need to "level the playing field." *J Pain Res.* 2016; 9: 1–2.
2. Callahan D. Managed care and the goals of medicine. *J Am Geriatr Soc.* 1998; 46: 385–388.
3. American College of Physicians, Ad Hoc Committee on Medical Ethics. American College of Physicians ethics manual, Part I: history of medical ethics, the physician and the patient, the physician's relationship to other physicians, the physician and society. *Ann Internal Med.* 1984; 101: 129–137.
4. Peppin JF. Marginalization of patients with chronic pain on chronic opioid therapy. *Pain Physician.* 2009; 12: 493–498.
5. Turk DC, Wilson HD, Cahana A. Treatment of chronic non-cancer pain. *Lancet.* 2011; 377: 2226–2235.
6. Institute of Medicine (IOM). *Relieving Pain in America: A Blueprint for Transforming Prevention, Care, Education, and Research.* Washington, DC: National Academies Press; 2011.
7. Ferrell BR. The role of ethics committees in responding to the moral outrage of unrelieved pain. *Bioethics Forum* 1997; 13: 11–16.
8. Mezei L, Murinson BB, Johns Hopkins Pain Curriculum Development Team. Pain education in North American medical schools. *J Pain.* 2011; 12: 1199–1208.
9. Peppin JF, Cheatle MD, Kirsh KL, McCarberg BH. The complexity model: a novel approach to improve chronic pain care. *Pain Med.* 2015; 16: 653–666.
10. Danmiller Pain Review Course with CME, 2003. Available at: https://cme.dannemiller.com/dvd-usb/pain/. Accessed January 25, 2016.
11. Upshur CC, Luckmann RS, Savageau JA. Primary care provider concerns about management of chronic pain in community clinic populations. *J Gen Intern Med.* 2006; 21: 652–655.
12. O'Rorke JE, Chen I, Genao I, Panda M, Cykert S. Physicians' comfort in caring for patients with chronic nonmalignant pain. *Am J Med Sci.* 2007; 333: 93–100.
13. Fassoulaki, A, Melemeni A, Staikou C, Triga A, Sarantopoulos C. Acute postoperative pain predicts chronic pain and long-term analgesic requirements after breast surgery for cancer. *Acta Anaesthesiol Belg.* 2008; 59: 241–248.

14. Peppin JF, Klim G, Burke J, Kirsh JL. A partial review of the appropriate use of opioid analgesics in the treatment of chronic pain: toward a model of good practice and rational pharmacotherapy. *Cri Rev Phys Rehab Med*. 2009; 21: 25–65.

15. Tsang A, Von Korff M, Lee S, et al. Common chronic pain conditions in developed and developing countries: gender and age differences and comorbidity with depression-anxiety disorders. *J Pain*. 2008; 9: 883–891.

16. Dworkind M, Yaffee MJ. Somatization and the recognition of depression and anxiety in primary care. *Am J Psychiatry*. 1993; 150: 734–741.

17. Von Korff M, Crane P, Lane M, et al. Chronic spinal pain and physical-mental comorbidity in the United States: results from the National Comorbidity Survey replication. *Pain*. 2005; 113: 331–339.

18. Rome H, Rome J. Limbically augmented pain syndrome (LAPS): kindling, corticolimbic sensitization, and the convergence of affective and sensory symptoms in chronic pain disorders. *Pain Med*. 2000; 1: 7–23.

19. Chapman CR, Tuckett RP, Song CW. Pain and stress in a systems perspective: reciprocal neural, endocrine, and immune interactions. *J Pain*. 2008; 9: 122–145.

20. van Dijk GM, Veenhof C, Schellevis F, et al. Comorbidity, limitations in activities and pain in patients with osteoarthritis of the hip or knee. *BMC Musculoskelet Disord* 2008; 9: 95.

21. AAPM Facts and Figures on Pain. American Academy of Pain Medicine. Available at: http://www.painmed.org/patientcenter/facts_on_pain.aspx#incidence. Accessed May 15, 2017.

22. Chrubasik S, Junck H, Zappe HA, Stutzke O. A survey on pain complaints and health care utilization in a German population sample. *Eur J Anaesthesiol*. 1998; 15: 397–408.

23. Chou R, Qaseem A, Snow V, et al. Diagnosis and treatment of low back pain: a joint clinical practice guideline from the American College of Physicians and the American Pain Society. *Ann Intern Med*. 2007; 147: 478–491.

24. Daniel M, Keefe FJ, Lyna P, et al. Persistent smoking after a diagnosis of lung cancer is associated with higher reported pain levels. *J Pain*. 2009; 10(3): 323–328.

25. Friedman R, Li V, Mehrotra D. Treating pain patients at risk: evaluation of a screening tool in opioid-treated pain patients with and without addiction. *Pain Med*. 2003; 4: 182–185.

26. National Institute of Health (NIH). Rehabilitation of persons with traumatic brain injury. *NIH Consensus Statement*. 1998; 16: 1–41.

27. Bjork JM, Grans SJ. Does traumatic brain injury increase risk for substance abuse? *J Neurotrauma*. 2009; 26: 1077–1082.

28. Hibbard MR, Uysal S, Kepler K, Bodgany J, Silver J. Axis I psychopathology in individuals with traumatic brain injury. *J Head Trauma Rehabil*. 1998; 13: 24–39.

29. Packard RC. Chronic post-traumatic headache: associations with mild traumatic brain injury, concussion, and post-concussive disorder. *Curr Pain Headache Rep*. 2008; 12: 67–73.

30. Nampiaparampil DE. Prevalence of chronic pain after traumatic brain injury. *JAMA*. 2008; 300: 711–719.

31. Okifuji A, Hare BD. The association between chronic pain and obesity. *J Pain Res*. 2015; 8: 399–408.

32. Khoueir P, Black MH, Crookes PF, et al. Prospective assessment of axial back pain symptoms before and after bariatric weight reduction surgery. *Spine J*. 2009; 9: 454–463.

33. Harding GT, Dunbar MJ, Hubley-Kozey CL, Stanish WD, Wilson JLA. Obesity is associated with higher absolute tibiofemoral contact and muscle forces during gait with and without knee osteoarthritis. *Clin Biomech*. 2016; 31: 79–86.

34. Chan G, Chen CT. Musculoskeletal effects of obesity. *Curr Opin Pediatr*. 2009; 21: 65–70.

35. Vitiello MV, Rybarczyk B, Von Korff M, Stepanski EJ. Cognitive behavioral therapy for insomnia improves sleep and decreases pain in older adults with co-morbid insomnia and osteoarthritis. *J Clin Sleep Med*. 2009; 5: 355–362.

36. Quartana PJ, Wickwire EM, Klick B, Grace E, Smith MT. Naturalistic changes in insomnia symptoms and pain in temporomandibular joint disorder: a crosslagged panel analysis. *Pain*. 2010; 149: 325–331.

37. Tan V, Cheatle MD, Mackin S, Moberg PJ, Esterhai JL. Goal setting as a predictor of return to work in a population of chronic musculoskeletal pain patients. *Int J Neurosci*. 1997; 92(3–4): 161–70.

38. Belo JN, Berger MY, Koes BW, Bierma-Zeinstra SM. Prognostic factors in adults with knee pain in general practice. *Arthritis Rheum*. 2009; 6: 143–151.

39. Linton SJ. A review of psychological risk factors in back and neck pain. *Spine*. 2000; 25: 1148–1156.

40. Turk DC, Okofuji A. Psychological factors in chronic pain: evolution and revolution. *J Consult Clin Psychol*. 2002; 70: 678–690.

41. Gallagher RM. Pain science and rational polypharmacy: an historical perspective. *Am J Phys Med Rehabil*. 2005; 84(suppl 3): S1–3.

42. Fitzgerald RJ. Medication errors: the importance of an accurate drug history. *Br J Clin Pharmacol*. 2009; 67: 671–675.

43. Dunbar S, Katz NP. Chronic opioid therapy for nonmalignant pain in patients with a history of substance abuse: report of 20 cases. *J Pain Symptom Manage*. 1996; 11: 163–171.

44. Hoffman MD, Shepanski MA, Mackenzie SP, Clifford PS. Experimentally induced pain perception is acutely reduced by aerobic exercise in people with chronic low back pain. *J Rehabil Res Dev*. 2005; 42: 183–190.

45. Peppin JF, Kirsh KL, Marcum S. The chronic pain patient and functional assessment: use of the 6-minute walk test in a multidisciplinary pain clinic. *Curr Med Res Opin*. 2014; 30: 361–365.

46. Antunes RS, Macedo BG, Amaral TS, Gomes HA, Pereira LSM, Rocha FL. Pain, kinesiophobia and quality of life in chronic low back pain and depression. *Acta Ortop Bras*. 2013; 21: 27–29.

47. Passik S, Kirsh KL, Casper D. Addiction-related assessment tools and pain management: instruments for screening, treatment planning, and monitoring compliance. *Pain Med*. 2008; 9: S145–S166.

48. American Pain Society. *Principles of Analgesic Use in the Treatment of Acute Pain and Cancer Pain*. Glenview, IL: Author, 2008.

49. Gourlay DL, Heit HA, Almahrezi A. Universal precautions in pain medicine: a rational approach to the treatment of chronic pain. *Pain Med*. 2005; 6: 107–112.

50. Starrels JL, Becker WC, Alford DP, Kapoor A, Williams AR, Turner BJ. Systematic review: treatment agreements and urine drug testing to reduce opioid misuse in patients with chronic pain. *Ann Intern Med*. 2010; 152: 712–720.

51. Ballak SB, Degens H, de Haan A, Jaspers RT. Aging related changes in determinants of muscle force generating capacity: a comparison of muscle aging in men and male rodents. *Ageing Res Rev*. 2014; 14: 43–55.

52. Weinert BT, Timiras PS. Invited review: theories of aging. *J Appl Physiol*. 2003; 95: 1706–1716.

53. Bolignano D, Mattace-Raso F, Sijbrands EJ, Zoccali C. The aging kidney revisited: a systematic review. *Ageing Res Rev*. 2014; 14: 65–80.

54. Tennant F, Hocum B. Pharmacogenetics and pain management. *Practical Pain Management*. 2015; 15: 1–11.

55. McNicol E, Horowicz-Mehler N, Fisk RA, et al. Management of opioid side effects in cancer-related and chronic noncancer pain: a systematic review. *J Pain*. 2003; 4: 231–256.

56. Cavalcanti IL, Carvalho AC, Musauer MG, et al. Safety and tolerability of controlled-release oxycodone on postoperative pain in patients submitted to the oncologic head and neck surgery. *Rev Col Bras Cir*. 2014; 41: 393–399.

57. Dietrich B, Ramchandran K, Von Roenn JH. Nausea and vomiting. *Psycho-Oncology*. 2015; 24: 199.

58. Smith SS, Laufer A. Opioid-induced nausea and vomiting. *Eur J Pharmacol*. 2014; 722: 67–78.

59. Baldessarini RJ, Tarazi FI. Drugs and the treatment of psychiatric disorders. In: Goodman LS, Hardman JG, Limbird LE, Gilman AG, eds. *Goodman & Gilman's the Pharmacologic Basis of Therapeutics.* 10th ed. New York: McGraw-Hill; 2001:485–520.

60. Pasricha PJ. Prokinetic agents, antiemetics, and agents used in irritable bowel syndrome. In: Goodman LS, Hardman JG, Limbird LE, Gilman AG, eds. *Goodman & Gilman's the Pharmacologic Basis of Therapeutics.* 10th ed. New York: McGraw-Hill; 2001:1021–1036.

61. Apfel CC, Korttila K, Abdalla M, et al. A factorial trial of six interventions for the prevention of postoperative nausea and vomiting. *N Engl J Med.* 2004; 350: 2441–2451.

62. Cherny N, Ripamonti C, Pereira J, et al. Strategies to manage the adverse effects of oral morphine: an evidence-based report. *J Clin Oncol.* 2001; 19: 2542–2554.

63. Barbour SY. Corticosteroids in the treatment of chemotherapy-induced nausea and vomiting. *J Natl Compr Canc Netw.* 2012; 10: 493–499.

64. Kanbayashi Y, Hosokawa T. Predictive factors for nausea or vomiting in patients with cancer who receive oral oxycodone for the first time: is prophylactic medication for prevention of opioid-induced nausea or vomiting necessary? *J Palliative Med.* 2014; 17: 83–687.

65. Smith HS, Peppin JF. Toward a systematic approach to opioid rotation. *J Pain Res.* 2014; 7: 589–608.

66. Tripathee S, Akbar T, Richards D, Themessl-Huber M, Freeman R. The relationship between sugar-containing methadone and dental caries: a systematic review. *Health Educ J.* 2013; 72: 469–485.

67. Donaldson M, Goodchild JH, Epstein JB. Sugar content, cariogenicity, and dental concerns with commonly used medications. *J Am Dental Assoc.* 2015; 146: 129–133.

68. Brondani M, Park PE. Methadone and oral health—a brief review. *Am Dental Hygienists Assoc.* 2011; 85: 92–98.

69. Graham CH, Meechan JG. Dental management of patients taking methadone. *Dental Update.* 2005; 32: 477–478, 481–482, 485.

70. Fallon M, Reale C, Davies A, et al. Efficacy and safety of fentanyl pectin nasal spray compared with immediate-release morphine sulfate tablets in the treatment of breakthrough cancer pain: a multicenter, randomized, controlled, double-blind, double-dummy multiple-crossover study. *J Supportive Oncol.* 2011; 9: 224–231.

71. Lintzeris N, Leung SY, Dunlop AJ, et al. A randomised controlled trial of sublingual buprenorphine–naloxone film versus tablets in the management of opioid dependence. *Drug Alcohol Dependence.* 2013; 131: 119–126.

72. Suzuki J, Mittal L, Woo SB. Sublingual buprenorphine and dental problems: a case series. *Prim Care Compan CNS Disord.* 2013; 15(5).

73. Argoff CE, Kopecky EA. Patients with chronic pain and dysphagia (CPD): unmet medical needs and pharmacologic treatment options. *Curr Med Res Opin.* 2014; 30: 2543–2559.

74. Pergolizzi JV Jr, Taylor R Jr, Nalamachu S, et al. Challenges of treating patients with chronic pain with dysphagia (CPD): physician and patient perspectives. *Curr Med Res Opin.* 2013; 30: 191–202.

75. Williams RE, Bosnic N, Sweeney CT, et al. Prevalence of opioid dispensings and concurrent gastrointestinal medications in Quebec. *Pain Res Manage.* 2008; 13: 395–400.

76. Kraichely R, Arora AS, Murray JA. Opiate-induced oesophageal dysmotility. *Aliment Pharmacol Ther.* 2010; 31: 601–606.

77. Mixides G, Liegi MG, Bloom K. Enteral administration of naloxone for treatment of opioids-associated intragastric feeding intolerance. *Pharmacotherapy.* 2004; 24: 291–294.

77a. Schmulson, Max J, Douglas A. Drossman. What Is New in Rome IV. *Journal of Neurogastroenterology and Motility.* 2017; 23(2): 151–163. PMC. Web. 7 Mar. 2018.

78. Pappagallo M. Incidence, prevalence, and management of opioid bowel dysfunction. *Am J Surg.* 2001; 182: S11–S18.

79. Slatkin N, Thomas J, Lipman AG, et al. Methylnaltrexone for treatment of opioid-induced constipation in advanced illness patients. *J Support Oncol.* 2009; 7: 39–46.

80. Nisbet A, Mooney-Cotter F. Comparison of selected sedation scales for reporting opioid-induced sedation assessment. *Pain Manage Nurs.* 2009; 10: 154–164.

81. Pasero C, McCaffery M. Section IV, Opioid Analgesics. In *Pain Assessment and Pharmacologic Management.* St Louis: Mosby/Elsevier; 2011:277–622.

82. Jarzyna D, Jungquist CR, Pasero C, et al. American Society for Pain Management: nursing guidelines on monitoring for opioid-induced sedation and respiratory depression. *Pain Manage Nursing.* 2011; 12: 118–145.

83. Saunders KW, Von Korff M, Campbell CI, et al. Concurrent use of alcohol and sedatives among persons prescribed chronic opioid therapy: prevalence and risk factors. *J Pain.* 2012; 13: 266–275.

84. Reich A, Szepietowski JC. Opioid-induced pruritus: an update. *Clin Exp Dermatol.* 2010; 35: 2–6.

85. Phan NQ, Siepmann D, Gralow I, Stander S. Adjuvant topical therapy with a cannabinoid receptor agonist in facial postherpetic neuralgia. *J Dtsch Dermatol Ges.* 2010; 8: 88–91.

86. Kjellberg F, Tramer MR. Pharmacological control of opioid-induced pruritus: a quantitative systematic review of randomized trials. *Eur J Anaesthesiol.* 2001; 18: 346–357.

87. Clegg A, Young JB. Which medications to avoid in people at risk of delirium: a systematic review. *Age Ageing.* 2011; 40: 23–29.

88. Sieber FE, Mears S, Lee H, Gottschalk A. Postoperative opioid consumption and its relationship to cognitive function in elderly hip fracture patients. *J Am Geriatr Soc.* 2011; 59: 2256–2262.

89. Mercadante S. Pathophysiology and treatment of opioid-related myoclonus in cancer patients. *Pain.* 1998; 74: 5–9.

90. Thwaites D, McCann S, Broderick P. Hydromorphone neuroexcitation. *J Palliat Med.* 2004; 7: 545–550.

91. Kullgren J, Le V, Wheeler W. Incidence of hydromorphone-induced neuroexcitation in hospice patients. *J Palliat Med.* 2013; 16: 1205–1209.

92. Caraceni A, Hanks G, Kaasa S, et al. Use of opioid analgesics in the treatment of cancer pain: evidence-based recommendations from the EAPC. *Lancet Oncol.* 2012; 13: e58–68.

93. Foreo M, Chan PSL, Restrepo-Garces CE. Successful reversal of hyperalgesia/myoclonus complex with low-dose ketamine infusion. *Pain Practice.* 2012; 12: 154–158.

94. Albanese A, Bhatia K, Bressman SB, et al. Phenomenology and classification of dystonia: a consensus update. *Move Disord.* 2013; 28: 863–873.

95. Moldofsky H. Sleep and pain. *Sleep Med Rev.* 2001; 5: 387–398.

96. Smith MT, Perlis ML, Smith MS, Giles DE, Carmody TP. Sleep quality and presleep arousal in chronic pain. *J Behav Med.* 2000; 23: 1–3.

97. Aurora RN, Kristo DA, Bista SR, et al. The treatment of restless legs syndrome and periodic limb movement disorder in adults—an update for 2012: practice parameters with an evidence-based systematic review and meta-analyses: an American Academy of Sleep Medicine Clinical Practice Guideline. *Sleep.* 2012; 35: 1039.

98. Blågestad T, Pallesen S, Lunde LH, Sivertsen B, Nordhus IH, Grønli J. Sleep in older chronic pain patients: a comparative polysomnographic study. *Clin J Pain.* 2012; 28: 277–283.

99. Webster LR, Cochella S, Dasgupta N, et al. An analysis of the root causes for opioid-related overdose deaths in the United States. *Pain Med.* 2011; 12(s2): S26–35.

100. Dahan A, Sarton E, Teppema L, et al. Anesthetic potency and influence of morphine and sevoflurane on respiration in mu-opioid receptor knockout mice. *Anesthesiology.* 2001; 94: 824–832. [Erratum in: *Anesthesiology.* 2001; 95: 819.]

101. Boom M, Niesters M, Sarton E, Aarts L, Smith TW, Dahan A. Non-analgesic effects of opioids: opioid-induced respiratory depression. *Curr Pharmaceut Design.* 2012; 18: 5994–6004.

102. Cashman JN, Dolins SJ. Respiratory and haemodynamic effects of acute postoperative pain management: evidence from published data. *Br J Anaesth*. 2004; 93: 212–223.

103. Doneh B. Epworth Sleepiness Scale. *Occup Med*. 2015; 65: 508.

104. Dahan A, Aarts L, Smith TW. Incidence, reversal, and prevention of opioid-induced respiratory depression. *Anesthesiology*. 2010; 112: 226–238.

105. Wheatley RG, Somerville ID, Sapsford DJ, Jones JG. Postoperative hypoxaemia: comparison of extradural, i.m. and patient-controlled opioid analgesia. *Br J Anaesth*. 1990; 64: 267–275.

106. Voscopoulos CJ, MacNabb CM, Freeman J, Galvagno SM Jr, Ladd D, George E. Continuous noninvasive respiratory volume monitoring for the identification of patients at risk for opioid-induced respiratory depression and obstructive breathing patterns. *J Trauma Acute Care Surg*. 2014; 77: S208–S215.

107. Tickoo R, Thaler HT, Saldivar R, Bushan A, Stover DE, Churak M. Assessing excessive daytime sleepiness by the Epworth Sleepiness Scale in ambulatory cancer patients on chronic opioid therapy for chronic cancer related pain. *Am J Respir Crit Care Med*. 2014; 189: A6698.

108. Jennings AL, Davies AN, Higgins JP, Gibbs JS, Broadley KE. A systematic review of the use of opioids in the management of dyspnoea. *Thorax*. 2002;57:939–944.

109. Rocker G, Young J, Donahue M, Farquhar M, Simpson C. Perspectives of patients, family caregivers and physicians about the use of opioids for refractory dyspnea in advanced chronic obstructive pulmonary disease. *Can Med Assoc J*. 2012; 184: E497–E504.

110. Wang D, Teichtahl H, Drummer O, et al. Central sleep apnea in stable methadone maintenance treatment patients. *Chest*. 2005; 128: 1348–1356.

111. Walker JM, Farney RJ, Rhondeau SM, et al. Chronic opioid use is a risk factor for the development of central sleep apnea and ataxic breathing. *J Clin Sleep Med*. 2007; 3: 455–461.

112. Lee-Iannotti J, Parish JM. The epidemic of opioid use: implications for the sleep physician. *J Clin Sleep Med*. 2014; 10: 645–646.

113. Webster LR, Choi Y, Desai H, Webster L, Grant BJB. Sleep-disordered breathing and chronic opioid therapy. *Pain Med*. 2008; 9: 425–432.

114. Alattar MA, Scharf SM. Opioid-associated central sleep apnea: a case series. *Sleep Breath*. 2009; 13: 201–206.

115. Davis MJ, Livingston M, Scharf SM. Reversal of central sleep apnea following discontinuation of opioids. *J Clin Sleep Med*. 2012; 8: 579–580.

116. Bruera E, Miller MJ. Non-cardiogenic pulmonary edema after narcotic treatment for cancer pain. *Pain*. 1989; 39: 297–300.

117. Sternbach G. William Osler: narcotic-induced pulmonary edema. *J Emerg Med*. 1983; 1: 165–167.

118. Osler W. Oedema of left lung—morphia poisoning. *Montreal Gen Hosp Rep*. 1880; 1: 291–292.

119. Skjervold B, Bathen J, Spigset O. Methadone and the QT interval: relations to the serum concentrations of methadone and its enantiomers (R)-methadone and (S)-methadone. *J Clin Psychopharmacol*. 2006;26:687–689.

120. Schatman ME. The role of the health insurance industry in perpetuating suboptimal pain management. *Pain Med*. 2011; 12: 415–426.

121. Kornick CA, Kilborn MJ, Santiago-Palma J, et al. QTc interval prolongation associated with intravenous methadone. *Pain*. 2003; 105: 499–506.

122. Miranda-Grajales H, Hao J, Cruciani RA. False sense of safety by daily QTc interval monitoring during methadone IVPCA titration in a patient with chronic pain. *J Pain Res*. 2013; 6: 375.

123. Cruciani RA, Sekine R, Homel P, et. al. Measurement of QTc in patients receiving chronic methadone therapy. *J Pain Symptom Manage*. 2005; 29: 385–391.

124. Krantz MJ, Lewkowiez L, Hays H, Woodroffe MA, Robertson AD, Mehler PS. Torsades de pointes associated with very-high-dose methadone. *Ann Intern Med*. 2002; 137: 501–504.

125. Ower K, Morley-Forster P, Moulin D. Fluctuating QTc interval in an asymptomatic patient treated with methadone for chronic pain. *J Opioid Manage.* 2005; 1: 73–76.

126. Gil M, Sala M, Anguera I, et al. QT prolongation and torsades de pointes in patients infected with human immunodeficiency virus and treated with methadone. *Am J Cardiol.* 2003; 92: 995–997.

127. Webster LR. Responsible Prescribing of Methadone for Pain Management: Safety First. Providers' Clinical Support System for Opioid Therapies (PCSS-O). Salt Lake City, April 14, 2015.

128. Pham JC, Banks MC, Narotsky DL, Dorman T, Winters BD. The prevalence of long QT interval in post-operative intensive care unit patients. *J Clin Monitoring Computing.* 2016; 30: 437–443.

129. Schwartz PJ, Crotti L, Insolia R. Long-QT syndrome from genetics to management. *Circulation: Arrhythmia and Electrophysiology.* 2012; 5: 868–877.

130. Krantz MJ, Martin J, Stimmel B, Mehta D, Haigney MC. QTc interval screening in methadone treatment. *Ann Intern Med.* 2009; 150: 387–395.

131. Cohen SP, Mao J. Concerns about consensus guidelines for QTc interval screening in methadone treatment. *Ann Intern Med.* 2009; 151: 216–217.

132. Jansson LM, Velez M. Neonatal abstinence syndrome. *Curr Opin Pediatr.* 2012; 24: 252–258.

133. Mawhinney S, Ashe RG, Lowry J. Substance abuse in pregnancy: opioid substitution in a Northern Ireland maternity unit. *Ulster Med J.* 2006; 75: 187–191.

134. Seligman NS, Almario CV, Hayes EJ, Dysart KC, Berghella V, Baxter JK. Relationship between maternal methadone dose at delivery and neonatal abstinence syndrome. *J Pediatr.* 2010; 157: 428–433.

135. Liu AJ, Jones MP, Murray H, Cook CM, Nanan R. Perinatal risk factors for the neonatal abstinence syndrome in infants born to women on methadone maintenance therapy. *Aust N Z J Obstet Gynaecol.* 2010; 50: 253–258.

136. Wong S, Ordean A, Kahan M. Substance use in pregnancy. *J Obstet Gynaecol Can.* 2011; 33: 367–384.

137. World Health Organization. Guidelines for the identification and management of substance use and substance use disorders in pregnancy. Available at: http://www.who.int/substance_abuse/publications/pregnancy_guidelines/en/. Accessed May 15, 2017.

138. Chu LF, Angst MS, Clark D. Opioid-induced hyperalgesia in humans: molecular mechanisms and clinical considerations. *Clin J Pain.* 2008; 24: 479–496.

139. Fishbain DA, Cole B, Lewis JE, Gao J, Rosomoff RS. Do opioids induce hyperalgesia in humans? An evidence-based structured review. *Pain Med.* 2009; 10: 829–839.

140. Ramasubbu C, Gupta A. Pharmacological treatment of opioid-induced hyperalgesia: a review of the evidence. *J Pain Palliat Care Pharmacother.* 2011; 25: 219–230.

141. Demarest SP, Gill RS, Adler RA. Opioid endocrinopathy. *Endocrine Practice.* 2015; 21: 190–198.

142. Gudin JA, Laitman A, Nalamachu S. Opioid related endocrinopathy. *Pain Med.* 2015; 16: S9–S15.

143. Smith HS, Elliott JA. Opioid-induced androgen deficiency (OPIAD). *Pain Physician.* 2012; 15(Suppl): E145–E156.

144. Kim CH, Garcia R, Stover J, Ritchie K, Whealton T, Ata MA. Androgen deficiency in long-term intrathecal opioid administration. *Pain Physician.* 2014; 17: E543–E548.

145. Birthi P, Nagar VR, Nickerson R, Sloan PA. Hypogonadism associated with long-term opioid therapy: a systematic review. *J Opioid Manag.* 2015; 11: 255–278.

146. Abs R, Verhelst J, Maeyaert J, et al. Endocrine consequences of long-term intrathecal administration of opioids. *J Clin Endocrinol Metab.* 2000; 85: 2215–2222.

147. Daniell HW. Hypogonadism in men consuming sustained-action oral opioids. *J Pain.* 2002; 3: 377–384.

148. Daniell HW. DHEAS deficiency during consumption of sustained-action prescribed opioids: evidence for opioid-induced inhibition of adrenal androgen production. *J Pain.* 2006; 7: 901–907.

149. Daniell HW. Opioid endocrinopathy in women consuming prescribed sustained-action opioids for control of nonmalignant pain. *J Pain*. 2008; 9: 28–36.

150. McWilliams K, Simmons C, Laird BJ, Fallon MT. A systematic review of opioid effects on the hypo-gonadal axis of cancer patients. *Supportive Care Cancer*. 2014; 22: 1699–1704.

151. Bawor M, Bami H, Dennis BB, et al. Testosterone suppression in opioid users: a systematic review and meta-analysis. *Drug Alcohol Dependence*. 2015; 149: 1–9.

152. Bliesener N, Albrecht S, Schwager A, Weckbecker K, Lichtermann D, Klingmüller D. Plasma testos-terone and sexual function in men receiving buprenorphine maintenance for opioid dependence. *J Clin Endocrinol Metab*. 2005; 90: 203–206.

153. Guay A, Seftel AD, Traish A. Hypogonadism in men with erectile dysfunction may be related to a host of chronic illnesses. *Int J Impot Res*. 2010; 22: 9–19.

154. Coluzzi F, Pergolizzi J, Raffa RB, Mattia C. The unsolved case of bone-impairing analgesics: the endocrine effects of opioids on bone metabolism. *Therapeutics Clin risk Management*. 2015; 11: 515–523.

155. Buckeridge D, Huang A, Hanley J, et al. Risk of injury associated with opioid use in older adults. *J Am Geriatr Soc*. 2010; 58: 1664–1670.

156. Fortin JD, Bailey GM, Vilensky JA. Does opioid use for pain management warrant routine bone mass density screening in men? *Pain Physician*. 2008; 11: 539–541.

157. Gozashti MH, Mohammadzadeh E, Divsalar K, Shokoohi M. The effect of opium addiction on thyroid function tests. *J Diabetes Metab Disord*. 2014; 13: 5.

158. Tennant F. The physiologic effects of pain on the endocrine system. *Pain and Therapy*. 2013; 2: 75–86.

159. Brennan MJ. The effect of opioid therapy on endocrine function. *Am J Med*. 2013; 126: S12–S18.

160. Patel IB, Bairy KL, Bhat SN, Shetty DJ, Chogtu B, Esha R. Adverse drug reactions and cost effectiveness of non-steroidal anti-inflammatory drugs, muscle relaxants, and neurotropic drugs in patients with low back pain. *Int J Basic Clin Pharmacol*. 2015; 4: 273–277.

161. Gilron I, Bailey JM, Tu D, Holden RR, Weaver DF, Houlden RL. Morphine, gabapentin, or their combination for neuropathic pain. *N Engl J Med*. 2005; 352: 1324–1334.

162. Papathanasiou T, Juul RV, Heegaard AM, Kreilgaard M, Lund TM. Combination of morphine and gabapentin leads to synergistic effects in a rat model of postoperative pain. Danish Society for Pharmacology, 7th annual meeting, 2015.

163. Chen C, Upward J, Arumugham T, Stier B, Davy M. Gabapentin enacarbil and morphine administered in combination versus alone: a double-blind, randomized, pharmacokinetic, and tolerability comparison. *Clin Therapeutics*. 2015; 37: 349–357.

164. Kukkar A, Bali A, Singh N, Jaggi AS. Implications and mechanism of action of gabapentin in neuropathic pain. *Arch Pharmacol Res*. 2013; 36: 237–251.

165. Watanabe T, Tanigawa T, Nadatani Y, et al. Risk factors for severe nonsteroidal anti-inflammatory drug-induced small intestinal damage. *Digestive Liver Dis*. 2013; 45: 390–395.

166. Ungprasert R, Cheungpasitporn W, Crowson CS, Matteson EL. Individual non-steroidal anti-inflammatory drugs and risk of acute kidney injury: a systematic review and meta-analysis of observa-tional studies. *Eur J Intern Med*. 2015; 26: 285–291.

167. Brune K, Patrignani R. New insights into the use of currently available non-steroidal anti-inflammatory drugs. *J Pain Res*. 2015; 20: 105–118.

168. US Food and Drug Administration, available at: http://www.fda.gov/Drugs/DrugSafety/ucm239821.htm. Accessed January 19, 2016.

169. US Food and Drug Administration, available at: http://www.fda.gov/Drugs/DrugSafety/ucm239821.htm. Accessed January 19, 2016.

170. Lancaster EM, Hiatt JR, Zarrinpar A. Acetaminophen hepatotoxicity: an updated review. *Arch Toxicol*. 2015; 89: 193–199.

171. Hochberg MC, Altman RD, April KT, et al. American College of Rheumatology 2012 recommendations for the use of nonpharmacologic and pharmacologic therapies in osteoarthritis of the hand, hip, and knee. *Arthritis Care Res.* 2012; 64: 465–474.

172. Chou R. ACP Journal Club: acetaminophen reduces pain in hip or knee osteoarthritis by a small amount, but not low back pain. *Ann Intern Med.* 2015; 163: JC10.

173. Moore RA, Derry S, Wiffen PJ, Straube S, Aldington DJ. Overview review: comparative efficacy of oral ibuprofen and paracetamol (acetaminophen) across acute and chronic pain conditions. *Eur J Pain.* 2015; 19: 1213–1223.

174. Chibnall JT, Tait RC, Harman B, Luebbert RA. Effect of acetaminophen on behavior, well-being, and psychotropic medication use in nursing home residents with moderate-to-severe dementia. *J Am Geriatr Soc.* 2005; 53: 1921–1929.

175. Alvarez CA, Mortensen EM, Makris UE, et al. Association of skeletal muscle relaxers and antihistamines on mortality, hospitalizations, and emergency department visits in elderly patients: a nationwide retrospective cohort study. *BMC Geriatr.* 2015; 15: 2.

176. American Geriatrics Society Expert Panel. American Geriatrics Society updated Beers Criteria for potentially inappropriate medication use in older adults. *J Am Geriatr Soc.* 2012; 60(4): 616–631.

177. Richards BL, Whittle SL, Buchbinder R. Muscle relaxants for pain management in rheumatoid arthritis. *Cochrane Database of Systematic Reviews* 2012, Issue 1. Art. No.: CD008922. DOI: 10.1002/14651858. CD008922.pub2.

178. Kurko TA, Saastamoinen LK, Tähkäpää S, et al. Long-term use of benzodiazepines: definitions, prevalence and usage patterns—a systematic review of register-based studies. *Eur Psychiatry.* 2015; 30: 1037–1047.

179. Dell'Osso B, Lader M. Do benzodiazepines still deserve a major role in the treatment of psychiatric disorders? A critical reappraisal. *Eur Psychiatry.* 2013; 28: 7–20.

180. Merskey H, Bogduk H, eds. *Classification of Chronic Pain: Descriptions of Chronic Pain Syndromes and Definitions of Pain Terms.* 2nd ed. Seattle, WA: IASP Press; 1994.

181. Goesling J, Clauw DJ, Hassett AL. Pain and depression: an integrative review of neurobiological and psychological factors. *Curr Psychiatry Rep.* 2013; 15: 1–8.

182. Bryson HM, Wilde MI. Amitriptyline. *Drugs Aging.* 1996; 8: 459–476.

183. Attal N, Cruccua G, Haanpaa M, et al. EFNS guidelines on pharmacological treatment of neuropathic pain. *Eur J Neurol.* 2006; 13: 1153–1169.

184. Wong K, Phelan R, Kalso E, Raja S, Gilron I. Antidepressant drugs for prevention of acute and chronic postsurgical pain. *Anesthesiology.* 2014; 121: 591.

185. Schatman ME. Medical marijuana and neuromysticism: the data spell the beginning of the end. *Painview.* 2015; 11: 24–25.

186. Schatman ME. Medical marijuana: the state of the science. http://www.topsfield-ma.gov/health/documents/MedicalMarijuana-TheScience.pdf. Accessed December 27. 2015.

187. Khorsan R, Coulter ID, Crawford C, Hsiao AF. Systematic review of integrative health care research: randomized control trials, clinical controlled trials, and meta-analysis. *Evid Based Complement Altern Med.* 2010; 2011: 1–10.

CHAPTER 6

AN OVERVIEW OF THE ABUSE POTENTIAL OF NONOPIOIDS

Sedatives, Hypnotics, and Stimulants

Christopher M. Herndon and Kelly N. Gable

INTRODUCTION

Use of substances for their sedative and anesthetic properties by humans dates back as far as 4500 BC. Opium and alcohol, as well as related tinctures and herbals, are referenced for their calming effects and ability to induce sleep.[1–3] Perhaps the oldest recorded texts reporting the pain-relieving and sedative effects of medicinals are the papyri of ancient Egypt.[4] It is here we learn of the use of *Papaver somniferum* (opium poppy), belladonna, and thyme.[4] Caffeine is likely the first stimulant used by humans. Caffeine-laden tea was used in China as early as the Shang dynasty. Cocoa (cacao) trees were cultivated by the Mayans as early as 1000 BC, and coffee bean consumption by Ethiopians is reported as early as the ninth century.[4] Along with the pertinent medical uses of these agents, references to their recreational benefit may give us a glimpse into our ancestors' first illicit medication use and substance use disorders.

The public health problem of nonmedical use of pharmaceuticals is growing at an alarming rate.[5,6] Data from the 2010 Drug Abuse Warning Network (DAWN, Center for Behavioral Health Statistics and Quality, no longer active) suggest that 1,173,654 unique emergency department (ED) visits were attributed to the nonmedical use of pharmaceuticals, representing approximately 25% of all drug-related ED visits nationwide.[7,8] This database established that while opioid analgesics were the most frequently cited drugs involved in ED presentation, cocaine, benzodiazepines (namely alprazolam), nonbenzodiazepine sedatives (zolpidem), stimulants (amphetamine derivatives, methylphenidate, cocaine), and centrally acting skeletal muscle relaxants (carisoprodol, cyclobenzaprine) also showed concerning increases in patterns of use. Most concerning is the preponderance of unique ED visits attributed to the misuse of multiple agents (typically opioids and benzodiazepines) and the associated morbidity and mortality.[7]

Today, numerous pharmacologic classes exist that fall under the broad classifications of sedative-hypnotics and stimulants. Medical indications for such agents include anxiety spectrum disorders; epilepsy; attention-deficit/hyperactivity disorder (ADHD); and narcolepsy, insomnia, and other sleep disorders. While the actual pharmacologic properties and chemical structures of these drugs can differ significantly, broad categorization for the purposes of this chapter will focus on central nervous system (CNS) depressants, CNS stimulants, and hallucinogens. Access to sedative-hypnotics and stimulants is widespread. Diversion occurs most commonly via friends and relatives with leftover prescriptions versus pharmacy theft or negligent prescribers.[9,10] However, the quantity of doses of these substances manufactured and prescribed should not be discounted. Units of methylphenidate sold in the United States almost doubled from the second quarter of 2012 to the second quarter of 2013.[11] Similarly, amphetamine/dextroamphetamine prescriptions increased by almost 50%.[12] Persons seeking to abuse commercially available pharmaceuticals frequently alter the dosage form to administer via inhalation, insufflation, injection, and even rectal administration to maximize the CNS effects of the drug.[7] Despite establishing controlled substance classifications to curb misuse and diversion of drugs, often the research conducted to assess the "addiction potential" or likeability of substances by abusers is performed using intact dosage forms, administered in the typical fashion (i.e., orally).[13]

REVIEW OF CNS PHARMACOLOGY

Psychoactive medications exert their effects almost entirely by impacting one of the following neurotransmitters: dopamine, norepinephrine, or serotonin. Drugs that enter the CNS often have powerful effects on mood, thinking, sensation, and behavior.[14] Dopamine, known as the pleasure-producing neurotransmitter,[15] is released naturally when we engage in pleasurable activities such as eating a meal, smoking a cigarette, or having sex. Dopamine-enhancing drugs can lead to increased feelings of pleasure, clearer thinking, and increased motivation. If dopamine is produced in excess, however, especially related to the misuse or overuse of specific drugs, it can lead to the development of disorganized and psychotic thinking, such as hearing voices and paranoia.[16,17] Norepinephrine is known as a stress hormone and a neurotransmitter that increases during times of fear. It affects the parts of the brain that control attention and focus.[18] Drug-induced increases in norepinephrine can also lead to an increase in blood pressure and pulse. Finally, serotonin is a neurotransmitter responsible for feelings of happiness and well-being. It is produced naturally and also synthesized directly from our diet (tryptophan) and from serotonin-enhancing drugs, such as antidepressants like fluoxetine.[19]

SEDATIVE-HYPNOTICS

The general classification of sedative-hypnotics encompasses several drug classes based on their general CNS depressant effects (Table 6.1). While several of these drug classes may not typically be referred to as sedative-hypnotics in their pharmacologic properties, for the purposes of this chapter they will be reviewed as such. Numerous prescription pharmaceuticals may cause sedation either by pharmacodynamic design or when used outside of typically prescribed parameters. These drug classes include benzodiazepines, barbiturates, nonbenzodiazepine sedatives, select antipsychotics, and select anticonvulsants. Misuse, abuse, and diversion have been reported in the literature for various medications from all of these classes, with benzodiazepines being the most prevalent.[20]

BENZODIAZEPINES

The benzodiazepines are a diverse class of medications with a wide variance for abuse potential (see Table 6.1). These agents exert their pharmacologic effect via potentiating gamma-aminobutyric acid (GABA), the primary inhibitory neurotransmitter in the CNS.[21] While numerous subtypes of the $GABA_A$ receptor exist, benzodiazepines are relatively nonselective and may bind to many of these receptor subtypes. Benzodiazepines are used clinically for the treatment of anxiety, panic disorder, alcohol abstinence syndromes (delirium tremens), insomnia, and refractory seizure disorders; they are used rarely as skeletal muscle relaxants.[22,23]

The abuse potential for benzodiazepines varies significantly based on the pharmacokinetics of the respective drug. As with most substances of abuse, the "desirability" of an individual substance largely depends on the speed in which it reaches maximum concentration within the CNS. Medications that reach peak CNS drug concentrations most quickly are usually the most popular for nonmedical use. Likely the most popular benzodiazepine of abuse is alprazolam (Xanax), a drug with an incredibly short time to peak CNS concentrations. Other common medications within this class with reported increased misuse potential include lorazepam (Ativan), triazolam (Halcion), and diazepam (Valium).[20]

Benzodiazepines are also used to enhance the euphoria and nonmedical effects of other substances of abuse.[23] Reports of heightened and prolonged euphoria when benzodiazepines are used concurrently with opioids and cocaine are common on drug abuse websites and blogs. Abusers of benzodiazepines report heightened euphoria when using nonmedically approved administration techniques. The most frequently reported methods include inhalation (smoking), insufflation (snorting), and lacing other illicit drugs with pulverized benzodiazepine tablets.[24]

There are numerous risks with frequent and ongoing abuse of benzodiazepines. All medications within this class are respiratory depressants, so there is a significant risk of mortality when overdose occurs. This risk of respiratory failure is greatly increased when these agents are used concurrently with other CNS/respiratory depressants such as opioids. Persons who are obese or have obstructive or central sleep apnea are more prone to negative consequences when using benzodiazepines for nonmedical purposes. Abrupt

TABLE 6.1 Representative sedative-hypnotic pharmaceuticals of abuse, desired nonmedical effects, aliases, and estimated street value

Drug	Nonmedical Effects	Alias*	Estimated Street Value (USD)* and Availability
Alprazolam	Sedation, anxiolysis, euphoria, assist with "coming down" from stimulants, enhance euphoria from other substances of abuse	Xanax, Xanbars, Handlebars, Z-bars, Totem poles, Footballs, Upjohns, School bus, Yellow boys, Planks, others	$2–$3 per 1.0 mg
Diazepam	Sedation, anxiolysis, euphoria, assist with "coming down" from stimulants, enhance euphoria from other substances of abuse	Valium, V, Downers, Foofoo, Howards, Tranks, Tags, Yellows, Blues, Flower Power, Valley Girl, Vallies, Scooby Doos, Scoobs, Valtoids	$0.50–$1 per 1.0 mg
Clonazepam	Sedation, anxiolysis, euphoria, assist with "coming down" from stimulants, enhance euphoria from other substances of abuse	Klonipin, KPin, K, Pin, Super Valium, K-cut	$0.50–$ per 1.0 mg
Phenobarbital	Sedation, anxiolysis, euphoria, assist with "coming down" from stimulants, enhance euphoria from other substances of abuse	Luminal, Purple hearts, goof balls	No information found on nonprescription cost. Commercially available in 15-mg, 16.2-mg, 30-mg, 32.4-mg, 60-mg, and 100-mg tablets.
Secobarbital	Sedation, anxiolysis, euphoria, assist with "coming down" from stimulants, enhance euphoria from other substances of abuse	Seconal, Reds, Red Birds, Red Devils, Lillys, F-40s, Pinks, Pink Ladies, Seggy	No information found on nonprescription cost. Commercially available in 100-mg capsules.
Butalbital	Sedation, anxiolysis, euphoria, assist with "coming down" from stimulants, enhance euphoria from other substances of abuse	Fioricet, Fiorinal	No information found on nonprescription cost. Commercially available in combination with either aspirin or acetaminophen and caffeine with 50-mg butalbital tablets.
Carisoprodol	Sedation, anxiolysis, euphoria, assist with "coming down" from stimulants, enhance euphoria from other substances of abuse	Soma, D's, Dance, Las Vegas Cocktail (with hydrocodone), Soma Coma	No information found on nonprescription cost. Commercially available in 250-mg and 350-mg tablets.

*Aliases and street values obtained from numerous blogs and discussion boards for persons seeking to abuse substances. The accuracy of aliases and street values cannot be confirmed.

discontinuation of benzodiazepines by persons frequently abusing these agents may precipitate seizures.[25,26]

Interpretation of urine drug screens when assessing for benzodiazepine use may be confusing if additional information is not provided with the laboratory report (see Chapter 11). Many of the frequently used/abused benzodiazepines are metabolized to active metabolites, and confusion can ensue during review when these are listed on the report. Diazepam is metabolized to numerous active and inactive metabolites, including temazepam and oxazepam, so the presence of these two substances should be expected in patients who are using diazepam. While detection time varies depending on the drug, generally benzodiazepines and their metabolites may be expected in the urine for 2 to 3 days following the last dose.[27,28]

NONBENZODIAZEPINE SEDATIVES

The nonbenzodiazepine sedatives are a diverse group of medications that are frequently prescribed for insomnia and anxiety (see Table 6.1). These include zolpidem (Ambien), eszopiclone (Lunesta), zaleplon (Sonata), and buspirone (BuSpar). Zolpidem, eszopiclone, and zaleplon interact with GABA receptors without fully binding these sites, in contrast to the benzodiazepines, and are prescribed medically for insomnia. Due to this mechanism of action, the abuse potential for these agents is relatively low, as is the risk for respiratory depressant effects. Dependence can occur with continued use of these agents, however. Buspirone, a nonbenzodiazepine anxiolytic, is pharmacologically distinct and exerts its mechanism of action by stimulating multiple serotonin receptors. Buspirone is frequently prescribed for anxiety when practitioners seek to avoid benzodiazepines in patients at elevated risk for misuse.[29–31]

All of these agents have relatively low abuse potential and reportedly low nonprescription value. A cursory review of some of the more prominent drug abuse discussion boards did reveal reports of adulteration of these agents, with varying reported effects.[24]

BARBITURATES

The barbiturates are a distinct class of medications that have a multitude of medical indications (see Table 6.1).[32] Many of the barbiturates are now only available parenterally and are largely reserved for procedure-related anesthesia and sedation. These medications exert their pharmacologic effect via the GABA receptor, similar to the benzodiazepines. While abuse of these agents has largely diminished due to the availability of more popular agents and decreased use in routine medical practice, a nonprescription market for these drugs continues to exist. The most commonly misused pharmaceuticals within this class include butalbital-containing products (Fioricet, Fiorinal), secobarbital (Seconal), and carisoprodol (Soma).[32–34] Carisoprodol is not a barbiturate by class, but it is metabolized to meprobamate and does have a high propensity for misuse.[34] While originally marketed as a nonaddicting skeletal muscle relaxant, carisoprodol has been reclassified as a controlled substance in the Federal Controlled Substance Act.[34–37] Websites discussing methods for abusing this agent suggest significant euphoria in doses between 750 and 1,000 mg.[24]

These medications do not have a significant nonprescription value, with the exception of carisoprodol. Reports of aberrant use include inhalation, insufflation, and lacing other substances of abuse with these agents.[24] Carisoprodol is commonly used in combination with opioids, which reportedly enhances euphoria. While less frequently cited, butalbital-containing products are also used with other substances of abuse to either counteract untoward effects or enhance euphoria.[38] Abrupt discontinuation of these agents in chronic users may result in seizures, and a medically supervised wean may be performed when necessary.

ANTIPSYCHOTICS

Until recently there were few reports of misuse, abuse, and diversion of the antipsychotics, but with the introduction of quetiapine (Seroquel), reports of its aberrant use have begun to surface.[24,39,40] Quetiapine is prescribed medically for schizophrenia, bipolar disorder, and refractory depression and is occasionally prescribed for insomnia. Like others in its class, quetiapine has an array of pharmacologic activities, including dopamine, serotonin, histamine, and alpha-receptor antagonism.[41] It has been proposed that these mechanisms make quetiapine an attractive adjuvant to other substances of abuse to enhance euphoria and attenuate the negative symptoms of "coming down," namely from cocaine or methamphetamine use.[39] Abusers report that crushing the tablets and snorting the powder produces an effect similar to that of small quantities of cocaine.[24] Off-label prescribing of this medication for the treatment of cravings has blossomed, but the inherent street value of quetiapine makes this a potentially troublesome proposition.[42]

ANTICONVULSANTS

Few reports of misuse of anticonvulsants appeared prior to the appearance of pregabalin (Lyrica).[43–45] Pregabalin, as well as its predecessor gabapentin, exerts its pharmacologic activity primarily by inhibiting a specific subtype of voltage-sensitive neuronal calcium channels.[46] At higher doses, both of these agents may modulate other neurotransmitter pathways, which may lead to the euphoric and hallucinogenic effects described by abusers. Reports of an opioid-like "high" have been described with large single doses of pregabalin.[24] Owing to its potential for abuse, even at medically prescribed doses, pregabalin is a controlled substance in the United States.[47] Aside from its potentially euphoric effects, pregabalin has also been reported to alleviate the withdrawal symptoms of both opioids and methamphetamine.[48]

Unlike pregabalin, gabapentin is relatively difficult to abuse without adulterating the dosage formulation because of its saturable active transport kinetics.[49] When taken orally, gabapentin is not absorbed in doses larger than 1,200 mg. Reports of gabapentin abuse predominantly involve removing the active medication from capsules and snorting the drug, thus bypassing the limited oral absorption phenomenon.[24,48] Abusers of gabapentin report euphoria and antianxiety properties as well as alleviation of symptoms associated with post-cocaine and methamphetamine dysphoria.[24,48] Currently gabapentin has a relatively negligible nonprescription resale value, likely due to the wide availability and noncontrolled status of the drug. In contrast, inmates have found gabapentin to be a recreational drug of choice and the value of this drug in prisons has skyrocketed.[50] Numerous prison systems have now either taken gabapentin off their medication formulary or reassigned it as a pseudo-controlled substance.

STIMULANTS

Drugs of abuse that result in CNS stimulation are a diverse group of agents with numerous pharmacologic mechanisms of action (Table 6.2). Cocaine, arguably the most commonly abused stimulant, is largely considered an illicit substance versus a pharmaceutical, although there are medical applications (local anesthetic for ophthalmic and nasal surgical procedures) for this compound, which warrants its discussion.[51] Cocaine is a potent neurostimulant with numerous pharmacologic activities.[52,53] It exerts its stimulant effects by inhibiting dopamine transport, thus increasing levels of this neurotransmitter in neuronal synapses. Cocaine is also active at a multitude of serotonin receptor sites, likely explaining its mood-elevating effects.[54] Cocaine is typically administered by mouth (rubbing the powder on the oral mucosa), insufflation, injection, and inhalation via smoking.[24] It is frequently used in conjunction with other substances of abuse to counteract untoward depressant effects while maintaining euphoria. Pharmaceutical stimulants are quickly replacing cocaine as a substance of choice given their relatively low cost, high potency, and perceived lower addiction potential.[55,56] While most pharmaceutical stimulants are amphetamine-like derivatives, other non–amphetamine-based drugs exist with varying risk for abuse.[57]

AMPHETAMINE DERIVATIVES AND METHYLPHENIDATE

Psychostimulants such as amphetamine and methylphenidate increase the release of dopamine and norepinephrine while also inhibiting the breakdown of these neurotransmitters (see Table 6.2). Amphetamine was synthesized in 1887 in Germany, and its stimulating effects were discovered in the early 1930s.[58] Amphetamine derivatives include dextroamphetamine/amphetamine mixed salts (Adderall), dextroamphetamine (Dexedrine), and lisdexamfetamine (Vyvanse).[59] Lisdexamfetamine is a prodrug designed to have less abuse potential than other amphetamines because it is not converted to its active form if it is inhaled or injected.[60] Methylphenidate products are the most widely prescribed stimulants for the treatment of ADHD, primarily targeting symptoms of inattention, hyperactivity, and impulsivity. Methylphenidate is considered to be a more potent stimulant than mixed amphetamine salts.[58] It has numerous trade names with varying release technologies and delivery routes, including Methylin, Ritalin, Concerta, Metadate, Focalin, and Daytrana. The onset of effects of psychostimulants is typically less than 1 hour.[58] Because of this quick onset of action, there is a higher abuse potential among college students using stimulants to improve study quality. Stimulants are often crushed and snorted in an effort to obtain a quick effect and potential euphoric rush.

TABLE 6.2 Representative pharmaceuticals of abuse with stimulant properties, desired nonmedical effects, aliases, and estimated street value

Drug	Desired Nonmedical Effects	Aliases*	Estimated Street Value (USD)* and Availability
Cocaine	Euphoria, enhanced sensation, enhanced cognition, increased energy	Big Flake, Crack, Icing, Line, Pearl, Snow White, Sleigh Ride, Snowcones, California Cornflakes, Foo Foo Dust, Girlfriend, Nose Candy, Nose Gin, Nose Powder, C, Coconut, Cola	$0.16 per 1.0 mg (usually purchased in "grams")
Lisdexamfetamine	Euphoria, concentration, energy	Vyvanse, V	$0.14–$0.20 per 1.0 mg for 70-mg tablets. Lower-strength tablets have negligible value. Commercially available in 20-mg, 30-mg, 40-mg, 50-mg, 60-mg, and 70-mg capsules.
Dextroamphetamine	Euphoria, concentration, energy	Dexedrine, ProCentral, Copilots, Go-pills, Pep-pills, Speed, Uppers	$0.50 per 1.0 mg. Commercially available in 5-mg, 10-mg. and 15-mg capsules (extended-release and sustained-release) and 1 mg/1 mL oral solution.
Dextroamphetamine and amphetamine salts	Euphoria, concentration, energy, enhancement of euphoria from other substances of abuse (opioids)	Adderall, Adderall XR, Ralls, Bennies, Amps, A-bombs, The A Train, Beans, Black Beauties, Dexies	$0.10 per 1.0 mg. Commercially available in dextroamphetamine and amphetamine mixed salts: 5 mg/1.25 mg, 10 mg/2.5 mg, 12.5 mg/3.125 mg, 15 mg/3.75 mg, 20 mg/5 mg, 25 mg/6.25 mg, and 30 mg/7.5 mg tablets and capsules, immediate-release and extended-release.

(Continued)

TABLE 6.2 Continued

Drug	Desired Nonmedical Effects	Aliases*	Estimated Street Value (USD)* and Availability
Methylphenidate	Euphoria, concentration, energy, enhancement of euphoria from other substances of abuse (opioids)	Ritalin, Concerta, Metadate, Methylin, Quillivant, Daytrana, Johnny, Pineapple, Mind Candy, Vitamin R, Rin Tin Tin, Loose Cannon, Bennies, Rits, West Coast, Truck Drivers	$0.30 per 1.0 mg. Commercially available in tablets (5, 10, 20 mg), chewable tablets (2.5, 5, 10 mg), extended-release tablets (10, 20, 30, 40, 50, 60 mg), powder for suspension, and transdermal patches.
Phentermine	Limited euphoria, energy, wakefulness, decreased appetite, counteract other substances of abuse (alcohol and opioids)	Adipex-P, Suprenza; no other aliases found although numerous reports of dosage-form alteration for abuse	$0.05 per 1.0 mg for 37.5-mg tablets or capsules. Commercially available in 15-mg, 30-mg, and 37.5-mg capsules, tablets, disintegrating tablets.
Diethylpropion	Limited euphoria, energy, wakefulness, decreased appetite, counteract other substances of abuse (alcohol and opioids)	Tenuate; no other aliases found although numerous reports of dosage-form alteration for abuse	No information found on nonprescription cost. Commercially available in 25-mg immediate-release tablets and 75-mg controlled-release tablets.
Benzphetamine	Limited euphoria, energy, wakefulness, decreased appetite, counteract other substances of abuse (alcohol and opioids)	Didrex, Regimex, Upjohns	$0.05 per 1 mg. Commercially available in 25-mg and 50-mg tablets.
Phendimetrazine	Limited euphoria, energy, wakefulness, decreased appetite, counteract other substances of abuse (alcohol and opioids)	Bontril; no other aliases found although numerous reports of dosage-form alteration for abuse	No information found on nonprescription cost. Commercially available in 35-mg immediate-release tablets and 105-mg sustained-release capsules.
Modafinil	Wakefulness, creativity, counteract other substances of abuse (alcohol and opioids)	Provigil, Alertec, Brain Viagra	$0.05 per 1.0 mg for 200-mg tablets. Commercially available as 100-mg and 200-mg tablets.

TABLE 6.2 Continued

Drug	Desired Nonmedical Effects	Aliases*	Estimated Street Value (USD)* and Availability
Armodafinil	Wakefulness, creativity, counteract other substances of abuse (alcohol and opioids)	Nuvigil; no other aliases found although numerous reports of dosage-form alteration for abuse	No information found on nonprescription cost. Commercially available in 50-mg, 150-mg, and 250-mg tablets.
Bupropion	Wakefulness, alleviate "coming down" effects of other stimulants, hallucinations at higher doses	Wellbutrin, Zyban, Budeprion SR, Aplenzin, Forfivo, Bupraban; no other aliases found although numerous reports of dosage-form alteration for abuse	No information found on nonprescription cost. Commercially available in 75-mg and 100-mg immediate-release tablets. Modified-release tablets are less desirable for abuse.

*Aliases and street values obtained from numerous blogs and discussion boards for persons seeking to abuse substances. The accuracy of aliases and street values cannot be confirmed.

Prior to the widespread availability of these more potent stimulants, appetite suppressants were used recreationally. Phentermine (Adipex-P, Qsymia with topiramate), benzphetamine (Didrex), diethypropion, and phendimetrazine (Bontril) have all been reported to possess abuse liability, but they have largely fallen out of favor due to the limited access to these medications and their comparatively lower potency compared to methylphenidate and mixed amphetamine salts.[61]

Pseudoephedrine is a sympathomimetic that is present as a naturally occurring alkaloid in plant species *Ephedra* (*ma huang*).[62] Structurally similar to amphetamine, pseudoephedrine possesses indirect noradrenergic agonist activity, as well as acting as a weak centrally acting stimulant. The principal medical use of pseudoephedrine is as a nasal decongestant; it is less frequently used as a mild antitussive. The abuse potential of unaltered pseudoephedrine is relatively low, although reports exist of students using high doses to self-medicate for AHDH symptoms. More concerning is the use of pseudoephedrine in the manufacture of illicit methamphetamine.[63] Due to the widespread use of large quantities of pseudoephedrine for this purpose, many governments have imposed strict monitoring and distribution processes to limit nonmedical use.[64,65] Even in areas that have not implemented such regulations, most pharmacy retailers have enacted policies to curb abusers from obtaining and diverting pseudoephedrine.

Modafinil (Provigil) and armodafinil (Nuvigil) are used medically to promote wakefulness in those with narcolepsy, sleep apnea, and shift work sleep disorder.[66,67] These agents have also been studied for opioid-induced somnolence. While it is unclear if they are truly problematic as substances of abuse, they do possess neuropharmacologic mechanisms that alleviate the dysphoric effects of "coming down" from methamphetamine. Methamphetamine users report on chat rooms that using these medications also helps with the cravings associated with methamphetamine withdrawal.[68–70] Traditionally modafinil and armodafinil were considered of low abuse potential and safer than their amphetamine and methylphenidate counterparts.[66,67] However, recent research points to changes in nigrostriatal dopamine transporter expression very similar to those seen with the amphetamine derivatives and methylphenidate. The website hosting forums for substance abusers, Bluelight, provides a glimpse into the relative abuse potential of these agents, with largely negative "reviews" from active users from a euphoria standpoint.[24]

OTHER/HALLUCINOGENS

Other medications with variable abuse potential include the cannabinoids nabilone (Cesamet) and dronabinol (Marinol) (Table 6.3). Dronabinol contains tetrahydrocannabinol (THC), whereas nabilone is a structurally similar analog that binds to the same receptor sites.[71,72] Dronabinol intake will result in positive cannabis screens on immunoassay-based urine and saliva drug screens,[73] but nabilone will not. While the use of cannabis as a recreational drug is discussed in detail elsewhere in this text, these two pharmaceuticals deserve specific mention here. There are few data regarding the abuse liability of these two agents, although anecdotal reports point to general disappointment in these two agents for recreational use among those who frequently use cannabis and other illicit substances.[74,75]

Ketamine, also known as "special K" by its abusers, was developed in the late 1960s as a derivative and theoretically safer anesthetic compared to its predecessor, phencyclidine (PCP).[76–78] This agent today is regaining popularity medically as an adjunctive inductive anesthetic, as an analgesic, for the treatment of some psychiatric disorders (i.e., treatment-resistant depression), and for pediatric conscious procedural sedation.[77] Its use medically is largely precluded by intense psychomimetic adverse effects, including vivid (often unpleasant) dreams and hallucinations.[77] These untoward effects are frequently prevented medically by co-administration with a benzodiazepine. Chronic recreational users of ketamine report intense euphoria and "out-of-body experiences" when taken concurrently with substances such as opioids and alprazolam.[79] The relative street value of ketamine, and thus its potential for diversion, is especially high compared to other medications discussed in this chapter.[79] Ketamine is available commercially as a parenteral compound, largely limited to use in hospitals and veterinary clinics, which limits prescribing directly to patients unless compounded for oral administration by specialty pharmacies.

CONCLUSIONS

The gradual conversion from so-called street drugs to pharmaceuticals as substances of choice among drug abusers has created a significant public health problem worldwide. Many of these substances are more potent than traditionally abused substances. Equally

Representative pharmaceuticals of abuse with hallucinogenic or other nonsedative, nonstimulant properties, desired nonmedical effects, aliases, and estimated street value

Drug	Desired Non-medical Effects	Aliases*	Estimated Street Value (USD)* and Availability*
Gabapentin	Euphoria, hallucinations, substance of abuse cravings, sedation	Neurontin, Horizant, Gralise, Quell, Gabs	No information found on nonprescription costs. Commercially available in 100-mg, 300-mg, 400-mg, 600-mg, and 800-mg tablets and capsules, both immediate- and controlled-release.
Ketamine	Hallucinations, dissociation, euphoria	Ketalar, K, Kitty, Ket, Special K, Super K, K2, Vitamin K, Jet, Blind Squid, Keller, Liquid K, Bump, Honey oil, Calvin Klein, Cat Valium, CK1 (mixed with cocaine), others	$0.10 per 1 mg (usually purchased in grams). Commercially available in 10 mg/mL, 50 mg/mL, and 100 mg/mL solution for injection.
Nabilone	Euphoria, enhanced effects of cannabis and other substances of abuse, vivid dreams	Cesamet, PMS-Nabilone, Blue and Whites	No information found on nonprescription costs. Commercially available in 1-mg oral capsules. Posted reports describe doses of 5–7 mg to achieve desired nonmedical effects.
Dronabinol	Euphoria, enhanced effects of cannabis and other substances of abuse, analgesia, anxiolysis	Marinol; no other aliases found. Active drug is suspended in sesame oil, limiting alteration of dosage form.	No information found on nonprescription costs. Commercially available in 2.5-mg, 5-mg, and 10-mg oral capsules.
Quetiapine	Euphoria, enhanced effects of stimulants and hallucinogens (cocaine and cannabis), alleviate "coming down" effects of substances of abuse, sedation	Seroquel, Squirrels, Suzie Q, Quells, Rosemary's Dolly, Q-ball (in combination with cocaine)	$5 per 400-mg tablet. No additional information for lower-strength formulations. Commercially available in 25-mg, 50-mg, 100-mg, 200-mg, 300-mg, and 400-mg immediate-release and extended-release tablets.

*Aliases and street values obtained from numerous blogs and discussion boards for persons seeking to abuse substances. The accuracy of aliases and street values cannot be confirmed.

concerning is the widely held misperception that these agents are safer for abuse given the lack of adulterants, the medical utility by prescription, and their availability, often with little to no money out of pocket, when diseases warranting their use are feigned.[80] The prevention of abuse of the prescription sedative-hypnotics and hallucinogens is fraught with difficulties given that many of the disorders these agents are used to treat are often not easy to diagnose objectively, so clinicians may be forced to rely on the patient's report of symptoms. Judicious prescribing, as well prescriber and law enforcement education, is paramount to curb the abuse of these substances and prevent their associated morbidity and mortality.

REFERENCES

1. Fields A, Tararin PA. Opium in China. *Br J Addict Alcohol Other Drugs*. 1970;64:371–382.

2. Hamarneh S. Pharmacy in medieval Islam and the history of drug addiction. *Med Hist*. 1972;16:226–237.

3. Kririkos PG, Papadaki S. A history of opium in antiquity. *J Am Pharm Assoc*. 1968;8:446–447.

4. Griffith FL. A medical papyrus from Egypt. *Br Med J*. 1893;1(1692):1172–1174.

5. Pade PA, Cardon KE, Hoffman RM, Geppert CM. Prescription opioid abuse, chronic pain, and primary care: a co-occurring disorders clinic in the chronic disease model. *J Subst Abuse Treat*. 2012;43:446–450.

6. Sweeney CT, Sembower MA, Ertischek MD, Shiffman S, Schnoll SH. Nonmedical use of prescription ADHD stimulants and preexisting patterns of drug abuse. *J Addict Dis*. 2013;32:1–10.

7. Cai R, Crane E, Poneleit K, Paulozzi L. Emergency department visits involving nonmedical use of selected prescription drugs in the United States, 2004–2008. *J Pain Palliat Care Pharmacother*. 2010;24:293–297.

8. Davis JM, Severtson SG, Bucher-Bartelson B, Dart RC. Using poison center exposure calls to predict prescription opioid abuse and misuse-related emergency department visits. *Pharmacoepidemiol Drug Saf*. 2013.

9. McCabe SE, West BT, Boyd CJ. Leftover prescription opioids and nonmedical use among high school seniors: a multi-cohort national study. *J Adolesc Health*. 2013;52(4):480–485.

10. Nordmann S, Pradel V, Lapeyre-Mestre M, et al. Doctor shopping reveals geographical variations in opioid abuse. *Pain Physician*. 2013;16:89–100.

11. Methylphenidate sales data. 2013. Accessed May 22, 2017.

12. Amphetamine/dextroamphetamine sales data. 2013. Accessed May 22, 2017.

13. Wightman R, Perrone J, Portelli I, Nelson L. Likeability and abuse liability of commonly prescribed opioids. *J Med Toxicol*. 2012;8:335–340.

14. Wise RA, Bozarth MA. Brain mechanisms of drug reward and euphoria. *Psychiatr Med*. 1985;3(4):445–460.

15. Valenta JP, Job MO, Mangieri RA, Schier CJ, Howard EC, Gonzales RA. Mu-opioid receptors in the stimulation of mesolimbic dopamine activity by ethanol and morphine in Long-Evans rats: a delayed effect of ethanol. *Psychopharmacology (Berl)*. 2013;22):389–400.

16. Brody AL, Mandelkern MA, Olmstead RE, et al. Ventral striatal dopamine release in response to smoking a regular vs. a denicotinized cigarette. *Neuropsychopharmacology*. 2009;34:282–289.

17. Le Foll B, Guranda M, Wilson AA, et al. Elevation of dopamine induced by cigarette smoking: novel insights from a [C]-(+)-PHNO PET study in humans. *Neuropsychopharmacology*. 2014;39(2):415–424.

18. McCorry LK. Physiology of the autonomic nervous system. *Am J Pharmaceut Educ*. 2007;71:78.

19. Young SN. How to increase serotonin in the human brain without drugs. *J Psychiatry Neurosci*. 2007;32:394–399.

20. Reynolds M, Fulde G, Hendry T. Trends in benzodiazepine abuse: 2007–2011. *Emerg Med Australas.* 2013;25:199–200.

21. Ben-Ari Y, Gaiarsa JL, Tyzio R, Khazipov R. GABA: a pioneer transmitter that excites immature neurons and generates primitive oscillations. *Physiol Rev.* 2007;87:1215–1284.

22. Campo-Soria C, Chang Y, Weiss DS. Mechanism of action of benzodiazepines on GABAA receptors. *Br J Pharmacol.* 2006;148:984–990.

23. Wick JY. The history of benzodiazepines. *Consult Pharm.* 2013;28(9):538–548.

24. Bluelight. 2013. http://www.bluelight.ru. Accessed November 22, 2013.

25. Jedeikin R, Menutti D, Bruderman I, Hoffman S. Prolonged respiratory center depression after alcohol and benzodiazepines. *Chest.* 1985;87:262–264.

26. Murray MJ, DeRuyter ML, Harrison BA. Opioids and benzodiazepines. *Crit Care Clin.* 1995;11:849–873.

27. Moeller KE, Lee KC, Kissack JC. Urine drug screening: practical guide for clinicians. *Mayo Clin Proc.* 2008;83:66–76.

28. Standridge JB, Adams SM, Zotos AP. Urine drug screening: a valuable office procedure. *Am Fam Physician.* 2010;81:635–640.

29. Hsu WY, Chiu NY. Intravenous zolpidem injection in a zolpidem abuser. *Pharmacopsychiatry.* 2013;46:121–122.

30. Licata SC, Mashhoon Y, Maclean RR, Lukas SE. Modest abuse-related subjective effects of zolpidem in drug-naive volunteers. *Behav Pharmacol.* 2011;22:160–166.

31. Victorri-Vigneau C, Feuillet F, Wainstein L, et al. Pharmacoepidemiological characterisation of zolpidem and zopiclone usage. *Eur J Clin Pharmacol.* 2013;69:1965–1972.

32. Morgan WW. Abuse liability of barbiturates and other sedative-hypnotics. *Adv Alcohol Subst Abuse.* 1990;9:67–82.

33. Gonzalez LA, Gatch MB, Forster MJ, Dillon GH. Abuse potential of Soma: the GABA(A) receptor as a target. *Mol Cell Pharmacol.* 2009;1:180–186.

34. Reeves RR, Carter OS, Pinkofsky HB, Struve FA, Bennett DM. Carisoprodol (Soma): abuse potential and physician unawareness. *J Addict Dis.* 1999;18:51–56.

35. Fass JA. Carisoprodol legal status and patterns of abuse. *Ann Pharmacother.* 2010;44:1962–1967.

36. Reeves RR, Burke RS. Carisoprodol: abuse potential and withdrawal syndrome. *Curr Drug Abuse Rev.* 2010;3:33–38.

37. Reeves RR, Burke RS, Kose S. Carisoprodol: update on abuse potential and legal status. *South Med J.* 2012;105:619–623.

38. Evans RW, Baskin SM. Why do migraineurs abuse butalbital-containing combination analgesics? *Headache.* 2010;50:1194–1197.

39. Oyemade A. Seroquel misuse/abuse. *Psychiatry (Edgmont).* 2010;7:15.

40. Sansone RA, Sansone LA. Is Seroquel developing an illicit reputation for misuse/abuse? *Psychiatry (Edgmont).* 2010;7:13–16.

41. Goldstein JM. Quetiapine fumarate (Seroquel): a new atypical antipsychotic. *Drugs Today (Barc).* 1999;35:193–210.

42. Tarasoff G, Osti K. Black-market value of antipsychotics, antidepressants, and hypnotics in Las Vegas, Nevada. *Am J Psychiatry.* 2007;164:350.

43. Gahr M, Franke B, Freudenmann RW, Kolle MA, Schonfeldt-Lecuona C. Concerns about pregabalin: further experience with its potential of causing addictive behaviors. *J Addict Med.* 2013;7:147–149.

44. Grosshans M, Lemenager T, Vollmert C, et al. Pregabalin abuse among opiate addicted patients. *Eur J Clin Pharmacol.* 2013;69:2021–2025.

45. Papazisis G, Garyfallos G, Sardeli C, Kouvelas D. Pregabalin abuse after past substance-seeking behavior. *Int J Clin Pharmacol Ther*. 2013;51:441–442.

46. Cai K, Nanga RP, Lamprou L, et al. The impact of gabapentin administration on brain GABA and glutamate concentrations: a 7T (1)H-MRS study. *Neuropsychopharmacology*. 2012;37:2764–2771.

47. Drug Enforcement Administration, Department of Justice. Schedules of controlled substances: placement of pregabalin into schedule V. Final rule. *Federal Register*. 2005;70:43633.

48. Tay KH. Gabapentin and opioid craving. *Pain Med*. 2009;10:774.

49. Dickens D, Webb SD, Antonyuk S, et al. Transport of gabapentin by LAT1 (SLC7A5). *Biochem Pharmacol*. 2013;85:1672–1683.

50. Reccoppa L, Malcolm R, Ware M. Gabapentin abuse in inmates with prior history of cocaine dependence. *Am J Addict*. 2004;13:321–323.

51. Brain PF, Coward GA. A review of the history, actions, and legitimate uses of cocaine. *J Subst Abuse*. 1989;1:431–451.

52. Kuhar MJ, Jaworski JN, Hubert GW, Philpot KB, Dominguez G. Cocaine- and amphetamine-regulated transcript peptides play a role in drug abuse and are potential therapeutic targets. *AAPS J*. 2005;7:E259–265.

53. Picetti R, Schlussman SD, Zhou Y, et al. Addictions and stress: clues for cocaine pharmacotherapies. *Curr Pharm Des*. 2013;19:7065–7080.

54. Haile CN, Mahoney JJ, 3rd, Newton TF, De La Garza R, 2nd. Pharmacotherapeutics directed at deficiencies associated with cocaine dependence: focus on dopamine, norepinephrine and glutamate. *Pharmacol Ther*. 2012;134:260–277.

55. Cassidy TA, McNaughton EC, Varughese S, Russo L, Zulueta M, Butler SF. Nonmedical use of prescription ADHD stimulant medications among adults in a substance abuse treatment population: early findings from the NAVIPPRO Surveillance System. *J Atten Disord*. 2015;19(4):275–283.

56. Curran GM, Ounpraseuth ST, Allee E, Small J, Booth BM. Trajectories in use of substance abuse and mental health services among stimulant users in rural areas. *Psychiatr Serv*. 2011;62:1230–1232.

57. Dalsgaard S, Mortensen PB, Frydenberg M, Thomsen PH. ADHD, stimulant treatment in childhood and subsequent substance abuse in adulthood—A naturalistic long-term follow-up study. *Addict Behav*. 2014 39(1):325–328.

58. McCann UD, Ricaurte GA. Amphetamine (or amphetamine-like)-related disorders. In: BJ Sadock, VA Sadock, P Ruiz, eds. *Kaplan and Sadock's Comprehensive Textbook of Psychiatry*. Philadelphia, PA: Lippincott, Williams, & Wilkins; 2009:1288–1295.

59. Simmler LD, Rickli A, Schramm Y, Hoener MC, Liechti ME. Pharmacological profiles of aminoindanes, piperazines, and pipradrol derivatives. *Biochem Pharmacol*. 2014;88:237–244.

60. Coghill DR, Caballero B, Sorooshian S, Civil R. A systematic review of the safety of lisdexamfetamine dimesylate. *CNS Drugs*. 2014;28:497–511.

61. Bray GA. Use and abuse of appetite-suppressant drugs in the treatment of obesity. *Ann Intern Med*. 1993 119(7, Part 2):707–713.

62. Laccourreye O, Werner A, Giroud JP, Couloigner V, Bonfils P, Bondon-Guitton E. Benefits, limits and danger of ephedrine and pseudoephedrine as nasal decongestants. *Eur Ann Otorhinolaryngol Head Neck Dis*. 2015;132:31–34.

63. Mazerolle L, McGuffog I, Ferris J, Chamlin MB. Pharmaceutical sales of pseudoephedrine: the impact of electronic tracking systems on methamphetamine crime incidents. *Addiction*. 2017;112:468–474.

64. Brandenburg MA, Brown SJ, Arneson WL, Arneson DL. The association of pseudoephedrine sales restrictions on emergency department urine drug screen results in Oklahoma. *J Okla State Med Assoc*. 2007;100:436–439.

64. Hendrickson RG, Cloutier RL, Fu R. The association of controlling pseudoephedrine availability on methamphetamine-related emergency department visits. *Acad Emerg Med*. 2010;17:1216–1222.

65. Murty S, Sangiry SS. Pseudoephedrine laws in the US—are we doing enough? *Ann Pharmacother*. 2006;40:1213–1215.

66. Garnock-Jones KP, Dhillon S, Scott LJ. Armodafinil. *CNS Drugs*. 2009;23(9):793–803.

67. Ballon JS, Feifel D. A systematic review of modafinil: potential clinical uses and mechanisms of action. *J Clin Psychiatry*. 2006;67:554–566.

68. Anderson AL, Li SH, Biswas K, et al. Modafinil for the treatment of methamphetamine dependence. *Drug Alcohol Depend*. 2012;120:135–141.

69. Mereu M, Bonci A, Newman AH, Tanda G. The neurobiology of modafinil as an enhancer of cognitive performance and a potential treatment for substance use disorders. *Psychopharmacology (Berl)*. 2013;229:415–434.

70. Raineri M, Gonzalez B, Goitia B, et al. Modafinil abrogates methamphetamine-induced neuroinflammation and apoptotic effects in the mouse striatum. *PLoS One*. 2012;7(10):e46599.

71. Lemberger L, Rubin A, Wolen R, et al. Pharmacokinetics, metabolism and drug-abuse potential of nabilone. *Cancer Treat Rev*. 1982;9(Suppl B):17–23.

72. Ward A, Holmes B. Nabilone. A preliminary review of its pharmacological properties and therapeutic use. *Drugs*. 1985;30:127–144.

73. Kulig K. Interpretation of workplace tests for cannabinoids. *J Med Toxicol*. 2017;13(1):106–110.

74. Lile JA, Kelly TH, Hays LR. Separate and combined effects of the cannabinoid agonists nabilone and Delta(9)-THC in humans discriminating Delta(9)-THC. *Drug Alcohol Depend*. 2011;116:86–92.

75. Ware MA, St Arnaud-Trempe E. The abuse potential of the synthetic cannabinoid nabilone. *Addiction*. 2010;105(3):494–503.

76. Bokor G, Anderson PD. Ketamine: an update on its abuse. *J Pharm Practice*. 2014;27:582–586.

77. Xu J, Lei H. Ketamine: an update on its clinical uses and abuses. *CNS Neurosci Therapeutics*. 2014;20:1015–1020.

78. Corazza O, Assi S, Schifano F. From "Special K" to "Special M": the evolution of the recreational use of ketamine and methoxetamine. *CNS Neurosci Therapeutics*. 2013;19:454–460.

79. Sassano-Higgins S, Baron D, Juarez G, Esmaili N, Gold M. A review of ketamine abuse and diversion. *Depression Anxiety*. 2016;33:718–727.

80. National Institute of Drug Abuse. https://www.drugabuse.gov/publications/drugfacts/prescription-over-counter-medications. Accessed May 22, 2017.

CHAPTER 7

PSYCHIATRY AND CHRONIC PAIN

An Associative Connection

Hani Raoul Khouzam

INTRODUCTION

Pain is considered a major global health problem affecting between 3% and 19% of the world's population.[1,2] Furthermore, chronic pain is one of the most reported complaints in the general medical setting, and its economic, psychological, social, and spiritual consequences make it one of the most common reasons for permanent disability. This led the World Health Organization (WHO) to endorse a worldwide global campaign toward pain reduction and elimination.[3,4] Chronic pain is widely accepted as a human phenomenon with statically and dynamically interacting biologic, psychological, social, and spiritual dimensions.[5] Further, the psychological dimension of chronic pain includes cognitive, mood, and behavioral manifestations and a high rate of co-occurring psychiatric disorders. Unfortunately, traditional psychiatric interventions, which could benefit many chronic pain sufferers, are frequently requested too late in the course of pain progression.

Nonetheless, psychiatric treatment for chronic pain has improved over the last five decades, during which there has been an increased tendency to include psychiatrists in the overall management of chronic pain. Identifying and addressing the various psychiatric components of chronic pain can significantly contribute to successful rehabilitation, recovery, and improved overall functioning.[6] Untreated psychiatric symptoms often exacerbate pain intensity, leading to increased disability and perpetuating a never-ending cycle of pain-related biologic, psychological, social, and spiritual dysfunctions.[6] This chapter provides an overview of the most common co-occurring psychiatric disorders in patients with chronic pain, including depression, anxiety disorders, posttraumatic stress disorder (PTSD), sleep disorders, personality disorders, and substance use disorders. In addition, the chapter will explore the expression of these disorders within the context of chronic pain, with a consideration of both diagnostic and treatment issues.[7]

PSYCHIATRY AND CHRONIC PAIN HISTORICAL ASSOCIATION

The word *psychiatry* derives its origin from both Greek and Latin and conveys care for mind, body, and spirit. In these two languages, psychiatry literally meant "a healing of the soul," and in the Latinized form of Greek, the word *psych* meant mind, breath, life, or soul.[8] The modern term *psychiatry* was coined by the German physician Johann Christian Real in 1808 and literally means the "medical treatment of the soul."[9,10] *Mens sana in corpore sano* is another often-mentioned Latin phrase, loosely translated as "a healthy mind in a healthy body."[11]

Chronic and persistent pain has been extensively recorded over time and across cultures as a human condition that inflicts unbearable suffering on the mind, body, and soul that can be relieved only by alleviating the physical, psychological, social, *and* spiritual burdens.[12] Pain is not merely a physical manifestation but, instead, a combination of psychiatric and physical symptomatology as described by Engel's System Theory.[13] Although pain may originate from an acute insult, Engel theorized that it can develop into an independent entity with primary psychological phenomenology.[13] In his widely cited article describing the "pain-prone patient," Engel delineated characteristics of people predisposed to the development of chronic pain, such as significant guilt, unsatisfied unconscious aggressive impulses, a history of defeat, and a propensity to develop pain after a real or imagined loss.[13]

PSYCHIATRY'S ROLE IN CHRONIC PAIN

In the 21st century, the definitions of psychiatry remain unresolved. Most widely accepted are those of WHO and the American Psychiatric Association (APA), which describe psychiatry as the branch of medicine that is focused on the diagnosis, treatment, and prevention of mental, emotional, and behavioral disorders.[14] Psychiatrists are usually referred to as physicians who specializes in mental health, including substance use disorders, and are qualified to assess and treat both the mental and physical aspects of psychological problems.[14]

Progress in pain research over the past five decades has improved diagnosis and treatment. That psychiatric factors play an important role in chronic pain has been demonstrated from a myriad of sources. It is of pivotal importance for psychiatrists to identify the effects of pain on the human soul and to collaborate with other mental health professionals and primary care providers in diagnosing, intervening, and treating pain to restore a healthy mind and body.[15,16] Pain is highly individualized, and chronic pain often impacts all aspects of patients' lives. They often report that pain interferes with their ability to engage in occupational, social, romantic, or recreational activities, resulting in withdrawal and dis-engagement.[17] This contributes to increased social isolation and feelings of worthlessness. In turn, this can precipitate a new onset of psychiatric disorders or worsen preexisting ones.[17] In clinical practice, the phenomenon of chronic pain has shown to be consistent with various psychiatric models of illness.[17] These models are useful in the diagnosis and management of chronic pain.[17]

In addition to addressing the biologic, psychological, and emotional needs of chronic pain patients, psychiatrists need to be active participants in the national debate of accurately diagnosing and effectively treating chronic pain while preventing opioid addiction.[18,19] This era of increased awareness concerning opioids and pain has engendered numerous reviews on how pain has been conceptualized in the past and how future directions should proceed for the theoretical foundation and treatment of chronic pain.[20,21]

CHRONIC PAIN EPIDEMIOLOGY

The National Institute of Health (NIH) has identified chronic pain as one of the costliest medical condition in the United States, costing a staggering estimated $100 billion each year.[20] Further, the Centers for Disease Control and Prevention (CDC) has reported that one in four individuals have had a day-long episode of severe pain within a 1-month period.[21] Pain accounts for over 80% of all physician visits, and approximately 54% of chronic pain patients have co-occurring psychiatric disorders, especially depression.[15,16,22] In the United States, pain medications are the second most prescribed agents, accounting for up to 12% of all outpatient prescriptions.[23]

PAIN DEFINITIONS

From a psychiatric perspective, pain needs to be constantly and carefully defined and interpreted in order to provide appropriate care. Psychiatrists can also assist healthcare providers in overcoming information deficiencies and biases to improve the diagnosis and treatment of patients, including the impact of psychiatric factors in the manifestation of pain.[15,16]

According to the International Association for the Study of Pain (IASP), pain is defined as "an unpleasant sensory and emotional experience associated with actual or potential tissue damage, or described in terms of such damage."[24] Generally, acute pain occurs as a consequence of a medical illness or a bodily physical injury, and usually subsides with the restoration of physical health or the resolution of the injury. It seldom leads to any new onset of psychiatric manifestation.[15,16,24] *Chronic* pain usually describes a category of per-sistent pain that lasts more than 6 months and continues longer than the expected duration of natural healing related to the original underlying disorder. Some sources in the medical literature classify pain as chronic if it persists more than 3 months.[24]

PAIN CLASSIFICATION

In clinical settings, classifications of pain are generally divided into two main categories: nociceptive or neuropathic.[25]

NOCICEPTIVE PAIN

This type of pain includes most cases of acute pain in which a strong, noxious stimulus impacts the skin or deep tissue. Although acute pain resolves after the noxious stimulus has been identified and removed, residual inflammatory and autoimmune mechanisms may lead to persistence of the nociceptive pain, which in turn may progress to chronic pain.[24,25] In addition, many patients with nociceptive pain conditions—such as musculoskeletal disorders, arthritis, migraines, tension headaches, and fibromyalgia—also have chronic pain.[24,25] Nociceptive pain is sometimes subclassified in the literature into either *somatic pain*, which is usually triggered by the fascia, skin dermatomes, muscles, and joint tender points, or *visceral pain* originating from the heart, lungs, gastrointestinal or genitourinary systems, or other organs such as the spleen or pancreas.[26] Clinicians are usually able to identify somatic pain due to the precise location of the somatosensory fibers in the spinal cord and brain.[26] In contrast, the localization of visceral pain is usually difficult due to the diffuse distribution and trajectory of the afferent visceral sensory fibers within the nervous system.[26]

NEUROPATHIC PAIN

This category of pain has a chronic course due to its manifestation of peripheral or central nervous system conditions, such as postherpetic neuralgia, diabetic neuropathy, phantom limb syndrome, and sciatica.[24] In contrast to the specific organ localization of nociceptive pain, neuropathic pain is often characterized by the patient's description of the pain.[24] Neuropathic pain is frequently described as burning, paroxysmal, stabbing, buzzing, or electric shocks, or as traveling along the spinal column to the extremities.[27]

NEUROPLASTIC CHANGES

Pain research studies have identified potential mechanisms for chronic pain in nociception, nerve conduction, regulation of spinal cord neurons, neuronal plasticity, and gene expression.[15,16,28] For example, there is evidence that neuroplastic change arising from poorly treated persistent pain can lead to sensitization, defined as an "increased responsiveness of neurons to their normal input or recruitment of a response to sub-threshold inputs."[16] Neuroplastic change is one possible explanation of the common phenomenon in chronic pain of altered pain perception, persistence of pain beyond tissue healing, and resistance to commonly used analgesics.[16] Nociceptive pain may respond to anti-inflammatory, analgesic pharmacologic agents.[16] In contrast, neuropathic pain often does not respond to these medications, and patients may require adjunctive treatment with psychopharmacologic agents, thus requiring adequate psychiatric input.[15,16]

NEUROPATHIC PAIN SCREENING TOOLS

The Leeds Assessment of Neuropathic Symptoms and Signs (LANSS) and its self-administered version (S-LANSS) are useful tools for assessing neuropathic pain.[29] The Neuropathic Pain Scale (NPS) is useful in evaluating neuropathic pain conditions.[30] The Pain Quality Assessment Scale (PQAS) is a generic instrument that differentiates between nociceptive and neuropathic pain conditions.[31] However, complex chronic pain conditions may have components of nociceptive, inflammatory, and neuropathic pain mechanisms.[30,31] Treatments may have different effects on the different pain mechanisms.[15,16,32]

CHRONIC PAIN AND PSYCHIATRY'S DIAGNOSTIC ISSUES

PSYCHIATRY'S INPUT

Initially, patients manage and interpret chronic pain in ways similar to acute pain. However, the persistence of pain can lead to new-onset psychiatric symptoms or exacerbate preexisting psychiatric conditions.[33] From a psychiatric perspective, these various pain definitions need to be constantly and carefully interpreted in order to assist healthcare providers in overcoming the tendency to separate pain that is triggered by underlying medical conditions from pain that is a manifestation of psychiatric factors.[25] Psychiatrists can serve as important patient advocates by gently challenging disproven assumptions with other healthcare providers—such as the notion that there is a difference between "real" and "imagined" pain.[34] In a practical and clinical context, patients' suffering always is real, whether or not a physical "cause" of pain is identified.[15,16,25]

The issue of chronic pain has not always been integrated within the various editions of the APA's *Diagnostic and Statistical Manual of Mental Disorders* (DSM). For instance, pain "determined" by emotional factors was classified in DSM-II among psychophysiological disorders.[35] DSM-III attempted to address chronic pain by introducing the concept of psychogenic pain disorder, in which pathophysiologic aspects were absent or insufficient to explain the length and the severity of pain, and in the diagnostic category of somatoform pain disorder, where psychological factors no longer were required in pain etiology.[36] DSM-III-R deleted the requirements that psychological factors be present or that the pain should result from another mental disorder.[37] Instead, the presence of "pain related problems of at least 6 months' duration" was introduced as the main criterion for "somatoform pain disorder." Even so, these diagnostic categories rarely are used in diagnosing or treating patients with chronic pain.[37]

To better define the diagnostic subgroup of somatoform disorders present in DSM-III-R, DSM-IV and DSM-IV-TR introduced the Pain Disorder category under somatoform disorders, which also included conversion disorder, hysteria, and body dysmorphic disorder—all characterized by the common feature of the presence of a physical symptom that is suggestive of a medical disorder not provoked by a medical disorder or by substance use.[38–40] Pain Disorder includes additional diagnostic subgroups: (1) Pain Disorder Associated with Psychological Factors, (2) Pain Disorder Associated with Both Psychological Factors and a General Medical Condition, and (3) Pain Disorder Associated with a General Medical Condition.[38–40] These diagnostic categories illustrate the entrenched concept of psychological and physical dualism and reinforce the mythology of "real pain" and "imaginary pain." They also may discourage the comprehensive treatment of patients with chronic pain.[38–40]

The diagnostic category of Pain Disorder was eliminated in DSM-5, which introduced a new diagnostic category of Somatic Symptoms and Related Disorders, identifying common features when, for example, patients have somatic symptoms associated with significant distress and impairment.[41] This diagnosis is made on the basis of signs and symptoms of somatic complaints—in addition to abnormal thoughts, feelings, and behaviors in response to these symptoms—rather than the absence of a medical condition that otherwise might explain the somatic complaints.[26] This improved diagnostic category will provide psychiatrists with a tool to enhance colleagues' understanding of the multidimensional nature of chronic pain and encourage comprehensive, interdisciplinary treatment.

CHRONIC PAIN ASSESSMENT AND PAIN SCALES

Pain assessment should include the use of validated tools, with attention to each patient's level of functioning, as a complement to traditional diagnostic approaches. A personalized, patient-centered assessment includes a determination of the pain's location, intensity, quality, onset, and duration, as well as factors that exacerbate or alleviate chronic pain.[42] It is important to inquire about patients' best, worst, and average pain intensities over a 24-hour time span.[42] Physically observable signs of pain—such as facial expression (especially grimacing), shortness of breath, heart palpitation, rapid pulse, and general body restlessness—are helpful, in conjunction with other assessment methods.[42] Patients with chronic pain and their caregivers should document the frequency, timing, and use of pain-relieving medications and other modalities, as well as their effectiveness in reducing pain.[42] A review of this information is a valuable tool in assessing the effectiveness of interventions at the time of their use.[42]

Despite the presence of several pain scales and instruments to improve assessment, none has proven be more accurate than others.[43] Consistent use of a particular scale over time with a given patient is more important than the use of any specific scale.[43] This allows for a valid assessment of the patient's pain and the effectiveness of therapies.[43] We will review some of the most common assessment tools.[44]

The Pain Beliefs Questionnaire (PBQ) assesses the patient's medical and psychological understanding about pain in the context of its impact on various coping behaviors.[27,45] The

Pain Self-Efficacy Questionnaire (PSEQ) assesses the patient's confidence in performing particular activities when experiencing pain;[46] higher scores are associated with higher levels of functioning.[46]

The Brief Pain Inventory (BPI), which evolved from the Wisconsin Brief Pain Questionnaire (WBPQ),[47] assesses pain severity and the degree of interference with function, using a 0-to-10 scale.[48] It can be self-administered, given in a clinical interview, or even administered over the telephone.[47] Most patients can complete the short version of the BPI in 2 or 3 minutes.[47] Chronic pain usually varies throughout the day and night, and therefore the BPI asks patients to rate their pain now and at its worst, using terms of "least and average" intensity over the last 24 hours.[47] Location of pain on a body chart and characteristics of the pain are documented.[49] The BPI also asks the patient to rate how much pain interferes with seven functional aspects of life: (1) general activity, (2) walking, (3) normal work, (4) relations with other people, (5) mood, (6) sleep, and (7) enjoyment of life.[49] In addition, the BPI asks patients to rate the relief they feel from the current pain treatment.[49]

The McGill Pain Questionnaire (MPQ) and the short-form MPQ (SF-MPQ) evaluate sensory, affective–emotional, evaluative, and temporal aspects of the patient's pain condition.[50,51] The SF-MPQ consists of 11 sensory (e.g., sharp, shooting) and four affective (e.g., sickening, fearful) verbal descriptors.[50,51] Patients are asked to rate the intensity of each descriptor on a scale from 0 to 3 (3 = severe).[50,51] The sensory, affective, and total pain index scores are calculated. Patients also rate their present pain intensity on a 0-to-5 scale.[50,51]

The Massachusetts General Hospital Pain Center's Pain Assessment Form (MGH-PCPAF) is another brief patient self-report form covering the essential issues needed for a self-report pain form.[46] This inventory is divided in three parts and includes 12 scales that examine the impact of pain on the patient's life, perceptions of others' responses to the patient's communications of pain, and the extent to which the patient participates in common daily activities.[52]

The selection of a given scale really depends on the practitioner. All these pain assessment tools can give good information, but none stands out as the "gold standard." The choice of scale or assessment tool to use should depend on the clinician's patient base, area of practice, type of practice, and needs.

CHRONIC PAIN PATIENTS' NARRATIVES

Communication and active listening are critical to appropriate assessment of any patient complaint.[53] This is even more important with patients who have chronic pain. Because there is no specific ancillary testing that can measure and locate chronic pain with precision, providers must rely on the patient's own description of the type, timing, and location of pain.[54] Reflective listening to the patient's narrative descriptions of the pain experience—including predisposing, existing, and perpetuating personal and environmental triggers—provides the best clues to the cause of the pain and is an important component of the initial evaluation. Given the unique training of psychiatrists in reflective listening, they could provide an invaluable contribution to their colleagues without psychiatric training. Eliciting patient narratives coupled with reflective listening lays the foundation for a comprehensive treatment plan that is based on a collaborative partnership between the patient and the healthcare providers.[8,15,16]

PSYCHIATRIC DISORDERS THAT CO-OCCUR WITH CHRONIC PAIN

The incidence of co-occurring psychiatric disorders is two to three times higher in chronic pain patients than in the general population.[15,16,55] The most common ones are depression, anxiety disorders, PTSD, sleep disorders, personality disorders, and substance use disorders.[15,16,55]

MAJOR DEPRESSIVE DISORDER IN PATIENTS WITH CHRONIC PAIN

The strong association between chronic pain and major depressive disorder (MDD) has been extensively reported in the literature, particularly in the context of the physiologic equivalence of physical pain and mental pain differentiated by anatomic localization.[15–17,39,40] The similarity in the neurophysiologic manifestations of physical and psychological pain may cause some physicians to diagnose "psychalgia" as a condition of severe depression.[59] Prevalence rates for MDD in patients with chronic pain vary widely, from 30% to 54% in studies that have used standardized diagnostic scales and 10% to 100% in studies that relied on self-reporting.[15,16] Diagnosing MDD in the chronic pain population can be an overwhelming endeavor because the two conditions share many features, such as fatigue, sleep disturbances, and cognitive deficits in memory and attention.[15,16] Many studies have identified high rates of MDD in chronic pain patients, with current and lifetime rates of this disorder of about 45% and 65%, respectively, in the chronic low back pain population.[16,57,58] Disabling chronic pain was present in 41% of those with MDD versus 10% of those without MDD. In addition, current and lifetime MDD rates are about 80% in the chronic upper extremity pain population.[15,16]

The functional consequences of co-occurring chronic pain and MDD are significant. Compared to pain patients without MDD, patients with co-occurring MDD and disabling chronic pain have a significantly poorer quality of life, an increased severity of somatic symptoms, a higher prevalence of panic disorder and PTSD, and a sixfold greater prevalence of anxiety.[15,16,57] The presence of MDD in patients with chronic pain is associated with decreased function, poorer treatment response, and increased healthcare costs.[60,61]

Moreover, MDD, anxiety, panic disorder, and PTSD are difficult to detect in a typical patient evaluation. This can lead to underdiagnosed and untreated comorbidities, thus aggravating the intensity of chronic pain.[62] Making an accurate diagnosis of MDD can be challenging in the setting of co-occurring chronic pain, especially in the context of establishing a valid correlation or a causal relationship between chronic pain and MDD in primary care settings and the general population.[62] It has even been suggested that sleep disorders can significantly cloud the diagnosis of MDD in the presence of chronic pain.[63]

Some progress has been achieved, particularly in terms of understanding the causal nature and the temporal relationship between chronic pain and depression.[15,16,56] Research has shown depression to be an antecedent to chronic pain, a consequence of chronic pain, and a concomitant biologic relative of chronic pain.[15,16,56] Based on this and other research, five research-based hypotheses have been proposed:

1. Antecedent hypothesis—depression precedes the development of chronic pain.
2. Consequence hypothesis—depression is a consequence and follows the development of pain.
3. Scar hypothesis episodes—depression occurring before the onset of pain predisposes individuals to a depressive episode following pain onset.
4. Cognitive-behavioral mediation hypothesis—cognitions mediate the relationship between chronic pain and the development of depression.
5. Common pathogenetic mechanisms hypothesis—depression and chronic pain share similar anatomic pathways and common dopamine, norepinephrine, and serotonin neurotransmitters.[16]

The common pathogenetic mechanism hypothesis suggests that shared neurotransmitters justify the clinical rationale of using psychopharmacologic agents, especially antidepressants and mood stabilizers, in the treatment of chronic pain, even in the absence of co-occurring MDD.[64] Despite the presence of the various common mechanisms between chronic pain and MDD, the evidence-based literature considers them as separate and distinct disorders because in many patients each condition exists in the absence of the other, and in many instances the onset of pain and that of depression do not coincide.[16] To accurately diagnose the presence of MDD in chronic pain, psychiatrists also need to assess carefully a category of patients who tend to attribute most of their symptoms to pain rather than to depression by generalizing most of their medical problems as being rooted in pain.[16] Others may find it more comfortable acknowledging somatic rather than psychiatric symptoms.[16] Some patients with chronic pain may also present with depressed mood, which may be related to an adjustment disorder with depressed mood rather than MDD.[16]

CHRONIC PAIN AND ANXIETY DISORDERS

Studies have shown high rates of anxiety disorders among chronic pain patients.[65] Reported anxiety disorders include panic disorder, agoraphobia, specific phobia, social phobia, and generalized anxiety disorder.[65] Although there is inconsistency in the chronic pain literature about specific anxiety disorders, it appears that panic disorder and generalized anxiety disorder are most commonly diagnosed.[15,16,66] The overall prevalence for anxiety disorders in chronic pain patients ranges from 16.5% to 28.8%.[15,16,65] Recent studies, however, suggest that anxiety disorders may be present in up to 60% of patients with chronic pain.[65,67]

Panic disorder and pain share several psychological vulnerabilities, such as hyperarousal, somatic cues, and attentional biases, which may underlie both the anxiety and pain conditions.[15,16,65,67] It also is possible that individuals use "worry" as a strategy for reducing somatic arousal associated with pain, making them more prone to develop generalized anxiety disorder.[15,16,65,67] Psychiatrists evaluating the co-occurrence of anxiety disorder in chronic pain patients need to be aware of the DSM-5 diagnostic criteria involved. In DSM-5 the diagnoses of agoraphobia, specific phobia, and social anxiety have been updated.[68] Panic attacks are now categorized as either expected or unexpected; furthermore, panic disorder and agoraphobia are no longer linked but are recognized as two separate disorders.[68]

CHRONIC PAIN AND PTSD

In DSM-5 PTSD has been removed as an anxiety disorder and moved to the new diagnostic classification of "trauma and stress-related disorders," which include reactive attachment and disinhibited social engagement, PTSD, acute stress disorder, adjustment disorder, and other trauma and stress-related disorders.[68]

Chronic pain and PTSD have been reported as common complications of experiencing a traumatic event, and their co-occurrence is likely more common than previously recognized. Although some earlier studies reported a 1.7% prevalence of PTSD among chronic pain patients, about 10% of veterans referred to a pain clinic and 10% of patients attending a multidisciplinary chronic pain center have been shown to meet criteria for PTSD.[69,70] Studies examining the prevalence of chronic pain in individuals with a primary diagnosis of PTSD have reported even higher co-prevalence rates.[70,71] In fact, pain is the most common physical complaint among patients who suffer from PTSD.[70,71] Research has also shown that 60% to 80% of veterans with PTSD have reported chronic pain conditions. Furthermore, patients with chronic pain related to trauma or PTSD experience more intense pain and affective distress, higher levels of life interference, and a greater degree of disability than chronic pain patients who have not experienced trauma or developed PTSD.[70,71] PTSD may go undiagnosed for a variety of reasons; for example, patients with chronic pain may attribute symptoms of sleep difficulties or mood and cognitive symptoms to pain.[70,71] This underscores the importance of a psychiatrist's involvement in the evaluation, assessment, and treatment of chronic pain.

CHRONIC PAIN AND SLEEP DISORDERS

Pain is a physical and emotional signal of bodily harm that strongly motivates an array of behaviors.[72] Sleep is also a behaviorally regulated drive and broadly serves to maintain homeostasis and optimize function across multiple physiologic systems.[72,73] Chronic impairments in the systems regulating pain and sleep can have a broad negative impact on health and well-being.[73] Sleep complaints are present in 67% to 88% of those with chronic pain, and at least 50% of individuals with insomnia suffer from chronic pain.[71] Furthermore, chronic pain and sleep disturbances share an array of physical and mental health comorbidities, such as obesity, type 2 diabetes, and depression.[16] The comorbidities of obesity and diabetes also have been shown to be related to chronic pain.[74,75]

Recent evidence-based studies support a reciprocal relationship between sleep disturbances and pain, but those relationships are not straightforward.[72,76] Insomnia is one such example.[72,76] Insomnia symptoms significantly increase the risk of developing future chronic pain disorders in previously pain-free individuals; however, existing pain is not a strong predictor of new-onset insomnia.[72,76]

CHRONIC PAIN AND PERSONALITY DISORDERS

Personality characteristics and personality disorders (PDs) have long been noted in the chronic pain population, with a prevalence ranging from 31% to 81%.[16,77] The relationship, however, between the physiologic and psychological mechanisms that underlies the interaction between chronic pain and PDs continues to pose a clinical challenge for healthcare providers.[77–82]

Patients with certain traits and PDs have a higher tendency to continue to worry and ruminate about their symptoms long after their initial acute pain episode resolves.[79] Other patients with PDs may overly rely on their clinicians and assume a passive role in their treatment, thereby decreasing the likelihood of a timely recovery. They may exhibit demanding behavior (borderline PD), self-absorbed behavior (narcissistic PD), or overtly entitled behavior (antisocial and borderline PDs).[15,16,77,78]

Current research has identified certain underlying biologic and psychological relationships between PDs and chronic pain.[83] Certain aspects of the gate control and the diathesis/stress models pain are also shared with PDs. These two models are summarized later in this chapter.[16] Based on the presence of direct and indirect links between PDs and chronic pain, it is important and clinically relevant for psychiatrists to understand and assess these links in the context of the diagnosis and management of PDs in patients with chronic pain.

CHRONIC PAIN AND SUBSTANCE USE DISORDERS

Although this topic is addressed in multiple other chapters, some additional comments are warranted. Numerous studies have identified high prevalence rates of substance use disorders in patients with chronic pain.[84] Some data suggest that approximately 32% of chronic pain patients may have co-occurring substance use disorders.[15,16,85,86] It is difficult to know the precise incidence of substance use disorders among chronic pain patients for a variety of reasons, including when aberrant medication-related behaviors develop as a complication of prescription opioid use.[84,88] Patients with a co-occurring substance use disorder (past and present) are also potentially more difficult to treat and are at higher risk for co-occurring depression, anxiety, and sleep disturbances.[84,85,87,88]

In the DSM-5 revised chapter "Substance-Related and Addictive Disorders," the diagnosis of substance use disorder is made for patients exhibiting maladaptive patterns of substance use leading to clinically significant impairment or distress.[88] The dangers of combining substances with addictive potential—including different classes of medication, alcohol, and illicit drugs—are often overlooked. For example, alcohol combined with pain-alleviating substances can increase the potential risks.[15,16,89] Benzodiazepines added to chronic opioid therapy (or, more commonly, when abused along with opioids) can increase the risk of death even when used as directed.[90,91]

Diagnosing a substance use disorder, distinguishing it from pseudoaddiction, and carefully evaluating a patient's suitability for opioid therapy are critical skills. Psychiatrists in general, and those with additional board certifications in addiction psychiatry, have an important role to play in preventing, identifying, and treating opioid use disorders and other substance use disorders in chronic pain patients.[89,92]

PSYCHIATRIC PAIN MODELS

Multiple psychiatric models have been proposed in regard to the human pain experience. Psychiatrists will find it clinically useful to explain them to patients with chronic pain and elicit their input as to which model fits best with their unique experience of pain. Examples of pain models include (1) gate control, (2) diathesis/stress, (3) biopsychosocial–spiritual, (4) cognitive-behavioral transactional, and (5) cognitive-behavioral fear avoidance.

GATE CONTROL MODEL

The gate control model was the first theory to suggest that pain is not simply a function of nerve impulses from sensory inputs directly to the brain.[93,94] There is a "gate mechanism" at the dorsal horn of the spinal cord, and the degree to which the gate is open determines the extent of the patient's pain experience. Factors that open the gate include depression, anxiety, fear, mental focus on injury/pain, sense of loss of control, negative thoughts, and social withdrawal.[93,94] Factors that close the gate include emotional control, relaxation, mental distraction, positive thoughts, sense of control, and engaging in pleasurable activities.[94]

DIATHESIS/STRESS MODEL

This multicausal developmental model posits that there is a window of vulnerability for developing pain.[93] Multiple risk factors over the course of development interact with stressors contributing to pain psychopathology.[93] Protective factors contributing to normal development prevent pain psychopathology.[93] The differential susceptibility hypothesis is a recent theory that stemmed from the diathesis/stress model.[93]

BIOPSYCHOSOCIAL–SPIRITUAL MODEL

This model represents a whole-person approach rather than a disease-focused model and was essential to the development of the therapeutic *interdisciplinary pain management teams*.[95] Pain is the product of interactions among biologic, psychological, social, and spiritual processes.[95] Variability in pain experiences is due to the range and interaction of these processes, which then modulate the patient's interpretation of pain symptoms.[96–99]

COGNITIVE-BEHAVIORAL TRANSACTIONAL MODEL

Pain is considered either as nonthreatening, which leads to engaging in adaptive behaviors to improve functioning, or as a threat and a catastrophe, which leads to development of fear of pain, avoidance, deconditioning, and subsequent increased pain.[100–102]

ADDRESSING PSYCHIATRIC DISORDERS IN CHRONIC PAIN

Successful management of chronic pain and co-occurring psychiatric disorders is usually based on a biopsychosocial–spiritual approach[103] that combines evidence-based pharmacotherapy with psychotherapy and social and spiritual interventions.[104,105] Cognitive-behavioral psychotherapy has had a long track record of success in addressing various aspects of chronic pain issues and psychiatric symptoms, including substance use disorders.[16,106–108] Other types of psychotherapy, such as motivational enhancement therapy, cognitive processing therapy, and acceptance commitment therapy, are useful for patients whose unique presentations may not respond to cognitive-behavioral therapy.[16,106–108] A graded, individually tailored physical exercise program can be added as an integral component of a holistic approach.[109] Finally, an exploration of the patient's core beliefs, especially as they relate to the meaning of physical and emotional pain and suffering, should be incorporated into the overall treatment framework.[15,16,96,110,111]

CHRONIC PAIN SELF-MANAGEMENT

The psychiatric approach to the chronic pain patient should facilitate self-care and personal advocacy by the patient and the patient's support system.[16,103] Patients should be provided with a careful and detailed education on the physiologic mechanisms underlying chronic pain and the risks, benefits, and efficacy of each recommended treatment.[112] Regular adherence with pharmacologic interventions for pain and co-occurring psychiatric disorders is critical, and providers need to communicate clearly this expectation.[113] However, if screening identifies the presence of an active substance use disorder or any substance-induced psychiatric disorder, psychiatric and addiction treatment should be integrated with the patient's ongoing chronic pain management program. The success of any chronic pain self-management program requires strong support from family, peers, and the primary chronic pain multidisciplinary treatment team.[114,115] The patient's support system can contribute to the success, for example, of graded exercise programs.[116] Peer support and self-help groups such as 12-step facilitation can benefit patients who do not feel comfortable in formal therapeutic settings.[116]

TREATMENT OF CO-OCCURRING PSYCHIATRIC DISORDERS

Psychiatrists can play a direct role in motivating patients with chronic pain to optimize their self-management of pain and depression, as well as indirectly conveying the same recommendation to patients' primary care providers.[15,16,56] The effectiveness of combining psychopharmacologic treatment with pain self-management programs can significantly reduce the psychiatric symptomatology and pain severity.[117] It is important to convey to patients that the improvement in their psychiatric conditions may not be immediate but, instead, probably will occur within 2 months of the start of treatment; further, psychiatric symptoms typically improve before the pain severity decreases.[117]

Education about anticipated side effects of psychiatric treatment—especially sexual dysfunction and weight gain—is critical to strengthen adherence and prevent premature discontinuation.[117] Benzodiazepines should be avoided, especially for patients taking therapeutic opioids for pain and those with a co-occurring substance use disorder.[117] Judicious use of opioids—especially for acute, nociceptive, inflammatory pain—and patient education can enhance the effectiveness of psychopharmacologic interventions.[117]

The integrated treatment for chronic pain and PTSD should include cognitive processing therapy or prolonged exposure therapy for the PTSD and cognitive-behavioral therapy for the chronic pain.[118] For patients with pain, PTSD, and a substance use disorder, treatment should also include combined relaxation training, relapse prevention, and seeking-safety therapy.[119] Appropriate antidepressants can achieve the dual benefits of improving PTSD symptoms and alleviating chronic pain intensity.[119] Although the co-occurrence of chronic pain, PTSD, and traumatic brain injury, especially in combat veterans, can make it difficult to pursue cognitively oriented psychotherapies, these highly structured approaches have shown efficacy in the general management of patients with traumatic brain injury.[119]

DIAGNOSING AND MANAGING SUBSTANCE USE DISORDERS

In the current opioid "epidemic," any active use of opioids is a matter of grave concern in patients with co-occurring psychiatric and addictive disorders and chronic pain.[15,16] Insufficient treatment of chronic pain in these patients is more likely to precipitate more substance use and more difficulty in treating addiction.[120] In addition, the pain reports of patients with an opioid use disorder in the setting of substance abuse counseling frequently are not believed.[121] It is of paramount importance for psychiatrists to be active advocates on behalf of these patients and to assure them that despite their addiction history, they will not be denied adequate treatment for their psychiatric disorder while being treated for their current and preexisting chronic pain.[121]

COLLABORATING WITH PRIMARY CARE PROVIDERS

The significant overall impact of chronic pain can adversely affect the patient's mood, personality characteristics, and social environment.[121] The complex multidimensional sequelae of chronic pain and the high prevalence of chronic pain in the primary care setting have increased the demand for psychiatric assistance in that setting.[121]

COMMUNICATION BETWEEN PSYCHIATRISTS AND PRIMARY CARE PROVIDERS

Psychiatrists can broaden and maximize their professional and clinical relationships with primary care providers by collaborating on chronic pain treatment.[122] Integrating treatment of psychiatric disorders in the same setting benefits their mutual patients and fits within the framework of a multidisciplinary treatment team.

Coordination is enhanced by having regular and timely face-to-face meetings (rather than via electronic medical records and emails) between the psychiatrist and the primary care provider to review the progression of treatment plans and to solicit opinions and feedback regarding the specific needs of patients.[122] Patients should be invited to participate in the planning and execution of their multidisciplinary treatment plans to enhance the therapeutic value of coordinating medical and psychiatric treatments.[122] The integration and coordination of mental health and primary care enhances patient and provider satisfaction alike.[122] It also contributes to improved outcomes and decreases healthcare costs.

PSYCHIATRISTS' ROLE IN DEVELOPING THE STEPPED-CARE APPROACH

The *stepped-care* model is a clinical approach for chronic pain management that guides the level of care based on patients' responses to treatment and their motivation to initiate and engage in self-care.[123–125] This model comprises three basic steps.

Step 1 is appropriate for the majority of patients seeking treatment for pain.[125] During Step 1, psychiatrists provide psychoeducation to their primary care colleagues with the goal of identifying and addressing specific concerns in order to enhance the patient's motivation to pursue self-care.[125] This education may include teaching techniques to manage the common fears that exertion, exercise, or sexual activity will worsen the intensity and level of pain.[125] These fears are decreased by clearly explaining the benefits of remaining active and by creating a plan for gradually returning to a safe level of activity.[125] Psychiatrists can introduce principles and practices of motivational interviewing and enhancement therapy to their primary care colleagues, which helps to modify the patient's expectations of a permanent cure for chronic pain, reinforce consistent self-care strategies, and develop realistic plans for managing pain exacerbations.[125]

Step 2 is reserved for patients who require a more active approach to their pain management because of pain and disability that persists for several weeks after their initial primary care appointment.[125] During this step, the patient is strongly encouraged to identify the specific difficulties or triggers that worsen pain levels.[125] This step requires the development and implementation of an individually tailored treatment plan.[125] The psychiatrist can make recommendations regarding individual or group therapy and pharmacologic, psychosocial, and spiritual interventions, which would require a more comprehensive psychoeducational program.[125]

Step 3 is recommended for patients who present with complex medical and psychosocial histories that are challenging to manage within a primary care setting.[125] These patients usually continue to experience significant levels of disability and distress despite comprehensive psychoeducational programs and the ongoing efforts of their primary care providers.[125] They typically require more extensive involvement by the psychiatric and pain management treatment team.[125]

ORGANIZATION OF PAIN MANAGEMENT TEAMS

Psychiatrists can facilitate chronic pain care by organizing providers with specific expertise in pain management and integrating them into multidisciplinary pain management teams.[126] The goal of the team is to provide a comprehensive assessment of chronic pain patients and coordinate and deliver an integrated, holistic treatment plan.[127] Because psychiatry plays an important and growing role in the management of chronic pain patients, psychiatrists with special interests in this field should strive to meet the training goals of the pain medicine fellowship established by the Accreditation Council for Graduate Medical Education.[128] Because of the recognition during the last few years that pain is a sensation influenced by cognitive, emotional, and psychological factors, an "irreversible symbiosis" has been established between pain medicine and psychiatry.[128] In addition, the American Board of Psychiatry and Neurology now offers a subspecialty certification in pain medicine.[129]

PSYCHOPHARMACOLOGIC TREATMENT OF CHRONIC PAIN

The role of psychopharmacologic agents in the treatment of co-occurring psychiatric disorders and chronic pain and the role of psychotropic medications in the management of chronic pain—even in patients without co-occurring psychiatric conditions—is beyond the scope of this review and may be addressed in other chapters. However, we will briefly discuss the use of antidepressants and mood stabilizers for treating these conditions.

ANTIDEPRESSANTS

The broad class of antidepressants includes tricyclic antidepressants, selective serotonin reuptake inhibitors, serotonin norepinephrine reuptake inhibitors, monoamine oxidase inhibitors, and other antidepressants such as mirtazapine, trazodone, and bupropion.[130,131] The pain-relieving properties of these medications are achieved using doses lower than those needed to treat depression. Unlike pain-relieving agents that are used only when needed, antidepressants must be taken every day regardless of pain level.[130,131] Although the exact mechanism by which antidepressants relieve pain is not fully understood, they are a mainstay in the treatment of many chronic pain conditions.[130,131] They offer an alternative to the opioid analgesics as a first-line treatment of chronic pain, thus avoiding many of the adverse and lethal effects associated with long-term use of opiates.[130,131] In addition, antidepressants improve co-occurring depression, anxiety, PTSD, insomnia, and other psychosomatic disorders.[130,131]

A comprehensive knowledge of dosing, side effects, and interactions with other medications is necessary for safe prescribing of antidepressants.[130,131] Despite their potential benefit for chronic pain, antidepressants can increase the risk of suicidality in children and adolescents with MDD and other psychiatric disorders.[132] Patients who are started on therapy should be observed closely for clinical worsening, suicidality, or unusual changes in behavior.[130,131] In addition, families and caregivers should be advised of the need for close observation of the patient and the need to establish lines of communication with the prescriber.[130,131]

MOOD STABILIZERS

Antiepileptic agents—such as gamma-aminobutyric acid (GABA), analog gabapentin and pregabalin, carbamazepine, oxycarbamazepine, sodium divalproate (and its many derivatives), topiramate, lamotrigine, zonisamide, and tiagabine—are sometimes used as mood stabilizers in patients with bipolar disorders.[132] They are also sometimes prescribed for chronic pain.[133,134] Like antidepressants, they should be taken every day even in the absence of pain when their use is otherwise indicated.[133,134] Careful monitoring of side effects and interactions with other medications remains of paramount importance in all clinical settings.[135] Some of the psychiatric medications that can be used in the treatment of co-occurring psychiatric disorders and chronic pain are summarized in Table 7.1.

CONCLUSIONS

The increased prevalence of chronic pain and co-occurring psychiatric conditions and the psychiatric sequelae of chronic pain—even in patients without preexisting psychiatric disorders—require accurate identification, diagnosis, treatment, and coordinated

TABLE 7.1 Psychiatric medications that can be used in the treatment of co-occurring psychiatric disorders and chronic pain

Co-occurring Psychiatric Disorders	Psychopharmacologic Agents
Major depressive disorder	Serotonin norepinephrine reuptake inhibitors, tricyclic antidepressants, trazodone, mirtazapine, nefazodone, bupropion
Major depressive disorder, anxiety disorders, PTSD	Selective serotonin reuptake inhibitors, serotonin norepinephrine reuptake inhibitors, tricyclic antidepressants, monoamine oxidase inhibitors
Major depressive disorder, sleep disorders	Tricyclic antidepressants, trazodone, mirtazapine, nefazodone
Mood disorders, bipolar disorders	Anticonvulsants

management. Although the biologic mechanisms associated with pain have long been long recognized, the biopsychosocial–spiritual approach to understanding and managing pain is increasingly endorsed. This approach emphasizes the importance of considering the unique interactions among the pain patient's biologic, psychological, social, and spiritual dimensions to better understand chronic pain syndromes. Because of their expertise in prevention, diagnosis, and treatment of mental illness, psychiatrists need to be involved in the overall management of chronic pain. Psychiatry's involvement in chronic pain treatment includes direct and indirect participation. The use of appropriate assessments and the integration of multidisciplinary treatment teams, in collaboration with the primary care provider and pain management specialists, can allow chronic pain patients to receive the most appropriate and uniquely tailored treatment. The associative connections between psychiatry and pain are an integral component of the human condition; psychiatrists need to adhere to their time-honored calling of healing the mind, the soul, and the body of patients in chronic pain.

ACKNOWLEDGMENTS

Sincere appreciation to Drs. Avak A. Howsepian and John F. Peppin for the opportunity to contribute and thankfulness to my wife Lynn and children Andrea, Andrew and Adam, my sisters Hoda and Héla, and my brother Hadi for their support and encouragement.

REFERENCES

1. Lohman D, Schleifer R, Amon JJ. Access to pain treatment as a human right. *BMC Med.* 2010;8:8.
2. Häuser W, Wolfe F, Henningsen P, Schmutzer G, Brähler E, Hinz A. Untying chronic pain: prevalence and societal burden of chronic pain stages in the general population-a cross-sectional survey. *BMC Public Health.* 2014;14:352.

3. Barsky AJ, Peekna HM, Borus JF. Somatic symptom reporting in women and men. *J Gen Intern Med.* 2001;16:266–275.

4. World Health Organization (WHO). WHO Guidelines for the Management of Chronic Pain in Adults. http://www.who.int/medicines/areas/quality_safety/Scoping_WHOGuide_non-malignant_pain_adults.pdf. Accessed May 30, 2017.

5. Turk DC, Flor H. Chronic pain: a biobehavioral perspective. In: Gatchel RJ, Turk DC, eds. *Psychosocial Factors in Pain: Critical Perspectives.* New York: Guilford Publications; 1999:18–34.

6. Howe CQ, Sullivan MD. The missing "P" in pain management: how the current opioid epidemic highlights the need for psychiatric services in chronic pain care. *Gen Hosp Psychiatry.* 2014;36(1):99–104.

7. Outcalt SD, Hoen HM, Yu Z, et al, Does comorbid chronic pain affect posttraumatic stress disorder diagnosis and treatment? Outcomes of posttraumatic stress disorder screening in Department of Veterans Affairs primary care. *J Rehabil Res Dev.* 2016;53(1):37–44.

8. Khouzam HR. The 21st century psychiatrists need to reestablish their identity as healers of the human psyche and not just pill pushers. *Contemp Behav Health Care.* 2016;2: 44–47.

9. Storrow HA. *Outline of Clinical Psychiatry.* New York: Appleton-Century- Crofts, 1969.

10. Binder DK, Schaller K, Clusmann H. The seminal contributions of Johann-Christian Reil to anatomy, physiology, and psychiatry. *Neurosurgery.* 2007;61:1091–1096.

11. Riva G, Serino S, Di Lernia D, Pavone EF, Dakanalis A. Embodied medicine: *mens sana in corpore virtuale sano. Frontiers Hum Neurosci.* 2017;11:120.

12. Bonica JJ. History of pain concepts and pain therapy. *Mt Sinai J Med.* 1991;58(3):191–202.

13. Engel GL. "Psychogenic" pain and the pain-prone patient. *Am J Med.* 1959;26:899–918.

14. American Psychiatric Association. https://www.psychiatry.org/patients-families/what-is-psychiatry. Accessed May 25, 2017.

15. Sharp J, Keefe B. Psychiatry in chronic pain: a review and update. *Curr Psychiatry Rep.* 2005;7:213–219.

16. Dersh J, Polatin PB, Gatchel RJ. Chronic pain and psychopathology: research findings and theoretical considerations. *Psychosom Med.* 2002;64:773–786.

17. Banks SM, Kerns RD. Explaining high rates of depression in chronic pain: a diathesis-stress framework. *Psychol Bull.* 1996;119:95–110.

18. Mercadante S. Pathophysiology of chronic pain. In Bruera E, Higginson I, von Gunten CF, Morita T, eds. *Textbook of Palliative Medicine and Supportive Care.* Boca Raton, FL: CRC Press; 2015:373–380.

19. Keefe FJ, Lumley MA, Buffington AL, et al. Changing face of pain: evolution of pain research in psychosomatic medicine. *Psychosom Med* 2002, 64:921–938.

20. Institute of Medicine, Board on Health Sciences Policy, Care, and Education Committee on Advancing Pain Research. *Relieving Pain in America: A Blueprint for Transforming Prevention, Care, Education, and Research.* 1st Ed. Washington, DC: National Academies Press; 2011. https://www.nap.edu/read/13172/chapter/1.

21. Centers for Disease Control and Prevention. New Report Finds Pain Affects Millions of Americans. https://www.cdc.gov/nchs/pressroom/06facts/hus06.htm. Accessed May 25, 2017.

22. National Center for Health Statistics. Data File Documentation, National Health Interview Survey, 2012. Hyattsville, MD: National Center for Health Statistics, Centers for Disease Control and Prevention; 2013. https://ftp.cdc.gov/pub/Health_Statistics/NCHS/NHIS/SHS/2015_SHS_Table_A-18.pdf. Accessed May 25, 2017.

23. Rasu RS, Vouthy K, Crowl AN, Stegeman AE, Fikru B, Bawa WA, Knell ME. Cost of pain medication to treat adult patients with nonmalignant chronic pain in the United States. *J Manag Care Spec Pharm.* 2014;20:921–928.

24. International Association for the Study of Pain. *IASP Taxonomy.* https://www.iasp-pain.org/Taxonomy. Accessed May 29, 2017.

25. Leo RJ, Pristach CA, Streltzer J. Incorporating pain management training into the psychiatry residency curriculum. *Acad Psychiatry*. 2003;27:1–11.

26. Mayou R, Kirmayer LJ, Simon G, et al. Somatoform disorders: time for a new approach in DSM-V. *Am J Psychiatry*. 2005;162(5):847–855.

27. Chapman CR, Casey KR, Dubner R, Foley KM, Gracely RH, Reading AE. Pain measurement: an overview. *Pain*. 1985;22:1–31.

28. Nekovarova T, Yamamotova A, Vales K, Stuchlik A, Fricova J, Rokyta R. Common mechanisms of pain and depression: are antidepressants also analgesics? *Frontiers Behav Neurosci*. 2014;8:99.

29. Bennett M. The LANSS Pain Scale: the Leeds assessment of neuropathic symptoms and signs. *Pain*. 2001;92:147–157.

30. Krause SJ, Backonja M-M. Development of a neuropathic pain questionnaire. *Clin J Pain*. 2003;19:306–314

31. Herr K. Pain assessment strategies in older patients. *J Pain*. 2011;12(3 Suppl 1):S3–S13.

32. Khouzam HR. Psychopharmacology of chronic pain: a focus on antidepressants and atypical antipsychotics. *Postgrad Med*. 2016; 128(3):323–330.

33. Gerrits MM, van Oppen P, van Marwijk HW, Penninx BW, van der Horst HE. Pain and the onset of depressive and anxiety disorders. *Pain*. 2014;155:53–59.

34. Katz J, Rosenbloom BN, Fashler S. Chronic pain, psychopathology, and DSM-5 somatic symptom disorder. *Can J Psychiatry*. 2015;60:160–167.

35. American Psychiatric Association. *Diagnostic and Statistical Manual of Mental Disorders*. Washington, DC, American Psychiatric Press; 1968:46–48.

36. American Psychiatric Association. *Diagnostic and Statistical Manual of Mental Disorders*, 3rd ed. Washington, DC: American Psychiatric Press; 1980.

37. American Psychiatric Association. *Diagnostic and Statistical Manual of Mental Disorders.*, 3rd ed., revised. Washington, DC, American Psychiatric Press; 1987:264–266.

38. King SA, Strain JJ. Somatoform pain disorder. In American Psychiatric Association. *Diagnostic and Statistical Manual of Mental Disorders*, 4th ed. Washington, DC: American Psychiatric Press; 1994.

39. American Psychiatric Association. *Diagnostic and Statistical Manual of Mental Disorders*, 4th ed. Washington, DC: American Psychiatric Press; 1994:458–462.

40. King SA, Stain JJ. Revising the category of somatoform pain disorder. *Hospital Community Psychiatry*. 1992;43:217–219.

41. American Psychiatric Association. *Diagnostic and Statistical Manual of Mental Disorders*, 5th ed. Washington, DC: American Psychiatric Press; 2015.

42. Peppin JF, Cheatle MD, Kirsh KL, McCarberg BH. The complexity model: a novel approach to improve chronic pain care. *Pain Med*. 2015;16:653–666.

43. Christo P, Fudin J, Gudin J. *Opioid Prescribing and Monitoring: How to Combat Opioid Abuse and Misuse Responsibly*. Montclair, NJ: Vertical Health, LLC; 2016.

44. Hjermstad MJ, Fayers PM, Haugen DF, et al. Studies comparing numerical rating scales, verbal rating scales, and visual analogue scales for assessment of pain intensity in adults: a systematic literature review. *J Pain Symptom Manage*. 2011;41:1073–1093.

45. Edwards LC, Pearce SA, Turner-Stokes L, Jones A. The Pain Beliefs Questionnaire: an investigation of beliefs in the causes and consequences of pain. *Pain*. 1992;51:267–272.

46. Williams RC. Toward a set of reliable and valid measures for chronic pain assessment and outcome research. *Pain*. 1988;35:239–251.

47. Daut RL, Cleeland CS, Flanery RC. Development of the Wisconsin Brief Pain Questionnaire to assess pain in cancer and other diseases. *Pain*. 1983;17:197–210.

48. Cleeland CS, Ryan KM. The Brief Pain Inventory. https://www.mdanderson.org/education-andresearch/departments-programs-and-labs/departments-and-divisions/symptom-research/symptomassessment-tools/BPI_UserGuide. Pdf. Accessed May 29, 2017.

49. Scott J, Huskisson EC. Graphic representation of pain. *Pain*. 1976;2:175–184.

50. Melzak R. The McGill Pain Questionnaire: major properties and scoring methods. *Pain*. 1975;1:277–299.

51. Reading AE, Everitt BS, Sledmere CM. The McGill Pain Questionnaire: a replication of its construction. *Br J Clin Psychol*. 1982;21:339–349.

52. Kerns RD, Turk DC, Rudy TE. The West Haven-Yale Multidimensional Pain Inventory (WHYMPI). *Pain*. 1985;23:345–356.

53. Matusitz J, Spear J. Effective doctor–patient communication: an updated examination. *Social Work in Public Health*. 2014;29:252–266.

54. Robinson ME, Staud R, Price DD. Pain measurement and brain activity: will neuroimages replace pain ratings? *J Pain*. 2013;14:323–327.

55. Kroenke K. Patients presenting with somatic complaints: epidemiology, psychiatric comorbidity and management. *Int J Methods Psychiatr Res*. 2003;12:34–43.

56. Khouzam HR. Psychopharmacology of chronic pain: a focus on antidepressants and atypical antipsychotics. *Postgrad Med*. 2016;128:323–330.

57. Simon GE, VonKorff M, Piccinelli M, et al. An international study of the relation between somatic symptoms and depression. *N Engl J Med*. 1999;341(18):1329–1335.

58. Gatchel RJ. Psychological disorders and chronic pain: cause and effect relationships. In: Gatchel RJ, Turk DC, eds. *Psychological Approaches to Pain Management: A Practitioner' s Handbook*. New York: Guilford Publications; 1996:33–54.

59. Clouston TS. *Clinical Lectures on Mental Diseases. Lecture III: States of Mental Depression-Melancholia (Psychalgia)*. Philadelphia: Henry C. Lea's Son & Co.; 1884:90–122.

60. Sharp TJ, Harvey AG. Chronic pain and posttraumatic stress disorder: mutual maintenance? *Clin Psychol Rev*. 2001;21:857–877.

61. Gerrits MM, van Oppen P, van Marwijk HW, Penninx BW, van der Horst HE. Pain and the onset of depressive and anxiety disorders. *Pain*. 2014;155:53–59.

62. Gureje O, Von Korff M, Simon GE, Gater R. Persistent pain and well-being: a World Health Organization study in primary care. *JAMA*. 1998;280:147–151.

63. Emery PC, Wilson KG, Kowal J. Major depressive disorder and sleep disturbance in patients with chronic pain. *Pain Res Manage*. 2014;19:35–41.

64. Fasick V, Spengler RN, Samankan S, Nader ND, Ignatowski TA. The hippocampus and TNF: common links between chronic pain and depression. *Neurosci Biobehav Rev*. 2015;53:139–159.

65. McWilliams LA, Cox BJ, Enns MW. Mood and anxiety disorders associated with chronic pain: an examination in a nationally representative sample. *Pain*. 2003;106:127–133.

66. Kessler RC, Petukhova M, Samson NA, Zaslavsky AM, Wittchen H-U. Twelve-month and lifetime prevalence and lifetime morbid risk of anxiety and mood disorders in the United States. *Int J Methods Psychiatr Res*. 2012;21:169–184.

67. Symreng I, Fishman SM. Anxiety and pain. *Pain Clinical Updates*. 2004;XII(7). http://iasp.files.cmsplus.com/Content/ContentFolders/Publications2/PainClinicalUpdates/Archives/PCU04-7_1390264411970_28.pdf. Accessed March 29, 2017.

68. American Psychiatric Association. *Diagnostic and Statistical Manual of Mental Disorders*, 5th ed. Arlington, VA: American Psychiatric Association Publishing; 2013.

69. Watts BV, Schnurr PP, Mayo L, Young-Xu Y, Weeks WB, Friedman MJ. Meta-analysis of the efficacy of treatments for posttraumatic stress disorder. *J Clin Psychiatry*. 2013;74(6):e541–550.

70. Jeffreys M. *Clinician's Guide to Medications for PTSD*. http://www.ptsd.va.gov/professional/treatment/overview/clinicians-guide-to-medications-for-ptsd.asp. Accessed March 29, 2017.

71. Khouzam HR, Donnelly NJ. Posttraumatic stress disorder, safe, effective management in the primary care setting. *Postgrad Med*. 2001;110:60–78.

72. Choiniere M, Racine M, Raymond-Shaw I. Epidemiology of pain and sleep disturbances and their reciprocal interrelationships. In: Lavigne G, Sessle B, Choiniere M, Soja P, eds. *Sleep and Pain*. Seattle, WA: IASP Press; 2007:267–284.

73. Lavigne G, Sessle B, Choiniere M, Soja P, eds. *Sleep and Pain*. Seattle, WA: IASP Press; 2007.

74. Narouze S, Souzdalnitski D. Obesity and chronic pain: systematic review of prevalence and implications for pain practice. *Regional Anesthesia Pain Med*. 2015 Mar 1;40(2):91–111.

75. Prados-Torres A, Calderón-Larranaga A, Hancco-Saavedra J, Poblador-Plou B, van den Akker M. Multimorbidity patterns: a systematic review. *J Clin Epidemiol*. 2014;67:254–266.

76. Lydic R, Baghdoyan HA. Neurochemical mechanisms mediating opioid-induced REM sleep disruption. In: Lavigne G, Sessle B, Choiniere M, Soja P, eds. *Sleep and Pain*. Seattle, WA: IASP Press; 2007.

77. Sansone RA, Whitecar P, Meier BP, Murry A. The prevalence of borderline personality among primary care patients with chronic pain. *Gen Hosp Psychiatry*. 2001;23:193–197.

78. Manchikanti L, Pampati V, Beyer C, Damron K. Do number of pain conditions influence emotional status? *Pain Physician*. 2002;5:200–205.

79. Workman EA, Hubbard JR, Felker BL. Comorbid psychiatric disorders and predictors of pain management program success in patients with chronic pain. *J Clin Psychiatry*. 2002;4:137–140.

80. Sansone RA, Sinclair JD, Wiederman MW. Borderline personality among outpatients seen by a pain management specialist. *Int J Psychiatry Med*. 2009;39:341–344.

81. Fischer-Kern M, Kapusta ND, Doering S, et al. The relationship between personality organization and psychiatric classification in chronic pain patients. *Psychopathology*. 2011;44:21–26.

82. Tragesser SL, Bruns D, Disorbio JM. Borderline personality disorder features and pain: the mediating role of negative affect in a pain patient sample. *Clin J Pain*. 2010;26:348–353.

83. Sansone RA, Sansone LA. Chronic pain syndromes and borderline personality. *Innovations Clin Neurosci*. 2012;9:10–14.

84. Pharmacists Recovery Network. usaprn.org. Accessed May 30, 2017.

85. Klipa D, Russeau JC. Pain and its management. In: Koda-Kimble MA, Young LY, Alldredge BK, et al, eds. *Applied Therapeutics: The Clinical Use of Drugs*. Philadelphia: Lippincott Williams & Wilkins; 2009:8.1–8.36.

86. Barry DT, Cutter CJ, Beitel M, Kerns RD, Liong C, Schottenfeld RS. Psychiatric disorders among patients seeking treatment for co-occurring chronic pain and opioid use disorder. *J Clin Psychiatry*. 2016;77:1413–1419.

87. Flannery B, Newlin D. Alcohol use disorders and their treatment. In: Smith HS, Passik SD, eds. *Pain and Chemical Dependency*. New York: Oxford University Press; 2008:131–136.

88. Norko MA, Lawrence Fitch W. DSM-5 and substance use disorders: clinicolegal implications. *J Am Acad Psychiatry Law*. 2014;42:443–452.

89. Khouzam HR. Help your patients beat cocaine addiction. The four dimensions of treatment. *Postgrad Med*. 1999;105:185–191.

90. Webster LR, Cochella S, Dasgupta N, et al. An analysis of the root causes for opioid-related overdose deaths in the United States. *Pain Med*. 2011;12(S2):S26–35.

91. Jones JD, Mogali S, Comer SD. Polydrug abuse: a review of opioid and benzodiazepine combination use. *Drug Alcohol Depend*. 2012;125:8–18.

92. Khouzam HR. Psychiatry residents' opinions of a substance abuse rotation in a VA hospital general internal medicine unit. *Substance Abuse*. 2000;21:149–154.

93. Moayedi M, Davis KD. Theories of pain: from specificity to gate control. *J Neurophysiol*. 2012;109: 5–12.

94. Melzack R, Wall PD. Pain mechanisms: a new theory. *Surv Anesthesiol*. 1967;11:89–90.

95. Duncan G. Mind-body dualism and the biopsychosocial model of pain: what did Descartes really say? *J Med Philosophy*. 2000;25:485–513.

96. Khouzam HR, Kissmeyer P. Antidepressant treatment, posttraumatic stress disorder, survivor guilt and spiritual awakening. *J Traumatic Stress*. 1997;10:691–696.

97. Apkarian AV, Sosa Y, Krauss BR, Thomas PS. Chronic pain patients are impaired on an emotional decision-making task. *Pain*. 2004;108:129–136.

98. Society for Neuroscience. News release: Feelings of hope create striking brain effects that could help alleviate serious afflictions like pain, Parkinson's disease, and depression; researchers' report. 2005. http://www.sfn.org/Press-Room/News-Release-Archives/2005/FEELINGS-OF-HOPE?returnId=%7B0C16364F-DB22-424A-849A-B7CF6FDCFE35%7D. Accessed May 31, 2017.

99. Wager TD, Rilling JK, Smith EE, et al. Placebo-induced changes in FMRI in the anticipation and experience of pain. *Science*. 2004;303;1162–1167.

100. Turk DC, Gatchel RJ. *Psychological Approaches to Pain Management: A Practitioner's Handbook*. 2nd ed. New York: Guilford Press. 2002.

101. Leeuw M, Goossens ME, Linton SJ, et al. The fear-avoidance model of musculoskeletal pain: current state of scientific evidence. *J Behav Med*. 2007;30:77–94.

102. Crombez G, Eccleston C, Van Damme S, Vlaeyen JW, Karoly P. Fear-avoidance model of chronic pain: the next generation. *Clin J Pain*. 2012;28:475–483.

103. Khouzam HR. Chronic pain and its management in primary care. *South Med J*. 2000;93:946–952.

104. Phillips H. How life shapes the brainscape. https://www.newscientist.com/article/mg18825274-900-how-life-shapes-the-brainscape/. Accessed May 31, 2017.

105. Benedetti F, Mayberg HS, Wager TD, Stohler CS, Zubieta JK. Neurobiological mechanisms of the placebo effect. *J Neurosci*. 2005;25:10390–10402.

106. Thoma N, Pilecki B, McKay D. Contemporary cognitive behavior therapy: a review of theory, history, and evidence. *Psychodynamic Psychiatry*. 2015;43:423–461.

107. Morley S, Williams A. New developments in the psychological management of chronic pain. *Can J Psychiatry*. 2015;60:168–175

108. Yu L, McCracken LM. Model and processes of acceptance and commitment therapy (ACT) for chronic pain including a closer look at the self. *Current Pain Headache Rep*. 2016;20:1–7.

109. Jayaseelan DJ, Post AA, Mischke JJ, Sault JD. Joint mobilization in the management of persistent insertional Achilles tendinopathy: a case report. *Int J Sports Phys Ther*. 2017;12:133–143.

110. Garschagen A, Steegers MA, Bergen AH, et al. Is there a need for including spiritual care in interdisciplinary rehabilitation of chronic pain patients? Investigating an innovative strategy. *Pain Pract*. 2015;15:671–687.

111. Taylor LE, Stotts NA, Humphreys J, Treadwell MJ, Miaskowski C. A biopsychosocial-spiritual model of chronic pain in adults with sickle cell disease. *Pain Manage Nurs*. 2013;14:287–301.

112. Balestrieri M, Williams P, Wilkinson G. Specialist mental health treatment in general practice: a meta-analysis. *Psychol Med*. 1988;18:711–717.

113. Byrne ZS, Hochwarter WA. "I get by with a little help from my friends": the interaction of chronic pain and organizational support on performance. *J Occup Health Psychol*. 2006;11:215–227.

114. Von Korff M, Moore JE, Lorig K, et al. A randomized trial of a layperson-led self-management group intervention for back pain patients in primary care. *Spine (Phila Pa 1976)*. 1998;23:2608–2615.

115. Brown C, Schulberg HC. The efficacy of psychosocial treatments in primary care. A review of randomized clinical trials. *Gen Hosp Psychiatry*. 1995;17:414–424.

116. Kingree JB. Twelve-step facilitation therapy. In: Miller PE, ed. *Interventions for Addiction: Comprehensive Addictive Behaviors and Disorders*. Vol. 3. Amsterdam: Academic Press; 2013:137–146.

117. Carleton RN, Abrams MP, Asmundson GJ, Antony MM, McCabe RE. Pain-related anxiety and anxiety sensitivity across anxiety and depressive disorders. *J Anxiety Disord*. 2009;23:791–798.

118. Hembree EA, Rauch SA, Foa EB. Beyond the manual: the insider's guide to prolonged exposure therapy for PTSD. *Cognitive Behav Pract*. 2004;10:22–30.

119. Jackson CE, Green JD, Bovin MJ, et al. Mild traumatic brain injury, PTSD, and psychosocial functioning among male and female US OEF/OIF Veterans. *J Traumatic Stress*. 2016;29:309–316.

120. Barry DT, Cutter CJ, Beitel M, Kerns RD, Liong C, Schottenfeld RS. Psychiatric disorders among patients seeking treatment for co-occurring chronic pain and opioid use disorder. *J Clin Psychiatry*. 2016;77:1413–1419.

121. Beitel M, Oberleitner L, Kahn M, et al. Drug counselor responses to patient pain reports: a qualitative investigation of barriers and facilitators to treating patients with chronic pain in methadone maintenance treatment. *Pain Med*. 2017;18(11):2152–2161.

122. Peterson BD, Pincus HA, Suarez A, Zarin DA. Datapoints: referrals to psychiatrists. *Psychiatr Serv*. 1998;49:449.

123. Von Korff M. Pain management in primary care: an individualized stepped-care approach. In: Gatchel RJ, Turk DC, eds. *Psychosocial Factors in Pain*. New York: Guilford Press; 1999:360–373.

124. Sobell MB, Sobell LC. Stepped care as a heuristic approach to the treatment of alcohol problems. *J Consult Clin Psychol*. 2000;68:573–579.

125. Dorflinger L, Moore B, Goulet J, et al. A partnered approach to opioid management, guideline concordant care and the stepped care model of pain management. *J Gen Intern Med*. 2014;29:870–876.

126. Dorflinger LM, Ruser C, Sellinger J, Edens EL, Kerns RD, Becker WC. Integrating interdisciplinary pain management into primary care: development and implementation of a novel clinical program. *Pain Med*. 2014;15:2046–2054.

127. Katon W, Robinson P, Von Korff M, et al. A multifaceted intervention to improve treatment of depression in primary care. *Arch Gen Psychiatry*. 1996;53:924–932.

128. Accreditation Council for Graduate Medical Education. ACGME Program Requirements for Graduate Medical Education in Pain Medicine. https://www.acgme.org/Portals/0/PFAssets/ProgramRequirements/530_pain_medicine_2016_1-YR.pdf. Accessed May 29, 2017.

129. American Board of Psychiatry and Neurology. https://www.abpn.com/become-certified/taking-a-subspecialty-exam/pain-medicine/ Accessed May 26 2017.

130. Saarto T, Wiffen PJ. Antidepressants for neuropathic pain. *Cochrane Database Syst Rev*. 2005;(3):CD005454.

131. Häuser W, Walitt B, Fitzcharles MA, Sommer C. Review of pharmacological therapies in fibromyalgia syndrome. *Arthritis Res Ther*. 2014;16:201.

132. Fabrazzo M, Tortorella A. Safety and tolerability of mood stabilizers. In: Spina E, Trifiro G, eds. *Pharmacovigilance in Psychiatry*. New York: Springer International Publishing; 2016:209–232.

133. Moore RA, Wiffen PJ, Derry S, McQuay HJ. Gabapentin for chronic neuropathic pain and fibromyalgia in adults. *Cochrane Database Syst Rev*. 2011;Mar 16. 3:CD007938.

134. Gilron I, Wajsbrot D, Therrien F, Lemay J. Pregabalin for peripheral neuropathic pain: a multicenter, enriched enrollment randomized withdrawal placebo-controlled trial. *Clin J Pain*. 2011;27:185–193.

135. Stone MB. The FDA warning on antidepressants and suicidality—why the controversy? *N Engl J Med*. 2014;371:1668–1671.

CHAPTER 8

MANAGING PAIN IN PATIENTS WITH A HISTORY OF A SUBSTANCE USE DISORDER

Challenges and Opportunities

Martin D. Cheatle

INTRODUCTION

Patients with chronic pain tend to be complex and typically present with myriad medical and psychiatric comorbidities that can influence not only their pain experience, but also their response to therapeutic interventions and their quality of life. Common comorbidities include sleep disturbance, depression, anxiety, development of secondary medical problems due to inactivity, functional disabilities, cognitive distortions, and, in a subgroup of patients, substance misuse and abuse. The number of patients who suffer from persistent or recurrent pain is staggering. In 2011, the Institute of Medicine (IOM; now the National Academy of Medicine) reported that the annual cost of chronic pain in the United States is estimated to be between $560 and $600 billion (this figure includes the cost of healthcare and lost productivity).[1] It has been estimated that almost 30% of adults in the United States suffer from chronic or recurrent pain, and the prevalence of pain is on the rise worldwide.[2] The IOM report on pain emphasized that disablement from chronic pain affects not only individuals but also families and society. To put the magnitude of chronic pain in perspective, pain is significantly more prevalent than cancer, heart disease, and diabetes combined. Likewise, the cost of pain to America—billions of dollars—is almost quadruple that of heart disease.[1]

The IOM report[1] challenged policymakers, clinicians, and scientists with several guiding principles:

- Effective pain management is "a moral imperative."
- Pain should be considered a disease with distinct pathology.
- There is a need for interdisciplinary treatment approaches.
- There is a serious problem of diversion and abuse of opioid drugs.

PAIN AND OPIOID ABUSE

Over the past several decades, pain management has become a very opioid-focused model of care. This was developed for a number of reasons, including adopting a unidimensional and unimodal approach to pain treatment; the focus and marketing of the pharmaceutical industry; convenience on the part of clinicians; and generalizing the opioid model used in the end-of-life cancer population to those with pain of noncancer origin.[3] This precipitated a dramatic increase in opioid prescribing for a variety of nonmalignant pain conditions, which led to a significant surge in the misuse and abuse of prescription opioid analgesics. The number of prescription opioid–related fatalities and the number of admissions to treatment facilities for opioid use disorders paralleled the increase in the sales of opioid analgesics from 1999 to 2010. In 2011, 488,004 emergency department visits were related to nonmedical use of opioids,[4] and there were 186,986 admissions to treatment facilities for opioid use disorders.[5] There were 38,329 pharmaceutical-related deaths in the United States in 2010, of which 16,651 were related to opioids alone, or related to other drugs, most commonly benzodiazepines.[6]

DEVELOPMENT OF AN OPIOID USE DISORDER

There is a misconception that long-term exposure to opioids will eventually lead to the development of opioid abuse or an opioid use disorder. However, addiction is multifaceted. It represents a confluence of biologic and genetic predisposition, interacting with the environment and the actual properties of the drug, filtered through brain mechanisms, and not just related to exposure over time. The issue of pain and substance use disorders is equally complex. Often patients with pain disorders have co-occurring psychiatric disorders; this is also very common in patients with substance use disorders. The drug's qualities, in terms of its tranquilizing effects and how rapidly it passes the blood–brain barrier, also interact with these factors.

Clinicians who care for patients with pain are faced with a very daunting treatment dichotomy. In a subgroup of patients with chronic nonmalignant pain, opioids can be extremely effective in reducing pain and improving function, mood, and general quality of life. However, another subgroup of patients with chronic pain, when exposed to opioids, can misuse or abuse opioids; in combination with their chronic pain, this can be devastating with respect to their quality of life.

PREVALENCE OF OPIOID ABUSE IN PATIENTS WITH CHRONIC PAIN

It has been estimated that 3% to 62% of patients with chronic nonmalignant pain who are prescribed long-term opioid therapy exhibit what is termed "problematic drug-taking behaviors."[7-10] These behaviors can include doctor shopping, requesting early refills, making multiple phone calls to the clinic regarding opioid therapy, frequenting the emergency department, lost prescriptions, and so forth. These behaviors are not necessarily markers for the development of an opioid use disorder but may reflect undertreatment of pain or what is called "chemical coping,"[11] where patients are using the opioids for self-treatment of their anxiety or mood disorders because opioids can have strong anxiolytic and antidepressant effects. Likewise, the estimated prevalence of substance use disorders in patients with chronic pain ranges from less than 1% to more than 40%.[12-16] These wide estimates reflect the complexity in rendering an accurate diagnosis in this population and is related to varying definitions of misuse, abuse, or substance use disorder.

An expert panel from ACTTION (Analgesic, Anesthetic, and Addiction Clinical Trials, Translations, Innovations, Opportunities, and Networks) completed a systematic review of the literature and made recommendations regarding the definition of misuse, abuse, and related events in opioid therapy.[17] This panel found significant limitations to the ICD-10 and DSM-IV-TR definitions of misuse and abuse. The panel recommended that *misuse* be defined as using a prescribed medication for the purpose for which it was therapeutically intended, but not as directed (e.g., a patient is prescribed two hydrocodone pills per day but uses three instead for pain relief and runs out early). *Abuse* is defined as using a therapeutic agent for a purpose for which it was not therapeutically intended (e.g., using an opioid to induce sleep, to reduce anxiety, to improve mood, or to obtain some type of euphoric state). *Addiction*, or what we now call substance use disorder, would include specific characteristics such as craving the use of an opioid for non–pain-relieving effects, losing control over medication use, incurring negative consequences from use, and using the medication compulsively despite the ensuing harm.

Several recent studies attempted to accurately assess the prevalence of opioid use disorder in patients with chronic noncancer pain receiving opioid therapy. One study by Boscarino et al.[15] used the DSM-5 criteria for diagnosing opioid use disorder in a large cohort of patients with chronic noncancer pain receiving opioid therapy. The prevalence of lifetime opioid use disorder was 34.9%; 21.7% of the group met criteria for moderate opioid use disorder, and 13.2% for severe opioid use disorder. In a subsequent study by the same group again employing the more sensitive DSM-5 criteria in another cohort of patients with chronic noncancer pain receiving long-term opioid therapy, an estimated 41.3% met criteria for a lifetime prevalence of any opioid use disorder.[16] In an older study, Jamison et al.[18] interviewed 248 patients at a methadone maintenance treatment program. Over 60% reported that they experienced chronic pain as a primary medical condition. The patients with pain reported more health problems and significant psychiatric comorbidities, and a history of prescription and nonprescription medication use. Forty-four percent of this population believed that being prescribed opioids for their pain contributed to the development of their substance use disorder. Vowles et al.[19] completed a systematic review of studies that assessed the rate of opioid misuse, abuse, and addiction in patients with chronic nonmalignant pain. The authors used the ACTTION[17] and IMMPACT (Initiative on Methods, Measurement, and Pain Assessment in Clinical Trials)[20] definitions of misuse, abuse, and addiction and calculated weighted separate means for low- and high-quality studies to address variability between studies. They estimated that misuse was present in 21.7% to 29.3% of the patients studied and opioid use disorder in 7.8% to 11.7%.

Volkow and McLellan,[21] in a recent review article, outlined a number of myths about opioids and addiction that were derived from questions submitted by physicians to the websites of the American Pain Society and the American Academy of Pain Management (now the Academy of Integrative Pain Management). These included the following:

- "Addiction is the same as physical dependence and tolerance."
- "Addiction is simply a set of bad choices."
- "Pain protects patients from addiction to their opioid medications."
- "Only long-term use of certain opioids produces addiction."
- "Only patients with certain characteristics are vulnerable to addiction."
- "Medication-assisted therapies are just substitutes for heroin or opioids."

Adhering to these misconceptions could lead clinicians to either underprescribe opioids to appropriate individuals, causing unneeded suffering, or overprescribe certain potentially high-risk opioids, contributing to the development of iatrogenic addiction. No class of opioids is "low risk," and no patient exposed to opioids is at no risk of misusing or abusing opioids. Volkow and McLellan concluded that "Addiction occurs in only a small percentage of persons exposed to opioids—even among those with preexisting vulnerabilities." They estimated that the rate of addiction, based on higher-quality studies, averaged less than 8%. However, given the high prevalence of chronic or recurrent pain in adults in the United States (approximately 100 million) and the fact that a substantial subset of this population is being prescribed opioids, even a rate of addiction of 8% to 11% is not inconsequential.

MANAGING PAIN IN THE PATIENT WITH PAIN AND A CO-OCCURRING OPIOID USE DISORDER

An effective treatment program for patients with chronic pain and a co-occurring opioid use disorder should be multimodal (Fig. 8.1) and should include psychological treatments, appropriate adjunctive pharmacologic agents, restorative exercise, and, in a subgroup of patients, medication-assisted therapy (MAT).

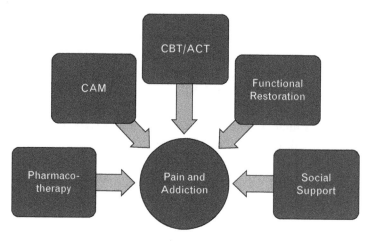

FIGURE 8.1 Multimodal approach to managing pain in a patient with addiction

PSYCHOSOCIAL AND COMPLEMENTARY AND ALTERNATIVE MEDICINE INTERVENTIONS

A number of psychosocial and complementary and alternative medicine (CAM) interventions can be helpful in treating patients who have a history of chronic pain and concomitant addiction. These include acupuncture, neurofeedback and biofeedback, massage therapy, 12-step programs, herbals, manipulation, mindfulness meditation, and yoga. These interventions have varying degrees of documented efficacy as it is difficult to perform randomized control trials, the gold standard for scientifically supported evidence-based practice. However, while a patient is in a period of recovery, these can provide pain relief and decrease the probability of a relapse. Two of the most widely employed psychosocial interventions for pain and addiction are 12-step programs and cognitive-behavioral therapy/acceptance and commitment therapy (CBT/ACT).

CBT/ACT

Individuals who suffer from pain often experience concomitant mood and anxiety disorders, as do those patients with a substance use disorder; it is likely that patients with both pain and a substance use disorder are particularly susceptible. Patients with chronic pain can engage in maladaptive behaviors (e.g., kinesiophobia, or fear of movement that will exacerbate pain; avoidance behaviors) and dysfunctional thinking patterns (e.g., catastrophizing, an irrational thought that a current or future situation is worse than it actually is). CBT is based on the assumptions that our emotions are related to self-talk and underlying beliefs and that when we are emotionally distressed our self-talk can become negative and irrational, thus perpetuating the negative affect. CBT includes a number of different strategies to help patients identify the maladaptive behaviors and/or dysfunctional thought patterns that may reduce their ability to adjust to and cope with their chronic pain.

The process of CBT typically involves specific skill acquisition—for example, mindfulness-based stress reduction, effective communication, cognitive restructuring, followed by skill consolidation, rehearsal, and relapse training.[22] Cognitive restructuring involves teaching patients to identify negative, dysfunctional thought patterns and to substitute more rational cognitions so they can reframe their view of pain. This encourages patients to be more proactive, rather than passive, and reinforces a sense of competence and self-efficacy.

CBT is cost-effective and has been demonstrated to be clinically efficacious/effective in a number of chronic pain disorders, including chronic low back pain,[23,24] arthritis,[25] lupus,[26] fibromyalgia,[27] and sickle cell disease.[28] For example, Bernardy et al.[29] performed a review of the effectiveness of CBT for fibromyalgia, a condition that is very refractory to various interventions. Twenty-three studies that met inclusion criteria with a total of 2,231 patients were evaluated. The CBT group was found to have superior results compared to groups receiving a control condition with respect to reducing negative mood, decreasing disability, and reducing pain, both at treatment completion and 6 months after treatment. There is also evidence that CBT not only improves mood and function in patients with fibromyalgia, but by reducing catastrophizing also can help to normalize pain-related brain responses in this population.[30]

A great deal of attention has been focused on the burgeoning rate of prescription opioid misuse/abuse and opioid-related fatalities. CBT can reduce the risk of misuse and abuse in high-risk patients on opioid therapy by improving sleep, anxiety, and mood disorders that can drive opioid misuse and also can enhance outcomes in patients with pain who have developed a substance use disorder. Morasco et al.[31] completed a pilot study examining the effectiveness of an eight-session integrated group CBT program for chronic pain and substance use disorder in patients infected with hepatitis C virus who had both chronic pain and a history of a substance use disorder. Results revealed an improvement in pain interference, reduction in cravings for alcohol and other substances, and a decrease in past-month alcohol and substance use. As in fibromyalgia, evidence is emerging that CBT not only alters dysfunctional thoughts and behaviors in patients with substance use disorder but also can normalize aberrant activity in the brain's reward circuitry and strengthen the brain's inhibitory control network, thus reducing craving and probability of relapse.[32]

ACT, a variation of CBT, is a directive and experiential type of therapy based on rational frame theory. The goal of ACT is to experience life mindfully and reinforce psychological flexibility. The core processes of ACT includes :contact with the present moment, self-as-context, defusion, acceptance, values, and committed action. ACT has been demonstrated to improve function in patients with pain both at the end of treatment and in the long term. Vowles et al.[33] evaluated the long-term outcome of a program of ACT in a cohort of patients with chronic pain. Three years after program completion, 64.8% of the patients had improved in physical and emotional functioning. ACT has also shown utility in treating substance use disorder compared to standard care.[34]

TWELVE-STEP PROGRAMS/SOCIAL SUPPORT

Twelve-step programs were first developed in 1935 with the goal to help individuals with alcohol use disorders maintain sobriety and reinforce abstinence. This concept was extended to include other substances of abuse, most notably narcotics. There is some anecdotal evidence that attending a 12-step program can reduce the rate of relapse; however, a 2006 Cochrane review[3] of 12-step programs in alcohol abuse concluded that there were no experimental studies demonstrating unequivocal support of the efficacy of these programs, as it has not been feasible to conduct randomized controlled trials with this type of intervention.[35] Despite the paucity of scientific evidence supporting efficacy, 12-step programs can offer a strong support system that may mitigate frequent relapses. One often-cited paper is by Dunbar and Katz,[36] who performed a retrospective review of a group of patients with chronic pain and a history of a substance use disorder exposed to opioid therapy. The patients who attended Alcoholics Anonymous or Narcotics Anonymous and had a good support system had a significantly lower rate of relapse. AA or NA might provide a source of support to individuals who otherwise do not have access to professional help or lack support in their life.

PHARMACOTHERAPY

While psychosocial interventions can be effective in reducing pain, improving function, and reducing the risk of opioid misuse/abuse or relapse, in a subgroup of patients with chronic pain who are susceptible to substance use disorder/relapse or those with a history of substance use disorder who cannot maintain sobriety, the careful use of appropriate adjunctive medications and analgesics (methadone, buprenorphine) may be necessary.

Two types of pharmacotherapy strategies may be helpful in managing both pain and substance use disorders adjunctive medications and MAT. The best course of treatment for patients who have chronic pain and an active opioid use disorder is to complete a medically supervised detoxification from opioids and then to use adjunctive medications for pain relief.

ADJUNCTIVE MEDICATIONS

Adjunctive medications include acetaminophen, nonsteroidal anti-inflammatories (NSAIDs), muscle relaxants, antidepressants, and antiepileptic drugs.

Acetaminophen is effective for noninflammatory pain and may be opioid-sparing; the long-term effects involving hepatotoxicity must be considered, especially with high daily doses.

NSAIDs have numerous side effects, related to the reduction of prostaglandin synthesis. Renal failure risk factors include preexisting glomerular disease, renal insufficiency, and states of effective volume depletion such as in congestive heart failure and cirrhosis, so it is best to avoid NSAIDs in these conditions. Other side effects include gastric toxicity, with an increased risk of bleeding in patients with a history of gastrointestinal problems (ulcers or bleeding), age greater than 60, high dose of NSAIDs, and concurrent use of glucocorticoids/anticoagulation therapy. NSAID use is also associated with an increased risk of myocardial infarction, stroke, heart failure, atrial fibrillation, and cardiovascular death, even in patients without a history of cardiovascular disease. In a meta-analysis, 280 trials of NSAIDs versus placebo and 474 trials of one NSAID versus another NSAID were examined. Results indicated that major vascular events were increased by one-third with use of selective COX-2 inhibitors (coxibs) or diclofenac and that ibuprofen also significantly increased major coronary events. Heart failure risk was doubled by all NSAIDs, and all NSAIDs increased gastrointestinal complications.[37] If NSAIDs are employed, they should be given at the lowest dose, in the lowest-risk patients, for the shortest amount of time.

There are a number of *muscle relaxants* available, most demonstrating similar efficacies. They should be used judiciously. For example, carisoprodol has a significant risk for abuse; dantrolene has a box warning for fatal hepatotoxicity; and tizanidine and chlorzoxazone can cause reversible hepatotoxicity, but this is rare.

The role of *antidepressants* in this setting may relate, in part, to the high prevalence of co-occurring depression and chronic pain. Improved mood may also improve the patient's perception of his or her pain and dysfunction. There is also evidence that tricyclic antidepressants and certain serotonin norepinephrine reuptake inhibitors (SNRIs) have analgesic properties, which may be related to modulating descending inhibitory pain pathways.

Antiepileptic drugs have been demonstrated to be the first-line agents for a myriad of neuropathic pain conditions (e.g., diabetic neuropathy, complex regional pain syndromes, chronic sciatica) and certain functional pain syndromes (e.g., fibromyalgia) and have also been employed in treating certain psychiatric disorders.

Use of these adjunctive medications alone or in combination can effectively manage pain in patients with a concomitant opioid use disorder, reducing the risk for relapse due to inadequate pain control. For example, in fibromyalgia, tricyclic antidepressants, SNRIs, and antiepileptic drugs have been shown to reduce pain, improve sleep, and lessen fatigue[38–39,40] and to improve comorbid mood and anxiety disorders.[41] In chronic low back pain, prevailing guidelines suggest use of NSAIDs and acetaminophen along with tricyclics as first-line pharmacologic options.[42] In the case of neuropathic pain conditions, antiepileptic drugs such as pregabalin and gabapentin have been shown to manage pain, and there is also evidence of efficacy from SNRIs.[43] There is some evidence that certain herbal medicines can relieve back pain, but this area of research requires additional well-controlled trials.[44] Other nonopioid adjunctive medication options include capsaicin cream and topical salicylates, or lidocaine patches.

MEDICATION-ASSISTED THERAPY

When patients are being considered for MAT, there are three options: methadone, buprenorphine, and naltrexone.

METHADONE

Methadone, a full mu-opioid agonist, blocks the N-methyl-D-aspartate receptor as well as monoamine reuptake, which may explain its efficacy in treating neuropathic pain disorders. The pharmacokinetic and pharmacodynamics effects of methadone have advantages over other opioids in that methadone is naturally long-acting and the development of tolerance is slow, thus potentially allowing lower dosing in the long term in nonaddicted pain patients. Patients on methadone maintenance therapy for an opioid use disorder who experience chronic pain will require higher dosing. Special precautions must be used when considering methadone, such as assessing via an electrocardiogram the patient's potential to have QT prolongation (torsades de pointes) and obstructive and central sleep apnea.[45] Methadone has a variable half-life from 8 to 130 hours but an analgesic effect of 4 to 8 hours. This can lead to an unpredictable buildup of methadone, which can increase the risk of unintentional overdose.[45–47] Prescribing methadone for pain does not require a special license from the US Drug Enforcement Administration; that is required only when it is being prescribed for substance use disorders.

BUPRENORPHINE FORMULATIONS

Buprenorphine, a partial mu-opioid agonist, has antagonist effects at the kappa receptors. The agonist effect on the mu-opioid receptor produces the analgesia, while the strong affinity at the kappa receptors reduces the abuse liability. Buprenorphine has been a highly effective treatment for opioid use disorder and as an alternative to methadone; it has been postulated as a relatively lower-risk medication compared to methadone in patients with pain and co-occurring opioid use disorder.[48] There is also some literature suggesting that buprenorphine can act as an antidepressant[49] and reduce suicidal ideation,[50] both of which are common in patients with pain and in patients with a substance use disorder (see below).

Buprenorphine comes in two forms: buprenorphine in combination with naloxone and buprenorphine alone. Both formulations have been approved for office-based opioid dependency treatment (which requires special certification), and certain formulations have been approved for on-label use for pain (which does not require a special license). Buprenorphine was originally developed as an injectable formulation used as a primary analgesic but was used off-label for the treatment of opioid withdrawal in heroin-dependent hospitalized patients.

Buprenorphine transmucosal film has been formulated in conjunction with naloxone and is indicated for the treatment of opioid dependence. It is used for heroin or other opioid use disorder, both for induction and maintenance therapy. A buprenorphine sublingual tablet has been approved for opioid use disorder with a particular focus on the induction phase of treatment. It has been used off-label for the treatment of chronic pain. Two newer formulations approved for management of moderate to severe pain are a transdermal patch and a buccal film indicated for the management of pain requiring around-the-clock, long-term opioid treatment. Finally, buprenorphine implants have been approved by the US Food and Drug Administration, and in recently available is a monthly subcutaneous injection for all treatment phases of opioid use disorder, from induction through maintenance. The effect of these latest delivery systems on pain has yet to be explored.

Naltrexone for extended-release injectable suspension has been effective for the treatment of opioid and alcohol use disorders. There is some emerging literature that low-dose oral naltrexone has been effective as an anti-inflammatory agent in reducing chronic pain[51] and in treating fibromyalgia.[52]

PAIN, SUBSTANCE USE DISORDERS, AND SUICIDE

There is robust evidence that there is a high prevalence of suicidal ideation in patients with pain.[53–56] A systematic review by Tang and Crane[57] revealed that the risk of successful suicide was doubled in patients with chronic pain as compared to controls. There is also very persuasive evidence that suicidal ideation and behavior is prevalent in patients with substance use disorders: (1) approximately 40% of patients seeking treatment for substance use disorders report a history of suicide attempts compared to the general population, (2) patients with alcohol use disorders are almost 10 times more likely to die by suicide, and (3) those who inject drugs are about 14 times more likely to commit suicide compared to the general population.[58–61]

Clinicians must remember that the vast majority of patients with chronic pain and patients with pain and substance use disorder are likely to have suicidal ideation. Appropriate screening should be conducted on a routine basis, and every clinic should develop an action plan to intervene if patients are actively suicidal.[62]

BARRIERS TO CARE

It has been well documented that interdisciplinary pain care is the most clinically and economically efficacious approach to managing patients with complex pain disorders and rarely causing iatrogenic complications.[63] The number of interdisciplinary pain centers in the United States has dwindled over the last decade, however, mostly due to changes in reimbursement.[64] Also, there is a mismatch between the number of adults in the United States who live with chronic pain (approximately 100 million)[2] and the number of board-certified pain clinicians (approximately 5,000); thus, the majority of patients with pain are being managed by primary care practitioners, who typically have a paucity of training in either pain or addiction.[65,66]

The Centers for Disease Control and Prevention's recent "Guidelines for Prescribing Opioids for Chronic Pain"[67] offers multiple recommendations for prescribing opioids. It states that "nonpharmacologic and non-opioid pharmacologic therapy are preferred for chronic pain." In practice, however, most individuals with chronic pain cannot afford or do not have access to these nonpharmacologic therapies (e.g., CBT/ACT, physical therapy, acupuncture).

CONCLUSION

Patients who suffer from both chronic pain and substance use disorders are exceedingly complex and present with numerous psychiatric and medical comorbidities. Ideally these patients would have access to a multimodal approach that would include appropriate pharmacotherapy, adjunctive medication and/or MAT targeting both pain and addiction, use of complementary and alternative medicine interventions, appropriate psychological interventions such as CBT and ACT, a program of functional restoration when appropriate, and maximizing social support through AA, NA, or other community resources. In practice, most of these therapies are not available to the majority of patients. Opioid misuse/abuse and diversion and undertreatment of pain and substance use disorders will continue until there is a fundamental change in the training of clinicians in pain medicine and addiction medicine, and value-based reimbursement for a holistic and evidence-based approach to pain and substance use disorders.[68] With the current national focus on the epidemic of opioid misuse and abuse and opioid-related fatalities, there is an opportunity to enact meaningful change in our training of future healthcare providers and in the delivery of pain and addiction treatment.

ACKNOWLEDGMENTS

MDC would like to acknowledge the support from Grant 1R01DA032776-01 from the National Institute on Drug Abuse, National Institutes of Health in the writing of this manuscript.

REFERENCES

1. Institute of Medicine. *Relieving Pain in America: A Blueprint for Transforming Prevention, Care, Education, and Research*. Washington, DC: National Academies Press; 2011.

2. Tsang AM, Von Korff S, Lee J, et al. Common chronic pain conditions in developed and developing countries: gender and age differences and comorbidity with depression-anxiety disorders. *J Pain*. 2008; 9(10):883–891.

3. Peppin JF, Cheatle MD, Kirsh K, McCarberg W. The complexity model: a novel approach to improve chronic pain care. *Pain Med*. 2015;16(4):653–666.

4. Substance Abuse and Mental Health Services Administration, Drug Abuse Warning Network, 2011: National Estimates of Drug-Related Emergency Department Visits. HHS Publication No. (SMA) 13-4760, DAWN Series D-39. Rockville, MD: Substance Abuse and Mental Health Services Administration; 2013.

5. Substance Abuse and Mental Health Services Administration, Center for Behavioral Health Statistics and Quality. *Treatment Episode Data Set (TEDS): 2001–2011. National Admissions to Substance Abuse Treatment Services*. BHSIS Series S-65, HHS Publication No. (SMA) 13-4772. Rockville, MD: Substance Abuse and Mental Health Services Administration; 2013.

6. Jones CM, Mack KA, Paulozzi LJ. Pharmaceutical overdose deaths, United States, 2010. *JAMA.* 2013;309(7):657–659.

7. Katz N, Sherburne S, Beach M, Rose RJ, et al. Behavioral monitoring and urine toxicology testing in patients receiving long-term opioid therapy. *Anesth Analg.* 2003;97(4):1097–1102.

8. Ballantyne JC, LaForge KS. Opioid dependence and addiction during opioid treatment of chronic pain. *Pain.* 2007;129(3):235–255.

9. Webster LR, Webster RM. Predicting aberrant behaviors in opioid-treated patients: preliminary validation of the Opioid Risk Tool. *Pain Med.* 2005;6:432–442.

10. Fleming M, Davis J, Passik S. Reported lifetime aberrant drug-taking behaviors are predictive of current substance use and mental health problems in primary care patients. *Pain Med.* 2008;9(8):1098–1106.

11. Passik SD, Kirsh KL. Chemical coping: the clinical middle ground. In: Smith HS, Passik SD eds. *Pain and Chemical Dependency.* New York: Oxford University Press; 2008:299–302.

12. Ives TJ, Chelminski PR, Hammett-Stabler CA, et al. Predictors of opioid misuse in patients with chronic pain: a prospective cohort study. *BMC Health Serv Res.* 2006;6:46.

13. Fishbain DA, Cole B, Lewis J, Rosomoff HI, Rosomoff RS. What percentage of chronic nonmalignant pain patients exposed to chronic opioid analgesic therapy develop abuse/addiction and/or aberrant drug-related behaviors? A structured evidence-based review. *Pain Med.* 2008;9:444–459.

14. Martell BA, O'Connor PG, Kerns RD, et al. Systematic review: opioid treatment for chronic back pain: prevalence, efficacy, and association with addiction. *Ann Intern Med.* 2007;146(2):116–127.

15. Boscarino JA, Rukstalis MR, Hoffman SN, et al. Prevalence of prescription opioid-use disorder among chronic pain patients: comparison of the DSM-5 vs. DSM-4 diagnostic criteria. *J Addict Dis.* 2011;30(3):185–194.

16. Boscarino JA, Hoffman SN, Han JJ. Opioid-use disorder among patients on long-term opioid therapy: impact of final DSM-5 diagnostic criteria on prevalence and correlates. *Subst Abuse Rehabil.* 2015;6:83–91.

17. Jamison RN, Kauffman J, Katz NP. Characteristics of methadone maintenance patients with chronic pain. *J Pain Symptom Manage.* 2000;19(1):53–62.

18. Smith SM, Dart RC, Katz NP, et al. Classification and definition of misuse, abuse, and related events in clinical trials: ACTTION systematic review and recommendations. *Pain.* 2013;154(11):2287–2296.

19. Vowles KE, McEntee ML, Julnes PS, Frohe T, Ney JP, van der Goes DN. Rates of opioid misuse, abuse, and addiction in chronic pain: a systematic review and data synthesis. *Pain.* 2015;156(4):569–576.

20. O'Connor AB, Turk DC, Dworkin RH, et al. Abuse liability measures for use in analgesic clinical trials in patients with pain: IMMPACT recommendations. *Pain.* 2013;154:2324–2334.

21. Volkow ND, McLellan AT. Opioid abuse in chronic pain—misconceptions and mitigation strategies. *N Engl J Med.* 2016;374(13):1253–1263.

22. Turk DC, Flor H. Etiological theories and treatments for chronic back pain. II. Psychological models and interventions. *Pain.* 1984;19(3):209–233.

23. Lamb SE, Hansen Z, Lall R, Castelnuovo E, Withers EJ, Nichols V. Group cognitive behavioral treatment for low-back pain in primary care: A randomized controlled trial and cost-effectiveness analysis. *Lancet.* 2010;375:916–923.

24. Linton SJ. A 5-year follow-up evaluation of the health and economic consequences of an early cognitive behavioral intervention for back pain: a randomized, controlled trial. *Spine.* 2006;31(8):853–858.

25. Keefe FJ, Caldwell DS. Cognitive behavioral control of arthritis pain. *Med Clin North Am.* 1997;81:277–290.

26. Greco CM, Rudy TE, Manzi S. Effects of a stress-reduction program on psychological function, pain, and physical function of systemic lupus erythematosus patients: a randomized controlled trial. *Arthritis Rheum.* 2004;51(4):625–634.

27. Thieme K, Flor H, Turk D. Psychological pain treatment in fibromyalgia syndrome: efficacy of operant behavioral and cognitive behavioral treatments. *Arthritis Res Ther.* 2006;8(4):R121.

28. Chen E, Cole SW, Kato PM. A review of empirically supported psychosocial interventions for pain and adherence outcomes in sickle cell disease. *J Pediatr Psychol.* 2004;29:1997–2009.

29. Bernardy K, Klose P, Busch AJ, Choy EH, Häuser W. Cognitive-behavioural therapies for fibromyalgia. *Cochrane Database Syst Rev.* 2013;(9):CD009796.

30. Lazaridou A, Kim J, Cahalan CM, et al. Effects of cognitive-behavioral therapy (CBT) on brain connectivity supporting catastrophizing in fibromyalgia. *Clin J Pain.* 2017;33(3):215–221.

31. Morasco BJ, Greaves DW, Lovejoy TI, Turk DC, Dobscha SK, Hauser P. Development and preliminary evaluation of an integrated cognitive-behavior treatment for chronic pain and substance use disorder in patients with the hepatitis C virus. *Pain Med.* 2016;17(12):2280–2290.

32. Zilverstand A, Parvaz MA, Moeller SJ, Goldstein RZ. Cognitive interventions for addiction medicine: understanding the underlying neurobiological mechanisms. *Prog Brain Res.* 2016; 224:285–304.

33. Vowles KE, McCracken LM, O'Brien JZ. Acceptance and values-based action in chronic pain: a three-year follow-up analysis of treatment effectiveness and process. *Behav Res Ther.* 2011;49(11):748–755.

34. Lee EB, An W, Levin ME, Twohig MP. An initial meta-analysis of Acceptance and Commitment Therapy for treating substance use disorders. *Drug Alcohol Depend.* 2015;155:1–7.

35. Ferri M, Amato L, Davoli M. Alcoholics Anonymous and other 12-step programmes for alcohol dependence. *Cochrane Database Syst Rev.* 2006 Jul 19;(3):CD005032.

36. Dunbar SA, Katz NP. Chronic opioid therapy for nonmalignant pain in patients with a history of substance abuse: report of 20 cases. *J Pain Symptom Manage.* 1996;11(3):163–171.

37. Coxib and Traditional NSAID Trialists' (CNT) Collaboration. Vascular and upper gastrointestinal effects of non-steroidal anti-inflammatory drugs: meta-analyses of individual participant data from randomised trials. *Lancet.* 2013;382(9894):769–779.

38. Arnold LM, Rosen A, Pritchett YL, et al. A randomized, double-blind, placebo-controlled trial of duloxetine in the treatment of women with fibromyalgia with or without major depressive disorder. *Pain.* 2005;119(1–3):5–15.

39. Mease PJ, Clauw DJ, Arnold LM, et al. Fibromyalgia syndrome. *J Rheumatol.* 2005;32(11):2270–2277.

40. Arnold LM, Russell IJ, Diri EW, et al. A 14-week, randomized, double-blinded, placebo-controlled monotherapy trial of pregabalin in patients with fibromyalgia. *J Pain.* 2008;9(9):792–805.

41. Arnold LM. Management of fibromyalgia and comorbid psychiatric disorders. *J Clin Psychiatry.* 2008;69(Suppl 2):14–19.

42. Chou R. Pharmacological management of low back pain. *Drugs.* 2010;70(4):387–402.

43. Namaka M, Leong C, Grossberndt A, et al. A treatment algorithm for neuropathic pain: an update. *Consult Pharm.* 2009;24(12):885–902.

44. Gagnier JJ, Oltean H, van Tulder MW, Berman BM, Bombardier C, Robbins CB. Herbal medicine for low back pain: a Cochrane Review. *Spine (Phila Pa 1976).* 2016;41(2):116–133.

45. Cheatle MD, Webster LR. Opioid therapy and sleep disorders: risks and mitigation strategies. *Pain Med.* 2015;16(Suppl 1):S22–26.

46. Webster LR. Eight principles for safer opioid prescribing. *Pain Med.* 2013;14(7):959–961.

47. Webster LR, Cochella S, Dasgupta N, et al. An analysis of the root causes for opioid-related overdose deaths in the United States. *Pain Med.* 2011;12(Suppl 2):S26–35.

48. Heit HA, Gourlay DL. Buprenorphine: new tricks with an old molecule for pain management. *Clin J Pain.* 2008;24(2):93–97.

49. Sher L. Buprenorphine and the treatment of depression, anxiety, non-suicidal self-injury, and suicidality. *Acta Psychiatr Scand.* 2016;134(1):84–85.

50. Yovell Y, Bar G, Mashiah M, et al. Ultra-low-dose buprenorphine as a time-limited treatment for severe suicidal ideation: a randomized controlled trial. *Am J Psychiatry.* 2016;173(5):491–498.

51. Younger J, Parkitny L, McLain D. The use of low-dose naltrexone (LDN) as a novel anti-inflammatory treatment for chronic pain. *Clin Rheumatol*. 2014;33(4):451–459.

52. Younger J, Noor N, McCue R, Mackey S. Low-dose naltrexone for the treatment of fibromyalgia: findings of a small, randomized, double-blind, placebo-controlled, counterbalanced, crossover trial assessing daily pain levels. *Arthritis Rheum*. 2013;65(2):529–538.

53. Braden JB, Sullivan MD. Suicidal thoughts and behavior among adults with self-reported pain conditions in the national comorbidity survey replication. *J Pain*. 2008; 9:1106–1115.

54. Ilgen MA, Zivin K, McCammon RJ, Valenstein M. Pain and suicidal thoughts, plans and attempts in the United States. *Gen Hosp Psychiatry*. 2008; 30: 521–527.

55. Ratcliffe GE, Enns MW, Belik SL, Sareen J. Chronic pain conditions and suicidal ideation and suicide attempts: an epidemiologic perspective. *Clin J Pain*. 2008;24:204–210.

56. Cheatle M, Wasser T, Foster C, Olugbodi A, Bryan J. Prevalence of suicidal ideation in patients with chronic noncancer pain referred to a behaviorally based pain program. *Pain Physician*. 2014;17(3):E359–367.

57. Tang NK, Crane C. Suicidality in chronic pain: a review of the prevalence, risk factors and psychological links. *Psychol Med*. 2006;36:575–586.

58. Roy A, Janal MN. Risk factors for suicide among alcohol-dependent patients. *Arch Suicide Res*. 2007;11:211–217.

59. Roy A. Characteristics of cocaine dependent patients who attempt suicide. *Arch Suicide Res*. 2009;13:46–51.

60. Roy A. Risk factors for attempting suicide in heroin addicts. *Suicide Life Threat Behav*. 2010; 40:416–420.

61. Wilcox HC, Conner KR, Caine ED. Association of alcohol and drug use disorders and completed suicide: an empirical review of cohort studies. *Drug Alcohol Depend*. 2004;76:S11–S19.

62. Cheatle MD. Depression, chronic pain, and suicide by overdose: on the edge. *Pain Med*. 2011;12(Suppl 2):S43–48.

63. Gatchel RJ, McGeary DD, McGeary CA, Lippe B. Interdisciplinary chronic pain management: past, present, and future. *Am Psychol*. 2014;69(2):119–130.

64. Schatman ME. Interdisciplinary chronic pain management: international perspectives. *ISAP Pain Clinical Updates*. 2012;XX(7):1–5.

65. Upshur CC, Luckmann RS, Savageau JA. Primary care provider concerns about management of chronic pain in community clinic populations. *J Gen Intern Med*. 2006;21(6):652–655.

66. Breuer B, Cruciani R, Portenoy RK. Pain management by primary care physicians, pain physicians, chiropractors, and acupuncturists: a national survey. *South Med J*. 2010;103(8):738–747.

67. Dowell D, Haegerich TM, Chou R. CDC Guideline for prescribing opioids for chronic pain—United States, 2016. *MMWR Recomm Rep* 2016;65(No. RR-1):1–49.

68. Cheatle MD. Facing the challenge of pain management and opioid misuse, abuse and opioid-related fatalities. *Expert Rev Clin Pharmacol*. 2016;9(6):751–754.

CHAPTER 9

OPIOID PRESCRIBING IN STIGMATIZED AND SPECIAL POPULATIONS

Kelly K. Dineen

INTRODUCTION

Caring for patients who may benefit from prescription opioids—such as those with chronic pain or those being treated for substance use disorders—has always been a complicated endeavor.[1] Long before the recent public health concerns surrounding opioids, the treatment of patients with opioids was associated with myriad negative historical, educational, cultural, legal, and social biases.[2,3] In the current cultural context of the opioid crisis, balancing the benefits and burdens of therapy is more complex than ever. Providers face enhanced and forceful cultural, professional, and legal incentives to avoid opioid prescribing altogether. Public policy has shifted to privileging the risks of addiction over the risks of untreated pain; moreover, prescribers are arguably incentivized to privilege the potential harm to themselves or third parties over harm to their own patients.

The idea that removing prescription opioids from care will reduce or eliminate opioid-related harms is elegant in its simplicity but dangerous in its oversimplification. In fact, in some situations this position facilitates increased harm to patients in the form of secondary complex pain syndromes, complications from self-medication with alcohol and illicit substances, increased isolation and decreased functional ability, and even death from combined substances or suicide. There simply are some patients who benefit from opioids.[4,5]

Oversimplification is a recurrent theme in public discourse around opioids. All too often, concerns about the treatment of pain and the prevention and treatment of substance use disorders are considered dichotomous; patients with these conditions are treated as mutually exclusive groups with disparate interests. As one garners public and policy attention, the other is minimized and discounted. The public spotlight is either focused on "legitimate" or "deserving" patients in pain (e.g., the *Decade of Pain Control and Research*) or on the "victims" of substance use disorder (e.g., the opioid epidemic). This approach has only succeeded in alienating some portion of people in need of care. Sometimes, the more nuanced realities of clinical complexity escape public discourse.

This is not as simple as one or even two public health crises—the problems of neglected pain, substance use disorders, and comorbid mental health disorders are part of a relational web of social, cultural, political, legal, and clinical needs that are inadequately and inappropriately addressed. Patients with one or more of these conditions are legitimate patients in need of better acceptance, access, and treatment options. The false dichotomy that prioritizes one condition as more deserving only perpetuates stigmatization and provider avoidance of anyone associated with opioid use.

These and other oversimplifications in this area likely contribute to decision-making errors by healthcare providers. Work on reducing errors in the decision-making process in medicine is now mainstream in medicine.[6,7] Much of that work focuses of understanding the cognitive processes involved and correcting for cognitive and affective biases.[8] However, less work has focused on the role of decision-making errors in the treatment of patients with pain or substance use disorders. This chapter will provide an overview of these issues in the context of decisions about prescribing opioids for patients in select populations.

The primary focus of this chapter is on a few of the many special populations of patients prone to increased harm because of oversimplification and broad-brush approaches to the opioid crisis: (1) patients with sickle cell disease (SCD), (2) patients with life-limiting conditions receiving palliative or hospice care, and (3) patients in chronic pain for whom chronic opioid therapy may improve function. With patients in each of these populations, patient-centered care in the context of the particular patient is critical but often difficult for providers in the current environment.

Even before the full weight of the current opioid crisis, inequities in care based on gender, race, culture, socioeconomic status, and age as well as the resulting healthcare disparities were well documented. In particular, patients in the first three groups have long experienced discounting, stigmatization, disbelief, and even hostility from others, including providers.[9,10] They may now face additional barriers. For patients with SCD—who are predominantly but not exclusively black—existing stigma likely intersects powerfully with racial bias, exacerbating their marginalization and resulting healthcare disparities.[11] According to Keith Wailoo, "given the prevalence of sickle cell disease among black Americans, vexing questions of race and stigma have shadowed the history of its medical treatment."[12] For patients with life-limiting conditions, providers' presumptions and biases may remain despite their condition; on the other hand, providers may reflexively minimize the potential for opioid-related harms in this group. Finally, the small group of individuals with chronic pain who benefited from ongoing opioid therapy may suffer significant harms if providers reduce or eliminate opioids without clinical justification because of legal or professional pressures.

PROVIDER DECISION-MAKING

Decision-making is a complex part of social cognition that evolves through experience; however, sometimes we sacrifice accuracy for efficiency.[13,14] All of us are subject to errors in decision-making, and we all have biases that can contribute to decision-making errors. No one can avoid assimilating some of the negative attitudes that are communicated regularly in society—what sociologists refer to as "negative loading" in the cycle of stigmatization that imprints a negative connotation on a trait or characteristic.[15] Some biases are explicit; attitudes or beliefs held consciously about a group of people may cause providers to favor patients who fit into more socially desirable constructs.[16] More commonly, however, these biases are implicit:[17] they are "unconscious and involuntary attitudes which lie below the surface of consciousness, but can influence affect, behavior, and cognitive processes." Croskerry describes decisional errors rooted in biases as "predictable deviations from rationality." To understand how biases contribute to decision-making errors, I will provide an overview of the basic decision-making process.

Decision-making has been studied for decades by myriad disciplines. The most prevalent framework in medicine is the dual process theory,[18] which traces its roots to the foundational work of Tversky and Kahneman.[19] Under this theory, decisions roughly fall into one of two domains: type 1 (intuitive, unconscious, fast, efficient) and type 2 (analytical, conscious, methodical).[20] Both modes serve important purposes, and the ability to shift quickly between them is a critical clinical skill.[21] Type 1, the default mode, is highly efficient but more prone to error than type 2, which involves metacognition (thinking about thinking). In type 1, we use shortcuts or rules of thumb, also known as heuristics, that fill in parts of missing information with attribute substitution to make frugal decisions.[22]

Type 2 processing includes deliberate reasoning using analytic frameworks or checklists, or when learning a new skill.[23] It is more labor-intensive but less susceptible to error—although errors can still occur under conditions of cognitive strain such as fatigue, which may lead to mistakes in selecting the correct analytic framework.[24] Type 2 processing is also useful as a device to correct for errors that may occur using type 1 processing. This technique is used in healthcare routinely. The use of checklists and the requirement to physically mark the operative site before surgery are common examples.

Type 1 processing can be subdivided into two types—impressionistic thinking and insightful intuition.[25] Insightful intuition includes when a type 2 process becomes a type 1 process through repetition and experience; for example, learning the route to a new house may require metacognition, but when the route is traveled repeatedly, it becomes second nature. In the clinical context, learning emergency protocols requires labor and metacognition initially, but they become type 1 processes through practice and repeated use. Impressionistic thinking, on the other hand, is highly susceptible to the influence of biases and error.

A full review of cognitive biases and errors is outside the scope of this chapter, but the most common biases include confirmation bias (looking only for the information that confirms our initial impressions), anchoring bias (focusing all clinical efforts on the first diagnostic impression), availability bias (overestimating the probability of a condition based on salience), and visceral biases (irrational decisions guided by powerful emotions such as indignation, disgust, and anger).[26] Situations that exacerbate the potential for decision-making errors are common when caring for patients who use opioids, such as multiple comorbidities, uncertainty, or lack of familiarity with a patient.[27] Errors are also more common when patients are in groups that are stigmatized and prone to stereotyping,[28] as is the case with patients in pain. Those errors can lead to worsening health disparities. Any of these errors can contribute to a range of harms to patients. Croskerry et al. offer a comprehensive review of decision-making in medicine and "debiasing" strategies to reduce error.[29] Providers are encouraged to study this issue and adapt these debiasing practices, from building awareness, to seeking a second opinion, to simply considering the opposite.[29] These are especially important when treating patients in highly stigmatized groups, such as those with SCD.

SICKLE CELL DISEASE

SCD is an umbrella term for autosomal recessive genetic blood disorders designated by the presence of hemoglobin S, a structurally abnormal, rigid version of hemoglobin.[30,31] Hemoglobin S causes red blood cells to adopt a sickle shape, leading to anemia, acute vaso-occlusive crises (VOCs), chronic inflammation, and chronic organ dysfunction.[32] VOCs—common in joints, extremities, and the chest—are exceedingly painful and involve hypoxia and tissue ischemia (poor oxygen delivery and tissue damage) and inflammatory cascades.[33] Repeated ischemia and inflammation from VOCs, along with infection, anemia, and infarctions, lead to a range of life-threatening complications such as acute chest syndrome, stroke, multisystem organ failure, and avascular necrosis.[34]

An estimated 100,000 people in the United States live with SCD.[35] Most but not all of them are black—this is because SCD occurs in individuals whose ancestors were from malarial regions, such as sub-Saharan Africa.[36] The legacy of racial politics in the United States and the history of eugenics-based policies still pervade policy and care for SCD patients, especially for adults with SCD.[37,38] Few treatments have been approved for SCD— which is often attributed to the lower priority afforded a perceived "black disease"—and those that have been approved have shown inconsistent results across the population. Thus, providers caring for these patients should make a special effort to avoid decision-making errors that may be rooted in biases around race and the SCD diagnosis.[39]

The survival rate and life expectancy for patients with SCD have improved dramatically over the last 50 years, primarily because of newborn screening, preventive measures in childhood, and specialized pediatric clinics for SCD. The progress is not the same for adults, though: most patients with SCD do not live past their 50s.[40] In fact, many pediatric providers resist transferring their young adult patients to adult providers because of the decrease in quality of care reported by patients. These shortcomings are demonstrated by the high utilization of acute care and increased morbidity and mortality in 18- to 30-year-olds.

Adults with SCD have long experienced stigma, disbelief, and discounting by providers.[41,42] Providers rate patients with SCD as among their most challenging.[43,44] The mistrust of patients with SCD is particularly strong with respect to opioids. While most providers expend tremendous energy to be thoughtful and present with their patients, I have seen some providers' undisguised frustration and even hostility with patients with SCD.

This often took the form of disbelief when patients reported that certain medications, such as codeine or hydrocodone, were ineffective, or when they suggested particular medications had been historically effective for their pain. It was not uncommon for providers to use derogatory names and to assume that patients with SCD asking for opioids were "addicts." Such behaviors may indicate that providers are morally disengaged from their own mistreatment of patients. This mistreatment by some providers is echoed by the reported experiences of many patients with SCD.[45]

Research now supports the claim by many patients that certain opioid medications are truly ineffective in relieving their pain. Genetic polymorphisms common in patients with SCD can lead to altered perceptions of pain or responses to opioids. For example, many people with SCD have CYP enzyme variations that result in the rapid metabolism of or even inability to convert hydrocodone, codeine, and tramadol into active analgesics.[46,47] In one study, nearly 50% of the study group were affected by variations in the CYP enzymes. Other research reveals complex mechanisms underlying opioid response in this population. This research is an important reminder to providers that mutual trust and a presumption of patient honesty are critical to carry out the ethical and professional obligation of caregiving and to improve the quality of care.

ACUTE PAIN AND DISPARITIES IN THE EMERGENCY DEPARTMENT

Some of the greatest difficulty in communicating with providers and some of the greatest delays in providing appropriate care to patients with SCD occur in the emergency department (ED).[44,48] This is a critical problem because severe pain associated with a VOC is the most common reason people with SCD seek emergency care; it is also the most common reason for hospital admissions. Despite high-quality evidence and unambiguous clinical guidelines, treatment for VOC is delayed relative to patients with other painful diagnoses in the ED. These delays are perplexing and may well be the direct result of biased decision-making. The evidence-based consensus for SCD patients with VOC is to provide appropriate and rapid treatment, which includes intravenous opioids, often at high doses, as well as around-the-clock opioids administered through patient-controlled anesthesia or through regular (rather than "as needed") doses.[49]

Qualitative work indicates the possible operation of bias with this population. Although the use of opioids during a VOC is evidence-based and necessary, patients with SCD report consistent disbelief by providers, suspicion of their request for opioids, and resulting treatment delays. In one study, a participant described her experiences this way:

> I feel like they look at all sicklers as drug seekers because you come in asking for a dose that a normal person who does not have sickle cell would not need. But this is a different type of pain, and I don't think that they really understand that … This is serious pain where you can't function. And so for them to be looking at you like: "Let's wait and see before we medicate you because that's a really high dose."

Another participant focused on the unnecessary delays, explaining:

> . . . and the same hospital that I go to yearly, every time I have a crisis, they will wait three or four days before they transfuse. They'll wait two or three days before they give me the appropriate amount of opiates . . . And once I start receiving that proper care it's like the fourth or fifth day.[42]

In a study by O'Connor et al.,[48] participants echoed the disbelief and suspicion by providers:

> The doctors and nurses need to have more considerations to the patients' pain. Some don't believe in the pain. We've [the patient and her sister] had the disease all our life. We know from the type of pain if it's due to anemia, dehydration, or pain crisis. We need doctors and nurses to be partners with us.

Another explained, "Many times I get comments from nurses and medics that I'm coming in to the hospital for medication for an addiction as their first thought. It would improve care if doctors didn't have that in their brain."

Providers' concerns about substance use disorders among patients with SCD are also not supported by evidence. Evidence suggests that the rate of substance use disorders in patients with SCD is close to the rate in the general population.[50] However, some providers—especially in the ED—dramatically overestimate both the actual prevalence and the long-term risks of addiction in this population while underestimating the level of pain and the immediate risks of treatment delay.[51] Further, ED providers who hold negative attitudes toward patients with SCD may be less likely to follow evidence-based guidelines for pain management.[52] Pat Croskerry, who is perhaps the international authority on medical decision-making errors, has addressed the particular challenges of the ED, writing:

> The single unifying theme underlying all aspects of patient safety is human cognition, and the primary output of cognition is decision making, the engine that drives all behaviours involved in patient care. Cognition is a precious resource in the emergency department, and we need to know it well.

More research is needed into the attitudes of ED personnel toward SCD patients and the delays in their treatment. Research so far reveals that nurses may hold more negative attitudes than physicians; providers who have a higher regard for patients with SCD also have a higher level of unease with their coworkers' poor treatment of these patients. Some pilot programs to correct attitudes with educational campaigns have had mixed results. Those that included first-person patient narratives may have more success.[53] This finding is consistent with social science work on stigma reduction that demonstrates that campaigns that humanize individuals with a stigmatizing condition and allow others to empathize are more effective than just providing information about a condition alone.[54]

CHRONIC PAIN

Acute pain management is not the only area of concern for patients with SCD. Although VOCs are intensely painful and can be life-threatening, recent research has revealed that many patients with SCD also suffer from neuropathic pain.[55] The nature of and types of pain experienced by patients with SCD are poorly understood, but the underlying pathophysiology is more complex than previously thought; in addition to acute pain crises, individuals with SCD may experience chronic pain of undetermined origin as well as neuropathic pain.[56] Adults with SCD report they experience pain more than 50% of the time.

Many adults with SCD require long-term opioid therapy to manage their pain. In the first national database survey of opioid use among people with SCD, Han et al. found that about 40% of patients with SCD took regular doses of opioids.[57] Those with higher rates of serious sequelae of SCD—including VOC, avascular necrosis, acute chest syndrome, and chronic heart failure—were also higher utilizers of chronic opioid therapy and at higher doses. Patients who had two or more acute hospital admissions per year were also likely to be higher utilizers and to take higher daily doses of opioids. While the median daily opioid dose (6.1 mg of oral morphine equivalents) was lower than reported doses in patients with other chronic pain syndromes, there was wide variability in dosing. The need for many patients with SCD to take opioids intermittently or chronically is evidence-based. Their doses may vary and may even be higher than those considered to be "maximums" in policies. Providers should not consider lack of response, or variable response, to opioids to be an aberrant drug-seeking behavior. Law enforcement officers as well as healthcare providers should carefully consider medication use in the context of the patient's diagnosis and overall treatment.

ONGOING HARMS OF BIAS

Beyond the harms of neglected pain and delayed treatment, decisions by providers that are rooted in bias rather than evidence contribute to ongoing harm in patients with SCD.[58] Ezenwa et al. found correlations between perceived stigma in patients with SCD and increased rates of anxiety, depression, fatigue, and anger.[59] The intersection of racial bias with other implicit biases toward patients in pain likely compounds the harms.[60] The role of racial bias in the treatment of patients with SCD is substantial and has health consequences. Haywood et al. found that 48.6% of patients surveyed perceived racism by providers, and this perceived racism was correlated with poor trust and nonadherence to providers' recommendations.[61]

Yet race alone does not explain the poor quality of care for patients with SCD: more likely, both racial and pain-based biases explain some of the quality-of-care issues. Compared with a national sample of African Americans, patients with SCD report statistically significant poorer perceptions of providers' listening skills, respect for them, and spending adequate time with them during the clinical encounter.[62] Other work shows that patients with SCD who perceive disease-based bias by providers, more than race-based bias, have a higher pain burden.[63] Important work by Hirsh et al. examined the intersection of race and clinical ambiguity, a defining feature of pain assessment in complex patients.[64] They discovered that ambiguity altered treatment decisions for white patients but not significantly for black patients, leading to the possibility that providers do not appropriately adjust for contextual, patient-centered information for black patients. This finding is consistent with other work in decision-making errors that indicates that conditions of uncertainty (or ambiguity) increase the risk of biased decisions.[65]

Research is needed on the impact of providers' attitudes, decision-making errors by providers, and patients' perceptions on health quality and outcomes. In the short term, there is evidence that knowledge of the cognitive processes involved in decision-making and the use of existing, simple debiasing techniques can help correct the issues. Another challenge is how best to disseminate evidence-based information so that it is assimilated into clinical attitudes and practice.

Providers and regulators should understand that at the time of this writing, the following statements about patients with SCD are supported by substantial evidence:

1. Patients have variable responses to opioids and often need *particular opioids* and at *higher doses* for pain control, especially during a VOC.
2. Patients may require chronic opioid therapy to maximize functioning.
3. There is no evidence that the rate of substance use disorder among SCD patients is any higher than in the general population. To the extent that patients are perceived to be "drug-seeking," the cause is most likely untreated pain.
4. Guidelines for daily opioid doses or mandates for particular opioids may not be appropriate in SCD patients.
5. There is no justification for delays in treatment of a VOC.

OPIOIDS IN PALLIATIVE CARE AND HOSPICE

Many patients with life-limiting conditions experience significant pain,[66] whether or not that pain is related to cancer. Approximately two-thirds of patients with cancer and half of patients with other life-limiting conditions experience significant pain.[67] As with other kinds of pain, beginning treatment with nonopioid medications is often appropriate, but assessment of the individual patient should always guide decisions. As patients approach the end of life, pain intensity increases and opioids are the standard of care. However, some patients do not receive them, especially in hospitals and nursing homes.[68]

Bailey et al.[68] retrospectively reviewed Veterans Administration hospital records of patients in their last days of life and found that while 81% of the patients had pain documented in their care plan, only 64% had an active order for opioids, and of those 64%, only 47% received an opioid in the last 24 hours of life. Older patients and black patients were less likely to have an order for pain medication or to receive pain medication. These findings may correspond to the documented disparities in pain treatment by age and race.[69]

Another study found that while 95% of patients in home hospice care received some medication for pain, black patients were less likely to have their pain assessed and Hispanics were less likely to receive opioids; patients over 85 years of age were also less likely to receive opioids. These findings are consistent with a large body of research on disparities in palliative care and hospice care.[70,71]

Although it is often assumed that patients with life-limiting conditions who receive opioids are immune from the harms associated with the opioid crisis, some have raised concerns that policies may lead to restricted opioid prescribing even for this population.[72] Others have questioned the frequent blanket exclusion of patients with life-limiting conditions from prescribing restrictions or regulatory requirements. Although the rates of diversion or substance use disorders are believed to be the same for this population as for others, guidelines for risk assessment in these populations are scant. A recent article calls into question whether this is an oversight or reflects an oversimplification of risks.[73] Even in hospice patients, for whom concerns about addiction are minimal, the presence of opioids in the home could lead to a risk of diversion by a third party; this could also leave the patient without the prescribed opioids.[74,75] Although some hospices screen for substance use disorders in patients and family members, they tend to do so informally.[76]

The use of standard risk assessments or Universal Precautions adapted for people with life-limiting conditions are appropriate to protect the patient and third parties in this setting. This is an even more important consideration as patients are referred to palliative care services earlier in their disease process—allowing additional time and opportunity for harms such as third-party diversion and the sequelae of possible underlying substance use disorders. If, for example, patients are referred to palliative care when their life expectancy is a year or more, the risks of substance use disorders are less tempered by their prognosis. Moreover, palliative care practitioners may have had less education on risk assessments and care for patients with substance use disorders precisely because of the presumption of very short life expectancies in this group of patients. In fact, a survey of palliative care fellows revealed that less than half of the respondents felt comfortable or knowledgeable dealing with these issues.[77]

While there is relatively little research in this area compared to other areas of opioid prescribing, these issues are ripe for discussion and policy development. Diversion of opioids presents a risk of harm to both the patient and third parties. Presuming that patients with life-limiting conditions are immune from the risks of opioids is a decision-making error in its own right. Treatment with opioids is appropriate for these patients, but the risks of diversion and other harms should also be assessed and mitigated.

OPIOIDS IN PATIENTS WITH CHRONIC PAIN

The use of long-term opioids for patients with chronic pain was one of the first targets of public policy and professional pressure as the rise in opioid-related harms emerged. Most experts now agree that there was a lack of careful prescribing by many providers. However, initial policy efforts amounted to a single focus on reducing prescription opioid use. Such policies were initially enacted to the exclusion of important harm-reduction measures, such as those aimed at reducing concomitant use of other substances, improving access to treatment for opioid use disorders, or promoting safe medication storage. There is also preliminary evidence that the reclassification of hydrocodone has decreased access to therapeutic opioids and increased provider avoidance.[78] Careful assessment, and reduction when appropriate, of chronic opioid therapy is critical because evidence suggests that the rate of some level of substance use disorder in persons on chronic opioid therapy is slightly higher than in the general population.[79] At the same time, there is newer evidence that the rush to reduction was inappropriate in the context of some patients' circumstances. According to Dr. Kurt Kroenke,

> . . . we all agree there is a national problem with prescription opioid use, including thousands of overdose deaths each year. However, most of the patients on chronic opioids do not misuse their medications, yet many are being pressured to discontinue their opioids, despite having taken them appropriately for years.[80]

Many people with chronic or persistent pain who are taking opioids believe that the medication has improved their functional abilities.[81] The legal and professional response, however, led to many providers reducing prescribing reflexively—a not irrational response to fears of legal scrutiny.

However, eliminating therapeutic opioids as an option for some patients may be dangerous in and of itself. There is certainly evidence that the public disproportionately blames prescription opioids and prescribers for the opioid-related public health crisis.[82] It is not surprising, then, that some evidence suggests that physicians have stopped or drastically reduced their opioid prescribing, even for patients for whom it improved function, as a response to increased regulatory pressures.[83]

A possibly related harm that has received less attention is the suicidality of patients with chronic pain. In 2014, Dr. Lynn Webster wrote about the harms that can result from the push to reduce even therapeutic opioid doses out of regulatory concerns.[84] He wrote of the suicide death of his patient Jack after his daily dose of opioids was reduced. Jack was on a large daily dose but had no history of misuse or abuse. His suicide note said he "couldn't live with the pain anymore." Webster reflected,

> I had to ask myself if my concern for my freedom and licensure had led to this tragedy. This was a moral dilemma for me. I could have continued to prescribe a high dose of opioid, but if he had died, even from a natural cause, the medical examiner might have said the death was an unintentional overdose from opioids. Jack might have even intentionally overdosed and no one would know. Deaths from opioids have become red flags for investigations. By contrast, Jack's death by suicide was not widely recognized by anyone beyond his family and me. I was tormented by the thought that he might have died because I was unable to help him escape extreme pain.

Though the issue is not well studied, this is certainly not an isolated incident.[85] A St. Louis reporter profiled a person who died by suicide after his access to pain care was cut off. His suicide note was a three-word text to his wife: "I'm so sorry."[86] A story on NPR detailed a group of chronic pain patients from Montana whose only access to chronic pain management with therapeutic opioids is in California, where they fly every 90 days to see a pain specialist and receive opioids. One of the patients is quoted as saying, "Had I stayed in Montana, I would have killed myself." A pain advocate, Barby Ingle, posted the following comment in response to the Centers for Disease Control and Prevention's proposed guidelines for opioid prescribing, describing the suicide deaths of several friends with chronic pain:

> I have lost at least 2 friends each month due to suicide. Many of them did it through intentional overdose . . . When they feel trapped, hopeless, and like they are not going to be able to get their medication due to barriers like the ones the CDC is proposing they give up. They are getting slammed off of their medications and decide death is a better option as they have no strength to fight the system to get what they need.[87]

Chronic pain is already an independent risk factor for suicide.[88–90] Campbell et al. found that 16.4% of a population of chronic pain patients taking opioids reported making a suicide attempt at some point in their life and 36.5% had recent or active suicidal ideation.[91] According to Madadi and Persaud, "opioid management tools for clinicians . . . have been created for assessing the risk of addiction, opioid misuse, and aberrant drug behaviors . . . assessing prior history of suicide attempts should be included in this assessment."[92] The idea that patients with chronic pain require regular screening for suicidality has not yet received widespread support. At the same time, many experts suggest that many of the overdose deaths attributed to accidental death may actually be suicides.[93,94] The results of these screenings should assist providers in assessing whether opioid use is appropriate at all and, if so, whether additional precautions should be taken—such as prescribing small quantities and requiring weekly visits, as are typical in psychiatry for at-risk patients.

Ongoing research and better data collection are crucial to reduce harms to patients with chronic pain. In the short term, providers must act to treat each patient individually in the context of his or her goals and needs. Suicidality should be assessed regularly, and these concerns are just as crucial to patients' well-being as other risk management tools used with opioid therapy.

CONCLUSION

Prescription opioids are only one tool is the provider's toolbox for treating pain. They are neither universally helpful nor universally harmful. Regarding them in either extreme light leads to harms for patient and third parties. There is always danger in oversimplification. Careful providers are increasingly discerning with their opioid prescribing. However, while caution in opioid prescribing is warranted, in some populations opioid use is essential to their care and functioning—such as many people with SCD, those with life-limiting conditions, and some patients with chronic pain. At the same time, prescribers should not reflexively prescribe opioids for patients with life-limiting conditions without taking into account the risk of diversion or substance use disorder in this population. Enhancing providers' awareness of their decision-making processes and the errors that may result from assumptions and biases may help reduce the risks of harm.

REFERENCES

1. Ling W, et al. Prescription opioid abuse, pain, and addiction: clinical issues and implications. *Drug Alcohol Rev.* 2011;30:300–305.

2. Institute of Medicine. *Relieving Pain in America: A Blueprint for Transforming Prevention, Care, Education, and Research.* Washington, DC: National Academies of Sciences; 2011:66–81.

3. Bergman AA, et al. Contrasting tensions between patients and PCPs in chronic pain management: a qualitative study. *Pain Med.* 2013;14:1689–1694.

4. Peppin JF, et al. The complexity model: a novel approach to improve chronic pain care. *Pain Med.* 2015;16:653–666.

5. Kroenke K, Cheville A. Management of chronic pain in the aftermath of the opioid backlash. *JAMA.* 2017;317(23):2365–2366.

6. Croskerry P, Singhal G, Mamede S. Cognitive debiasing 1: Origins of bias and theory of debiasing. *BMJ Quality Safety.* 2013;22:ii58.

7. Epstein RM, et al. Self-monitoring in clinical practice: a challenge for medical educators. *J Cont Educ Health Prof.* 2008;28(1):5–13.

8. Croskerry P. Our better angels and black boxes. *Emerg Med J.* 2016;33(4):242–244.

9. Pack-Mabien A, Labbe E, Herbert D, Haynes J. Nurses' attitudes and practices in sickle cell pain management. *Appl Nurs Res.* 2001;14(4):187–192.

10. Dineen KK. Moral disengagement of medical providers: another clue to the continued neglect of treatable pain? *Houston J Health Law Policy* 2013;13:163–202.

11. Green CR, Anderson KO, Baker TA, et al. The unequal burden of pain: confronting racial and ethnic disparities in pain. *Pain Med.* 2003;4:277–294.

12. Wailoo K. Sickle cell disease—a history of progress and peril. *N Engl J Med.* 2017;376(9):805–807.

13. Tait RC, et al. Provider judgments of patients in pain: seeking symptom certainty. *Pain Med.* 2009;10:11.

14. Lee D. Decision-making: from neuroscience to psychiatry. *Neuron.* 2013;78:233.

15. Sayce L. Beyond good intentions. Making anti-discrimination strategies work. *Disability & Society.* 2003;18(5):625–642.

16. Maina IW, Johnson TJ. A decade of studying implicit racial/ethnic bias in healthcare providers using the implicit association test. *Social Science & Medicine* 2017 May 4 [E-pub ahead of print].

17. Matthew DB. *Just Medicine: A Cure for Racial Inequality in American Medicine.* New York: NYU Press; 2015;39.

18. Marewski JN, Gigerenzer G. Heuristic decision-making in medicine. *Dialogues Clin Neurosci.* 2012;14:77.

19. Tversky A, Kahneman D. Judgment under uncertainty: heuristics and biases. *Science.* 1974;185:1124.

20. Saposnik G, Redelmeir D, Ruff CC, Tobler PN. Cognitive biases associated with medical decisions: a systemic review, *BMC Medical Informatics and Decision Making.* 2016;16:138.

21. Epstein RM, Gramling R. What is shared in shared decision-making? Complex decisions when the evidence is unclear. *Med Care Res Rev.* 2012;70:94S.

22. Gigerenzer G, Gaissmaier W. Heuristic decision-making. *Ann Rev Psychol.* 2011;62:451–454.

23. Sunstein CR. Moral heuristics and moral framing. *Minnesota Law Rev.* 2004;88:1556.

24. Croskerry P. From mindless to mindful practice—cognitive bias and clinical decision-making. *N Engl J Med.* 2013;368:2445–2448.

25. Reyna VF, Brainerd CJ. Dual processes in decision-making and developmental neuroscience: a fuzzy-trace model. *Devel Rev.* 2011;31:180–186.

26. Dineen KK. Addressing prescription opioid abuse concerns in context: synchronizing policy solutions to multiple complex health problems. *Law Psychol Rev.* 2016;40(1).

27. Wilson TD, Brekke N. Mental contamination and mental correction: unwanted influences on judgments and evaluations. *Psychol Bull.* 1994;116:117.

28. Teal CR, et al. Helping medical learners recognise and manage unconscious bias toward certain patient groups. *Medical Educ.* 2012;46:80.

29. Croskerry P, Singhal G, Mamede S. Cognitive debiasing 2: Impediments to and strategies for change. *BMJ Quality and Safety.* 2013;22:ii65–ii72.

30. Husain M, Hartman AD, Desai P. Pharmacogenomics of sickle cell disease: steps toward personalized medicine. *Pharmacogenomics Personalized Med.* 2017;10:261–265.

31. McClish DK, Smith WR, Levenson JL, et al. Comorbidity, pain, utilization, and psychosocial outcomes in older versus younger sickle cell adults: the PiSCES project. *BioMed Research Intl.* 2017 March 28 [E-pub ahead of print].

32. van Tuijn CFJ, Sins JWR, Fijnvandraat K, Biemond BJ. Daily pain in adults with sickle cell disease—a different perspective. *Am J Hematol.* 2017;92:179–186.

33. Owusu-Ansah A, Ihunnah CA, Walker AL, Ofori-Acquah SF. Inflammatory targets of therapy in sickle cell disease. *Transl Res.* 2016;167(1):281–297.

34. Ware RE, Abboud MR. Sickle cell disease. *Lancet.* 2017;390(10091):311–323.

35. Molokie RE, Wilkie DJ. Opioid doses and acute care utilization outcomes for adults with sickle cell disease: ED versus acute care unit. *Am J Emerg Med.* 2018;36(1):88–92.

36. Ciribassi R, Patil CL. We don't wear it on our sleeves: sickle cell disease and the (in)visible body parts. *Social Sci Med.* 2016;148:131–138.

37. Wailoo K. *Dying in the City of Blues: Sickle Cell Anemia and the Politics of Race and Health.* Chapel Hill: University of North Carolina Press; 2001.

38. Goldsmith JC, Bonham VL, Joiner CH, Kato GJ, Noonan AS, Steinberg MH. Framing the research agenda for sickle cell trait: building on the current understanding of clinical events and their potential implications. *Am J Hematol.* 2012;87(3):340–346.

39. Creary M, Eisen A. Acknowledging levels of racism in the definition of "difficult." *Am J Bioethics.* 2013;13(4):16–18.

40. DeBaun MR, Telfair J. Transition and sickle cell disease. *Pediatrics.* 2012;130(5):926–935.

41. Resnik D, Rehm M, Rich B. Pain and sickle cell anemia. *Hastings Center Rep.* 2001;31(3):29–30.

42. Williams-Gray B, Senreich E. Challenges and resilience in the lives of adults with sickle cell disease. *Social Work in Public Health.* 2015;30:88–105.

43. Bergman EJ, Diamond NJ. Sickle cell disease and the "difficult patient" conundrum. *Am J Bioethics.* 2013;13(4):3–10.

44. Freiermuth CE, Haywood C, Silva S, et al. Attitudes towards patients with sickle cell disease in a multicenter sample of emergency department providers. *Adv Emerg Nurs J.* 2014;36(4):335–347.

45. Todd KH, Green C, Bonham VL, Haywood C, Ivy E. Sickle cell disease–related pain: crisis and conflict. *J Pain.* 2006;7(7):453–458.

46. Yee MM, Josephson C, Hill CE, et al. Cytochrome P450 2D6 polymorphisms and predicted opioid metabolism in African American children with sickle cell disease. *J Pediatr Hematol Oncol.* 2013;35(7):e301–305.

47. Ballas S. Pathophysiology and principles of management of the many faces of the acute vaso-occlusive crisis in patients with sickle cell disease. *Eur J Haematol.* 2014;95:113–123.

48. O'Connor S, Hanes D, Lindsey A, Weiss M, Petty L, Overcash J. Attitudes among healthcare providers and patients diagnosed with sickle cell disease: frequent hospitalizations and stressors. *Clin J Oncol Nurs.* 2015;18:(6):675–680.

49. Yawn BP, Buchanan GR, Afenyi-Annan AN, et al. Management of sickle cell disease: summary of the 2014 evidence-based report by expert panel members. *JAMA.* 2014;312(10):1033–1048.

50. Brown SE, Weisberg EF, Balf-Soran G, Sledge WH. Sickle cell disease patients with and Without extremely high hospital use: pain, opioids, and coping. *J Pain Symptom Manage*. 2015;49(3):539–547.

51. Elander J, Lusher J, Bevan D, Telfer P. Pain management and symptoms of substance dependence among patients with sickle cell disease. *Social Sci Med*. 2003;57:1683–1696.

52. Glassberg JA, Tanabe P, Chow A, et al. Emergency provider analgesic practices and attitudes toward patients with sickle cell disease. *Ann Emerg Med*. 2013;62:293–302.

53. Haywood C, Lanzkron S, Hughes MT, et al. A video-intervention to improve clinician attitudes toward patients with sickle cell disease: the results of a randomized experiment. *J Gen Intern Med*. 2011;26(5):518–523.

54. Heijnders M, Van Der Meij S. The fight against stigma: an overview of stigma-reduction strategies and interventions. *Psychol Health Med*. 2006;11:353–363.

55. Nogrady B. Life beyond the pain. *Nature*. 2014;515:S8–9.

56. Han J, Saraf SL, Zhang X, et al. Patterns of opioid use in sickle cell disease. *Am J Hematol*. 2016; 91(11):1102–1106.

57. Han J, Zhou J, Saraf SL, Gordeuk VR, Calip GS. Characterization of opioid use in sickle cell disease. *Pharmacoepidemiol Drug Safety*. 2017 August 16 [E-pub ahead of print].

58. Jenerette CM, Brewer C. Health-related stigma in young adults with sickle cell disease. *J Nat Med Assoc*. 2010;102(11):1050–1055.

59. Ezenwa M, Yao Y, Molokie R, et al. The association of sickle cell-related stigma with physical and emotional symptoms in patients with sickle cell pain. *J Pain*. 2016;7:4S.

60. Wyatt R. Pain and ethnicity. *AMA J Ethics*. 2013;15(5):449–454.

61. Haywood C, Lanzkron S, Bediako S, et al. Perceived discrimination, patient trust, and adherence to medical recommendations among persons with sickle cell disease. *J Gen Intern Med*. 2014;29(12):1657–1662.

62. Haywood C, Bediako S, Lanzkron S, et al. An unequal burden: poor patient–provider communication and sickle cell disease. *Patient Education and Counseling*. 2014;96(2):159–164.

63. Haywood C, Diener-West M, Strouse J, et al. Perceived discrimination in health care is associated with a greater burden of pain in sickle cell disease. *J Pain Symptom Manage*. 2014;48(5):934–943.

64. Hirsh AT, Hollingshead NA, Ashburn-Nardo L, Kroenke K. The interaction of patient race, provider bias, and clinical ambiguity on pain management decisions. *J Pain*. 2015;16(6):558–568.

65. Graber ML, et al. Cognitive interventions to reduce diagnostic errors: a narrative review. *BMJ Quality and Safety*. 2011;21:535.

66. Groninger H, Vijayan J. Pharmacologic management of pain at the end of life. *Am Fam Physician*. 2014;90(1):26–32.

67. Cea ME, Ried C, Inturris C, Witkin LR, Prigerson HG, Bao Y. Patients 65 years or older receiving hospice care in the U.S. *J Pain Symptom Manage*. 2016;52(5):663–672.

68. Bailey FA, Williams BR, Goode PS, et al. Opioid pain medication orders and administration in the last days of life. *J Pain Symptom Manage*. 2012;44(5):681–691.

69. Teno JM, Plotzke M, Christian T, Gozalo P. Examining variation in hospice visits by professional staff in the last 2 days of life. *JAMA Intern Med*. 2016;176(3):364–370.

70. Johnson KS. Racial and ethnic disparities in palliative care. *J Palliat Med*. 2013;16(11):1329–1334.

71. Sharma RK, Freedman VA, Mor V, et al. Association of racial differences with end-of-life care quality in the United States. *JAMA Intern Med*. 2017;177(12):1858–1860.

72. Wilson C. Opioid campaigns' impact on advanced cancer and hospice and palliative care: an invited commentary. *Rehab Oncol*. 2017;35(2):94–98.

73. Copenhaver DJ, Karvelas NB, Fishman SM. Risk management for opioid prescribing in the treatment of patients with pain from cancer or terminal illness: inadvertent oversight or taboo? *Anesthesia Analgesia*. 2017;125(5):1610–1615.

74. Covington-East C. Hospice appropriate Universal Precautions for opioid safety. *J Hospice Palliat Care.* 2017;19(3):256–260.

75. Venkat A, Kim D. Ethical tensions in the pain management of an end-stage cancer patient with evidence of opioid medication diversion. *HEC Forum.* 2016;28(2):95–101.

76. Sacco P, Cagle JG, Moreland ML, Camlin EAS. Screening and assessment of substance use in hospice care: examining content from a national sample of psychosocial assessments. *J Palliat Med.* 2017;20(8):850–856.

77. Childers J, Arnold R. Managing opioid misuse in palliative care settings: how prepared do hospice and palliative medicine fellows feel? *J Pain Symptom Manage.* 2011;41(1):227–228.

78. Webster LR, Grabois M. Current regulations related to opioid prescribing. *Phys Med Rehab.* 2015;7:S236–2447.

79. Cheatle M, Comer D, Wunsch M, Skoufalos A, Reddy Y. Treating pain in addicted patients: recommendations from an expert panel. *Population Health Management.* 2014;17(2):79–89.

80. Kronemyer B. Pain experts: opioids useful in some patients for managing chronic pain. *Pain Medicine News,* December 14, 2017.

81. Manchikanti L, Kaye AM, Knezevic NN, et al. Responsible, safe, and effective prescription of opioids for chronic non-cancer pain: American Society of Interventional Pain Physicians (ASIPP) guidelines. *Pain Physician* 2017;20(2S):S3–S9.

82. Blendon R, et al. The opioid abuse crisis is a rare area of bipartisan consensus. *Health Affairs Blog.* September 12, 2016. http://healthaffairs.org/blog/2016/09/12/the-opioid-abuse-crisis-is-a-rare-area-of-bipartisan-consensus/.

83. Kates-Carney C. Montana's "Pain Refugees" Leave State To Get Prescribed Opioids. *NPR Health Shots.* July 20, 2016. http://www.npr.org/sections/health-shots/2016/07/20/481771231/montanas-pain-refugees-leave-state-to-get-prescribed-opioids.

84. Webster L. Pain and suicide: the other side of the opioid story. *Pain Med.* 2014;15:345.

85. Anson P. Are CDC opioid guidelines causing more suicides? *Pain News Network.* May 27, 2016. http://www.painnewsnetwork.org/stories/2016/5/27/are-cdcs-opioid-guidelines-causing-more-suicides.

86. Messenger T. The opioid dilemma catches Wildwood couple in its web. *St. Louis Post Dispatch.* February 28, 2016. http://www.stltoday.com/news/local/columns/tony-messenger/messenger-the-opioid-dilemma-catches-wildwood-couple-in-its-web/article_a426108b-67b8-514d-bdf7-37c57247a375.html

87. Ingle B. Comment to proposed guidelines for prescribing opioids for chronic pain. https://www.regulations.gov/document?D=CDC-2015-0112-0291.

88. Ilgen MA, et al. Noncancer pain conditions and risk of suicide. *JAMA Psychiatry.* 2013;70:692–697.

89. Kanzler KE, et al. Suicidal ideation and perceived burdensomeness in patients with chronic pain. *Pain Practice.* 2012;12:602–604.

90. DeCaria SK, Patel V. Relationship of chronic pain and suicide. In: Anitescu M, Benzon H, Wallace M, eds. *Challenging Cases and Complication Management in Pain Medicine.* Springer; 2018.

91. Campbell G, Bruno R, Darke S, et al. Prevalence and correlates of suicidal thoughts and suicide attempts in people prescribed pharmaceutical opioids for chronic pain. *Clin J Pain.* 2016;32(4):292–301.

92. Madadi P, Persaud N. Suicide by means of opioid overdose in patients with chronic pain. *Current Pain & Headache Reports.* 2014;18:460.

93. Rockett IRH, Regier MD, Kapusta ND, et al. Leading causes of unintentional injury mortality: United States, 2000–2009. *Am J Public Health.* 2012;102(11):e84–92.

94. Stone DM, Holland KM, Bartholow B, Logan JE, McIntosh WL, Rockett IRH. Deciphering suicide and other manners of death associated with drug intoxication: a Centers for Disease Control and Prevention consultation meeting summary. *Am J Public Health.* 2017;107(8):1233–1239.

CHAPTER 10

THE DEMISE OF INTERDISCIPLINARY CHRONIC PAIN MANAGEMENT AND ITS RELATIONSHIP TO THE SCOURGE OF PRESCRIPTION OPIOID DIVERSION AND ABUSE

Michael E. Schatman

INTRODUCTION: INTERDISCIPLINARY PAIN MANAGEMENT PROGRAMS

Of all approaches to the treatment of chronic pain, none has a stronger evidence basis for efficacy, cost-effectiveness, and lack of iatrogenic complications than interdisciplinary pain management programs (IPMPs).[1-9]

While the composition of interdisciplinary treatment teams may vary to a certain degree, Okifuji et al. noted that the typical treatment provided includes three common elements: (1) medication management, (2) graded physical exercise, and (3) cognitive and behavioral techniques for pain and stress management.[2] Typically, the team includes a physician (ideally a physical medicine and rehabilitation specialist or someone with expertise in chronic pain and its treatment), physical and occupational therapists, pain psychologists, a biofeedback therapist, a vocational counselor, and a therapeutic recreation therapist, in addition to a nurse case manager and a business support manager.[10]

Although calls have been made for including complementary and alternative medicine (CAM) practitioners on the team, doing so is not typical in traditional programs.[11]

Containing costs is certainly a concern, although more importantly, systematic reviews of CAM for chronic pain performed by scientists trained in systematic review methodology (as opposed to those performed by CAM practitioners published in CAM journals) have not demonstrated particularly strong supportive evidence.[12]

IPMPs have traditionally been heavily psychoeducational, with an emphasis on teaching self-management skills that allow patients to "treat themselves" as opposed to receiving passive treatment. Much of the psychoeducational content is typically presented in group settings, as such group presentations are clearly more cost-effective than providing psychoeducational content on an individual basis; research indicates that group treatment is well accepted by patients with chronic pain.[13,14] The content of these sessions can vary based upon the patients' needs, as well as the orientation and goals of the psychologist. Typically, topics include self-management strategies and general wellness issues such as nutrition and tobacco cessation.[15]

There are few reliable data about which individual psychological approach is best in this setting, although it is generally accepted that cognitive-behavioral approaches are most effective.[16,17] However, "cognitive-behavioral therapy" (CBT) can refer to numerous types of interventions, and the psychologist should tailor the cognitive-behavioral interventions to the patient's unique needs. Furthermore, as individual psychological intervention is an expensive component of interdisciplinary programs, the number of sessions provided to a patient should be based upon his or her specific needs rather than a standardized protocol.

Perhaps the greatest strength of IPMPs lies in their treatment of the whole person: they recognize that chronic pain is a complex phenomenon that is unlikely to respond to a simplistic unimodal approach.[18] Few would suggest that a traditional biomedical approach is sufficient in terms of treating all of the pain-related problems that patients with chronic pain experience.[19] A complex medical condition cannot be treated simply by writing a prescription—this faulty belief is responsible, at least in part, for the opioid crisis the United States currently faces. In 1999, Gallagher wrote, "The biomedical model has limited outcome validity in chronic pain treatment" and "The history of pain medicine is replete with failures of the biomedical model."[20p558,p559] While Gallagher's approach to the treatment of the disease of chronic pain was a biopsychosocial rather than a biomedical one, perhaps an emphasis should be placed on a top-down "socio-psycho-biological," rather than a biopsychosocial, approach.[21] IPMPs are ideally psychosocially driven, which may explain their formidable clinical efficacy.[22]

BARRIERS

Despite their substantial evidence basis, a confluence of factors has contributed to a dramatic reduction in the number of IPMPs in the United States over the past two decades. In 1999, Anooshian et al. reported that there were more than a thousand such programs in the United States, but by 2012 this number dropped to under 100 outside those in Department of Veterans Affairs Medical Centers.[23,24] This represents a severe and disturbing trend, particularly given the results of a study indicating that the number of IPMPs in the rest of the industrialized world is increasing rapidly.[24] Much has been written about the demise of IPMPs in the United States because of the insurance industry, which, for the most part, now refuses to pay for this type of treatment in most parts of the country.[25–28] Insurance companies' rejection of IPMPs, at first glance, appears to be perplexing. Although numerous studies and reviews have lent support for the efficacy of these programs for functional restoration, there is certainly no reason to believe that private insurers have any concern for their enrollees' well-being.[3,29–33] As insurance companies are motivated solely by the "business ethic" of cost containment and profitability, they deny any fiduciary obligation to the individuals they insure.[34,35] It may appear that health insurers are unaware that IPMPs have also been empirically established as cost-effective as well as clinically efficacious.[5] In fact, one study determined that they resulted in lifetime savings of over a quarter of a million dollars per patient.[36] Just in terms of the expense of medications, these programs have been found to reduce costs by an average of $6 to $10 per day per patient—which can certainly add up over a lifetime of chronic pain. Furthermore, the iatrogenic complications associated with medications routinely used to treat chronic pain, such as opioids and nonsteroidal anti-inflammatory drugs, are well established.[37] However, the American health insurance system is unique, as insurers are aware that their enrollees will switch carriers every 3 or 4 years.[38] Accordingly, insurers are willing to gamble, hoping to avoid the cost of an IPMP with the hope that subsequent carriers will pay the costs of "treatment as usual"—which may translate to systemic opioid analgesics. Given the costs of drug rehabilitation, this can certainly result in quite a risk—yet we have no evidence that health insurance companies are averse to risk in regard to this issue. While the 2006 study that suggested that a quarter of a million dollars per patient can be saved by enrolling them in interdisciplinary programs represented methodologically sound science, more current data are necessary in order to reliably ascertain the extent of such savings a decade later.[36] Unfortunately, the demise of IPMPs in the United States has, logically, also resulted in the demise of research regarding such treatment—at least in the United States.

Although the insurance industry is primarily culpable for the demise of IPMPs in the United States, it should not bear all of the blame. The hospital industry has been complicit, since hospitals have chosen to close programs that they no longer see as profitable. Of course, health insurance carriers' refusal to pay for IPMPs in the vast majority of the United States has made it difficult to maintain their viability, since hospitals historically house IPMPs. However, hospitals have chosen to close programs due to their desire to maximize the profitability of every square foot of space.[39] Regarding hospitals' lack of support for IPMPs, John Loeser wrote, "For large American hospitals, especially those associated with a medical school, revenue generation is the major determinant of what services the institution will offer . . . [IPMPs are] not seen as a value compared to cosmetic surgery."[40ppv–vi]

Over the past 20 years, generally well-intentioned healthcare providers and organizations have attempted to make IPMPs more cost-effective by reducing the number of hours during which patients receive treatment and removing certain key elements of programs. Traditional interdisciplinary programs provided a considerable amount of treatment, with a 1992 meta-analysis indicating that programs averaged 7 weeks in duration, during which patients were provided with an average of 96 hours of treatment.[3] However, numerous programs provided far more hours of treatment, with the authors of a meta-analysis identifying courses of treatment as extensive as 264 hours.[39] A systematic review found that programs that offered more than 100 hours of treatment produced superior outcomes compared to briefer programs.[7] Although no studies of the "ideal" duration and intensity exist, data clearly indicate that when insurance carriers began to demand that programs "carve out" services, outcomes began to deteriorate.[41] These data are not surprising, given that like Rome, chronic pain is not "built in a day"—we cannot realistically expect most of our patients to learn to manage their pain effectively in a truncated program. As healthcare insurers are not more open to covering interdisciplinary treatment, we are beginning to see the development of programs that are intentionally designed as carve-outs. Instead of providing 4 to 6 weeks of 35-hour-per-week treatment, these programs may, for example, provide 12 hours of treatment per week for only 3 weeks. Although there are not yet any published data on the efficacy of these "planned carve-out programs," anecdotally, their success rates in regard to restoration of functional capacities and return-to-work rates pale when compared to those of traditional programs. It is unlikely that hospitals would be interested in opening these types of carve-outs if they were not profitable, as their tendency is to abandon unprofitable services.[42] Hopefully, the data on the relative lack of efficacy of these programs will eventually be published, subsequent to which insurers may choose not to cover even the watered-down versions of what were once the most clinically effective and cost-effective treatment approaches for many types of chronic pain.

Some have proposed other types of primarily educational programs for the treatment of chronic pain, including "pain schools" or "back schools."[43,44] A number of these programs can theoretically be considered "interdisciplinary," in that they involve the provision of education from physical therapists and behavioral health specialists.[45] Although empirically supported as a useful component of a traditional IPMP, their evidence basis as a standalone treatment since their initial development in the 1960s has not been particularly compelling.[46,47] Complicating the question of their empirical support is a lack of consensus regarding what constitutes a "back school," as packaged elements of such have been found to vary widely.[48]

Professional pain organizations, such as the American Academy of Pain Medicine (AAPM), are trying to revive IPMPs in the United States.[49] For example, in the past 2 years a vibrant AAPM Interdisciplinary Shared Interest Group has been developed, and the members are working on a white paper on IPMP that will be published in the Academy's journal, *Pain Medicine*.[50] Furthermore, at the AAPM's 2016 annual meeting, thought leaders in the field presented a symposium entitled "The Past, Present, and Future of Interdisciplinary Pain Management."[51] Although some of the organization's members are hopeful that these efforts to revive interdisciplinary treatment in the United States will result in a positive outcome, others believe that until chronic pain (as well as health more broadly) is treated through a national health system, these efforts will be merely symbolic and spurious.[27] As severely as the for-profit insurance industry is vilified, there is still no evidence to suggest that it can be coerced into providing coverage for this safe, efficacious, cost-efficient, yet expensive treatment approach.[27]

THE CONSEQUENCES OF THE DEMISE OF INTERDISCIPLINARY PAIN MANAGEMENT

With the demise of IPMPs in the United States, the treatment of chronic pain has become progressively more fragmented and ineffective, leaving pain care in a state of crisis.[52–54] Since this situation began almost a decade ago, the situation has only become graver. There are fewer IPMPs available, and pain care providers have been compelled to increase the frequency with which they provide "technophilic" approaches such as spine surgeries involving the implantation of hardware, interventional procedures, and, of course, the prescription of opioid pain medications—irrespective of their lack of evidence bases and iatrogeneses.[55–57] Although the overutilization of all technophilic approaches to chronic pain has been strongly criticized, the crisis of abuse, diversion, overdose, and death associated with opioids has caused the media and regulatory agencies to mount an attack on the pharmaceutical industry, physicians, and, indirectly, patients with chronic pain.[58] While some of the measures that have been taken to curb the opioid abuse epidemic have been thoughtfully developed and implemented, others have been ill advised and short-sighted.[59] The unintended consequences from these efforts include an increased incidence of oligoanalgesia of patients who lack realistic treatment alternatives, an increase in heroin abuse, and the very real possibility of increases in suicide among undertreated patients suffering from chronic pain, particularly given the data indicating that patients with poorly controlled pain are twice as likely to commit suicide as those in a control group.[60–63]

Simplistically speaking, with the demise of IPMPs in the United States, physicians have had to rely upon less effective and more iatrogenically problematic treatments of their patients—one of which is certainly chronic opioid therapy. Not only do interdisciplinary programs provide a safer and clinically more effective alternative to opioids, but they have also been empirically associated with reducing patients' reliance on opioids.[64] Indeed, IPMPs—particularly those with national reputations—have historically focused upon detoxification from opioids as an important goal of treatment.[65–67] Empirical data have indicated that patients who complete interdisciplinary programs while taking reduced levels of opioids demonstrate superior outcomes based upon a number of criteria, including return-to-work rates, indemnity, and healthcare utilization.[68] These data are important not only in terms of enhancing chronic pain sufferers' quality of life, but also in terms of reducing the likelihood of opioid diversion. Abusers are considerably more likely to obtain their prescription opioids from friends and family members versus legally receiving prescriptions themselves.[69,70] As interdisciplinary approaches represent an effective means of reducing opioid prescription and use among patients with chronic pain, they also have the unintended yet very positive consequence of fewer opioids becoming available for diversion.

Not surprisingly, the decrease in access to IPMPs in the United States coincided with the dramatic increase in opioid prescription and the myriad associated problems that have ensued. Poitras notes that the change in general pain management practices during this period resulted in "a substantial and predictable impact on the available supply of prescription opioids available for diversion."[71p34] This is not to suggest that the American prescription opioid crisis had been caused purely by the demise of interdisciplinary programs. Rather, the disappearance of these programs should be considered a contributory factor in the crisis of diversion and abuse and the associated destruction of lives. Poitras blames the opioid abuse epidemic on "economic medicalization," claiming that corporations' desires to create profits resulted in a dramatic increase in the number of legally prescribed opioids, which were ultimately illegally diverted.[71] As discussed earlier in this chapter, healthcare insurers and hospitals were largely responsible for the demise of IPMPs in the United States due the lack of profitability of these programs. Accordingly, the insurance and hospital industries have been indirectly responsible for the opioid diversion and abuse crisis due to economic medicalization of their own. The detrimental impact of corporatization on the well-being of patients with chronic pain has been addressed extensively in the literature.[25–28,72–74]

When IPMPs began to close, physicians who had relied upon them lost a critical resource in their toolbox for treating their more challenging patients with chronic pain. Working with these patients has been described as "time-consuming, frustrating, and emotionally draining."[75] Due to the challenge of changing patients' "stubborn and counterproductive" beliefs about their pain—which is a significant focus of interdisciplinary programs—physicians attempting to treat chronic pain in isolation often feel frustrated and helpless.[76] Although no formal investigations of how physicians view the demise of IPMPs have been published to date, anecdotally, many physicians report feeling disheartened: they relied upon these clinics as a therapeutic option for patients they had been unable to effectively manage on their own. Many have chosen to discontinue treating chronic pain altogether in their practices.[77,78] Perhaps equally distressing is the fact that physicians who have continued to treat patients with chronic pain had been forced to rely only upon opioid analgesics—thereby resulting in more prescriptions, and thus more diversion and abuse. Many physicians do not *want* to prescribe opioids with greater frequency and at higher dosages. Indeed, myriad providers do so with great trepidation due to increased regulatory scrutiny and sanction.[79,80] But what choice did they have, now that interdisciplinary care has become impossible to access for the vast majority of Americans?

It is likely not a coincidence that the initial and perhaps most severe problems with opioid diversion in the United States have occurred in rural Appalachia, a socioeconomically disadvantaged area in which pain treatment—as well as medical treatment more broadly—has lagged behind most of the more developed areas of the country. As a result, this region has had the unpropitious distinction of being the nation's leader in prescription opioid diversion, abuse, and overdose deaths.[81,82] In a study of barriers to effective pain care in Appalachia, the physician-identified barriers included lack of specialty care by pain physicians, limited access to healthcare due to financial burdens, and patients' reluctance to make necessary behavioral and lifestyle changes.[83] Despite findings that rural denizens are more likely to suffer from chronic pain than are their nonrural counterparts, rural pain sufferers—for a variety of reasons—have fewer options for treatment than do individuals living in more populated regions.[84–86] For example, lower levels of health literacy in rural areas, a shortage of mental health professionals, and a strong stigma regarding reception of mental health services may make CBT unrealistic and/or inaccessible for many pain sufferers in Appalachia.[87–91] This is relevant because CBT has been found to have one of the strongest evidence bases for the treatment of chronic pain; it also has been shown to reduce prescription opioid use and abuse among patients with chronic pain.[92,93] Empirical data also indicate that other components of interdisciplinary pain care are disproportionately unavailable in rural regions, which are faced with severe shortages of interdisciplinary treatment team members such as physical and occupational therapists, nurses, and vocational counselors.[94–96]

Given that the demise of IPMPs has been financially driven, in impoverished areas such as Appalachia, where many residents lack health insurance and rely upon Medicaid, IPMPs are essentially nonexistent.[97,98] Reliance upon Medicaid for health coverage was empirically associated with increased OxyContin claims in Appalachian Kentucky from 1999 to 2001.[99] Illicit dealers have been found to rely upon indigent Medicaid recipients as a primary source for diverted prescription opioid analgesics.[100] Compounding the problem, data show that rural denizens have higher levels of disease processes and their lifestyle choices make them more likely to develop painful conditions.[101] A review of the programs in the United States accredited by the Commission on Accreditation of Rehabilitation Facilities showed that the 59 accredited outpatient IPMPs are all located in urban and suburban areas; there are none in Appalachia.[102] Even though some of the IPMPs in the United States are not accredited by this commission, the current majority do have such accreditation, so this provides a strong estimation of the disparity between rural and nonrural access. Thus, even if the appropriate personnel to staff interdisciplinary programs were available in Appalachia, unfortunate financial realities would preclude their viability. Accordingly, pain management in Appalachia is more likely to be provided by primary care physicians, and this has been a problematic situation, as they tend to lack the training, skills, and resources to manage chronic pain in an effective, comprehensive manner.[88,103,104] Thus, primary care physicians in isolated rural areas like Appalachia are more likely to rely upon opioids to treat chronic pain in their patients just because there are rarely safer and more clinically effective alternatives.

Another unfortunate consequence of the lack of insurance coverage in rural areas such as Appalachia is the fact that many patients rely upon emergency departments (EDs) for their pain management needs.[105] A 2008 qualitative study found that while almost half of ED physicians saw diversion of opioids obtained in the ED as a possibility, 80% would not discriminate against "frequent flyers" (patients regularly presenting to the ED with pain complaints).[106] Despite being "annoyed" by patients presenting with pain, the authors determined that ED physicians found it easier to " 'simply write a prescription for the patient and give them what they wanted' " because it took " 'ten times longer to research a chart, find out how many visits they've had, find out how many prescriptions they've had, sit down, talk to the patient, or confront them with the information, and discuss it with them and then share their concerns.'"[106p257]

While investigators have not systematically studied the relationship between uninsured rural patients' use of the ED and the prevalence of diversion, one can speculate that such a relationship does indeed exist. A study by Jonas et al.[107] strengthens the concern that areas without interdisciplinary care are more likely to experience problems with prescription opioid diversion and abuse. They found that in areas with severe economic disparities such as Appalachia, OxyContin has actually become a form of currency that is associated with increased social capital.

SUMMARY AND CONCLUSIONS

Diversion of opioid analgesics would obviously not occur if there were no demand for these drugs. It is likely impossible to determine the degree to which diversion serves to feed non–pain-related addiction versus the iatrogenic dependence of persons with chronic pain. No matter who the recipient of diverted opioid analgesics is, the consequences can be deadly. Opioid abuse and addiction are certainly not new to the United States, with reports of wide-spread prevalence dating back to the Civil War. Opiates were used to treat not only the pain of the physically wounded but "shell shock" as well.[108] It has been estimated that by the turn of the 20th century, there were approximately 900,000 opioid addicts in the United States, the majority of whom became addicted during medical treatment.[109] Savage has noted that the following wave of opioid addiction affected the poor immigrant population and was not related to medical treatment.[110] With this shift, addiction became more of a criminal and social problem as opposed to a medical condition.[111] In 1980, Porter and Jick wrote a letter to the *New England Journal of Medicine* suggesting that opioid addiction was rare in patients treated for pain with opioid analgesics.[112] Perhaps physicians *wanted* to believe that addiction was rare among legitimate pain patients, as opioids provided (and continue to provide) a seemingly simple solution to the very complex problem of chronic pain.

Interdisciplinary management of chronic pain certainly would not be a panacea for the epidemic of prescription opioid diversion and abuse that had been witnessed in the United States. However, is the temporal contiguity of the well-documented development of the opioid abuse and diversion crisis and the progressive demise of interdisciplinary pain management merely a coincidence? Likewise, is Appalachia's notoriety as "ground zero" for the abuse and diversion epidemic related to the lack of interdisciplinary pain treatment resources? As physicians through the United States have, for the most part, lost the option of referring patients with pain to IPMPs, opioids had become the only apparent option. Heavy prescribers have not necessarily been pleased by their contribution to the abuse and diversion epidemic, but without the availability of interdisciplinary programs, what other choices did they have for ameliorating some of the suffering of their patients with chronic pain? Tragically, the future of interdisciplinary care in the United States is bleak—unless government intervention (as is being realized through the Department of Veterans Affairs' recent commitment to interdisciplinary care) occurs on a broad basis. It is unlikely that such bold intervention by the government will serve to "fix" the diversion and abuse crisis. However, given the data indicating that patients receiving interdisciplinary pain care are less likely to be prescribed opioid analgesics, the resurrection of this person-centered approach to the disease of chronic pain would potentially help stem the very unfortunate tide.[41,112,113]

REFERENCES

1. Turk DC, Swanson K. Efficacy and cost-effectiveness treatment for chronic pain: an analysis and evidence-based synthesis. In: Schatman ME, Campbell A, eds. *Chronic Pain Management: Guidelines for Multidisciplinary Program Development.* New York: Informa Healthcare; 2007:15–38.

2. Okifuji A, Turk DC, Kalauoklani D. Clinical outcome and economic evaluation of multidisciplinary pain centers. In: Block AR, Kramer EF, Fernandez E, eds. *Handbook of Pain Syndromes: Biopsychosocial Perspectives.* Mahwah, NJ: Lawrence Erlbaum Associates; 1999:77–97.

3. Flor H, Fydrich T, Turk DC. Efficacy of multidisciplinary pain treatment centers: a meta-analytic review. *Pain.* 1992;49:221–230.

4. Turk DC, Okifuji A. Treatment of chronic pain patients: clinical outcomes, cost effectiveness, and cost-benefits of multidisciplinary pain centers. *Crit Rev Phy Rehab Med.* 1998;10:181–208.

5. Turk DC. Clinical effectiveness and cost-effectiveness of treatments for patients with chronic pain. *Clin J Pain.* 2002;18:355–365.

6. Hoffman BM, Papas, RK, Chatkoff DK, Kerns RD. Meta-analysis of psychological interventions for chronic low back pain. *Health Psychol.* 2007;26:1–9.

7. Guzman J, Esmail R, Karjalainen L, Malmivaara A, Irvin E, Bombardier C. Multidisciplinary rehabilitation for chronic low back pain: a systematic review. *BMJ.* 2001;322:1511–1516.

8. Guzman J, Esmail R, Karjalainen L, Malmivaara A, Irvin E, Bombardier C. Multidisciplinary bio-psycho-social rehabilitation for chronic low back pain. *Cochrane Database Syst Rev.* 2002;1:CD000963.

9. Schonstein E, Kenny DT, Keating J, Koes BW. Work conditioning, work hardening and functional restoration for workers with back and neck pain. *Cochrane Database Syst Rev.* 2003;1:CD001822.

10. Stanos SP. Developing an interdisciplinary multidisciplinary chronic pain management program: nuts and bolts. In: Schatman ME, Campbell A, eds. *Chronic Pain Management: Guidelines for Multidisciplinary Program Development.* New York: Informa Healthcare; 2007:151–172.

11. Tan G, Jensen MP. Integrating complementary and alternative medicine into multidisciplinary chronic pain management. In Schatman ME, Campbell A, eds. *Chronic Pain Management: Guidelines for Multidisciplinary Program Development.* New York: Informa Healthcare; 2007:75–99.

12. Rubinstein SM, van Middelkoop M, Kuijpers T, et al. A systematic review on the effectiveness of complementary and alternative medicine for chronic non-specific low-back pain. *Eur Spine J.* 2010;19:1213–1228.

13. Holmes CP, Gatchel RJ, Adams LL, et al. An opioid screening instrument: long-term evaluation of the utility of the Pain Medication Questionnaire. *Pain Pract.* 2006;6:74–88.

14. Artner J, Kurz S, Cakir B, Reichel H, Lattig F. Intensive interdisciplinary outpatient pain management program for chronic back pain: a pilot study. *J Pain Res.* 2012;5:209–216.

15. Chen J. Outpatient pain rehabilitation programs. *Iowa Orthopaedic J.* 2006;26:102.

16. Nash VR, Ponto J, Townsend C, Nelson P, Bretz MN. Cognitive behavioral therapy, self-efficacy, and depression in persons with chronic pain. *Pain Manag Nurs.* 2013;14:e236–243.

17. Gatchel RJ, McGeary DD, McGeary CA, Lippe B. Interdisciplinary chronic pain management: past, present, and future. *Am. Psychol.* 2014;69:119–130.

18. Peppin JF, Cheatle M, Kirsh KL, McCarberg BH. The complexity model: a novel approach to improve chronic pain care. *Pain Med.* 2015;16:653–666.

19. Schatman ME. Psychological assessment of maldynic pain: the need for a phenomenological approach. In: Giordano J, ed. *Maldynia: Multidisciplinary Perspectives on the Illness of Chronic Pain.* New York: Taylor & Francis; 2011:157–182.

20. Gallagher RM. Primary care and pain medicine: a community solution to the public health problem of chronic pain. *Med Clin North Am.* 1999;83:555–583.

21. Carr DB, Bradshaw YL. Time to flip the pain curriculum? *Anesthesiology.* 2014;120:112–114.

22. Chou R, Loeser JD, Owens DK, et al. Interventional therapies, surgery, and interdisciplinary rehabilitation for low back pain: an evidence-based clinical practice guideline from the American Pain Society. *Spine.* 2009;34:1066–1077.

23. Anooshian J, Streltzer J, Goebert D. Effectiveness of a psychiatric pain clinic. *Psychosomatics.* 1999;40:226–232.

24. Schatman ME. Interdisciplinary chronic pain management: international perspectives. *Pain: Clin Updates.* 2012;20:1–5.

25. Schatman ME. The demise of multidisciplinary pain management clinics? *Practical Pain Manag.* 2006;6:30–41.

26. Schatman ME. The demise of the multidisciplinary chronic pain management clinic: bioethical perspectives on providing optimal treatment when ethical principles collide. In: Schatman ME, ed. *Ethical Issues in Chronic Pain Management.* New York: Informa Healthcare; 2007:43–62.

27. Schatman ME. The role of the health insurance industry in perpetuating suboptimal pain management: ethical implications. *Pain Med.* 2011;12:415–426.

28. Schatman ME. Corporate commoditization in pain medicine: increased profits translate to increased suffering. In: Giordano J, ed. *Augmenting Human Painlessness.* New York: Springer; 2018.

29. Johansson C, Dahl J, Jannert M, Melin L, Andersson G. Effects of a cognitive-behavioral pain-management program. *Behav Res Ther.* 1998;36:915–930.

30. Becker N, Sjogren P, Bech P, Olsen AK, Eriksen J. Treatment outcome of chronic non-malignant pain patients managed in a Danish multidisciplinary pain centre compared to general practice: a randomised controlled trial. *Pain.* 2000;84:203–211.

31. Dysvik E, Vinsnes AG, Eikeland OJ. The effectiveness of a multi-disciplinary pain management programme managing chronic pain. *Int J Nurs Pract.* 2004;10:224–234.

32. Patrick LE, Altmaier EM, Found EM. Long-term outcomes in multidisciplinary treatment of chronic low back pain: results of a 13-year follow-up. *Spine.* 2004;29:850–855.

33. Oslund S, Robinson RC, Clark TC, et al. Long-term effectiveness of a comprehensive pain management program: strengthening the case for interdisciplinary care. *Proc (Bayl Univ Med Cent).* 2009;22:211–214.

34. Craig L. Why a first party insurer is not a fiduciary. *Mealey's Litigation Rep.* 1999;13:21.

35. Richmond DR. Trust me: insurers are not fiduciaries to their insured. *Kentucky Law J.* 1999-2000;88:1–32.

36. Gatchel R J, Okifuji A. Evidence-based scientific data documenting the treatment and cost-effectiveness of comprehensive pain program for chronic nonmalignant pain. *J Pain.* 2006;7:779–783.

37. Cunningham JL, Rome JD, Kerkvliet JL, Townsend CO. Reduction in medication costs for patients with chronic nonmalignant pain completing a pain rehabilitation program: a prospective analysis of admission, discharge, and 6-month follow-up medication costs. *Pain Med.* 2009;10:787–796.

38. Keckley PH, Coughlin S. 2012 Survey of U.S. Health Care Consumers: Five-Year Look Back. Deloitte University Press. http://dupress.com/articles/2012-survey-of-u-s-health-care-consumers-five-year-look-back/. Accessed June 2, 2016.

39. Chen HF, Bazzoli GJ, Hsieh HM. Hospital financial conditions and the provision of unprofitable services. *Atl Econ J.* 2009;37:259–277.

40. Loeser JD. Foreword. In: Schatman ME, Campbell A, eds. *Chronic Pain Management: Guidelines for Multidisciplinary Program Development.* New York: Informa Healthcare; 2007:v–vi.

41. Robbins RJH, Gatchel CN, Gajraj N, et al. A prospective one-year outcome study of interdisciplinary chronic pain management: compromising its efficacy by managed care policies. *Anesthesia Analgesia.* 2003;9:156–162.

42. Iezzoni LI. Reinvigorating the quality improvement incentives of hospital prospective payment. *Med. Care.* 2009;47:269–271.

43. Greiff R. Pain school "Knowledge for Life" makes life easier for people with chronic pain. *Ann Rheumatic Dis.* 2014;73(Suppl 2):170–171.

44. Peters S, Faller H, Pfeifer K, Meng K. Experiences of rehabilitation professionals with the implementation of a back school for patients with chronic low back pain: a qualitative study. *Rehab Res Practice.* 2016;2016:6720783.

45. Meng K, Seekatz B, Roband H, Worringen U, Vogel H, Faller H. Intermediate and long-term effects of a standardized back school for inpatient orthopedic rehabilitation on illness knowledge and self-management behaviors: a randomized controlled trial. *Clin J Pain*. 2011;27:248–257.

46. Olason M. Outcome of an interdisciplinary pain management program in a rehabilitation clinic. *Work*. 2004;22:9–15.

47. Straube S, Harden M, Schröder H, et al. Back schools for the treatment of chronic low back pain: possibility of benefit but no convincing evidence after 47 years of research—systematic review and meta-analysis. *Pain*. 2016;157:2160.

48. Waddell G, Burton AK. Occupational health guidelines for the management of low back pain at work: evidence review. *Occup Med (Lond)*. 2001;51:124–135.

49. American Academy of Pain Medicine. http://www.painmed.org/. Accessed May 15, 2017.

50. American Academy of Pain Medicine. Interdisciplinary Pain Medicine Shared Interest Group. http://www.painmed.org/membercenter/interdisciplinary-pain-medicine-shared-interest-group/. Accessed May 15, 2017.

51. American Academy of Pain Medicine. 2017 Annual Meeting. http://www.painmed.org/annualmeeting/annual-meeting-archive/. Accessed May 15, 2017.

52. Giordano J, Schatman, ME. A crisis in pain care: an ethical analysis. Part 1: Facts, issues, and problems. *Pain Physician*. 2008;11:483–490.

53. Giordano J, Schatman ME. A crisis in chronic pain care: an ethical analysis. Part 2: Proposed structure and function of an ethics of pain medicine. *Pain Physician*. 2008;11:589–595.

54. Giordano J, Schatman ME. A crisis in chronic pain care: an ethical analysis. Part 3: Toward an integrative, multi-disciplinary pain medicine built around the needs of the patient. *Pain Physician*. 2008;11:771–784.

55. PRNewswire. Top 5 global spinal implant companies maintaining position but competition rising rapidly. December 8, 2012. http://www.prnewswire.com/news-releases/top-5-global-spinal-implant-companies-maintaining-position-but-competition-rising-rapidly-78763487.html. Accessed May 11, 2013.

56. Abbott ZL, Nair KV, Allen RR, Akuthota VR. Utilization characteristics of spinal interventions. *Spine J*. 2012;12:35–43.

57. Manchikanti L, Abdi S, Atluri S, et al. American Society of Interventional Pain Physicians (ASIPP) guidelines for responsible opioid prescribing in chronic non-cancer pain. Part I: Evidence assessment. *Pain Physician*. 2012;15(3 Suppl):S1–65.

58. Deyo RA, Mirza SK, Turner JA, Martin BI. Overtreating chronic back pain: time to back off? *J Am Board Fam Med*. 2009;22:62–68.

59. Schatman ME. Pain medicine: profession or business? *Medscape Neurology*. 2011. http://www.medscape.com/viewarticle/742692. Accessed May 20, 2013.

60. Motov SM, Khan ANGA. Problems and barriers of pain management in the emergency department: are we ever going to get better? *J Pain Res*. 2009;2:5–11.

61. Burch ADS. After war on "pill mills," heroin emerges as substitute. *Bellingham Herald*. May 16, 2013. http://www.bellinghamherald.com/2013/05/16/3011608/after-war-on-pill-mills-heroin.html. Accessed May 20, 2013.

62. American Academy of Pain Medicine. AAPM speaks on the use of opioids in the treatment of chronic pain. http://www.painmed.org/files/aapm-statement-on-opioids-chronic-pain-fda.pdf. Accessed May 20, 2013.

63. Tang NK, Crane C. Suicidality in chronic pain: a review of the prevalence, risk factors and psychological links. *Psychol Med*. 2006;36:575–586.

64. Hubbard JE, Tracy J, Morgan SF, McKinney RE. Outcome measures of a chronic pain program: a prospective statistical analysis. *Clin J Pain*. 1996;12:330–337.

65. Townsend CO, Rome JD, Bruce BK, Hooten WM. Interdisciplinary pain rehabilitation programs. In: Ebert M, Kerns R, eds. *Behavioral and Psychopharmacologic Pain Management.* New York: Cambridge University Press; 2011:114–128.

66. Gatchel RJ, Haggard R, Thomas C, Howard KJ. Biopsychosocial approaches to understanding chronic pain and disability. In: Moore RJ, ed. *Handbook of Pain and Palliative Care: Biobehavioral Approaches for the Life Course.* New York: Springer; 2012;1–16.

67. Stanos S. Focused review of interdisciplinary pain rehabilitation programs for chronic pain management. *Curr Pain Headache Rep.* 2012;16:147–152.

68. Kidner CL, Mayer TG, Gatchel RJ. Higher opioid doses predict poorer functional outcome in patients with chronic disabling occupational musculoskeletal disorders. *J Bone Joint Surg Am.* 2009;91:919–927.

69. American Association for the Treatment of Opioid Dependence. AATOD end of year report, 2005. www.aatod.org/pdfs/End_of_Year_Report_2005.pdf. Accessed May 25, 2013.

70. Shei A, Rice JB, Kirson NY, et al. Sources of prescription opioids among diagnosed opioid abusers. *Curr Med Res Opin.* 2015;31:779–784.

71. Poitras G. OxyContin, prescription opioid abuse and economic medicalization. *Medicolegal Bioethics.* 2012;2:31–43.

72. Benjamin WW. Corporatization threatens the ethos of medicine. *Minn Med.* 1989;72:273–292.

73. Schatman ME. Pain and corporatization: more special interests, more disparities, more vulnerability. *Pain Med.* 2011;12:632–633.

74. Meghani SH. Corporatization of pain medicine: implications for widening pain care disparities. *Pain Med.* 2011;12:634–644.

75. Weisberg MB, Clavel AL. Why is chronic pain so difficult to treat? Psychological considerations from simple to complex care. *Postgrad Med.* 1999;106:141–164.

76. Kenny DT. Constructions of chronic pain in doctor–patient relationships: bridging the communication chasm. *Patient Educ Couns.* 2004;52:297–305.

77. Libby RT. Treating doctors as drug dealers: the DEA's war on prescription painkillers. *Policy Anal.* 2005;545:1–27.

78. American Pain Foundation. Washington State: community health clinic access crisis. October 7, 2011. https://www.documentcloud.org/documents/271365-2-american-pain-foundation-report-pf-reportoct.html. Accessed May 26, 2013.

79. McCracken LM, Boichat C, Eccleston C. Training for general practitioners in opioid prescribing for chronic pain based on practice guidelines: a randomized pilot and feasibility trial. *J Pain.* 2012;13:32–40.

80. Kirsh KL, Passik SD, Rich BA. Failure to treat pain. In: Deer TR, Leong MS, Buvanendran A, et al., eds. *Comprehensive Treatment of Chronic Pain by Medical, Interventional, and Integrative Approaches: The American Academy of Pain Medicine Textbook on Patient Management.* New York: Springer Science & Business Media; 2013:1053–1058.

81. Hall AJ, Logan JE, Toblin RL, et al. Patterns of abuse among unintentional overdose fatalities. *JAMA.* 2008;300:2613–2620.

82. Centers for Disease Control and Prevention. Unintentional poisoning deaths—United States, 1999–2004. *MMWR Morb Mortal Wkly Rep.* 2007;56:93–96.

83. Remster EN, Marx TL. Barriers to managing chronic pain: perspectives of Appalachian providers. *Osteopath Fam Physician.* 2011;3:141–148.

84. Hoffman PK, Meier BP, Council JR. A comparison of chronic pain between an urban and rural population. *J Community Health Nurs.* 2002;19:213–224.

85. Breuer B, Pappagallo M, Tai JY, Portenoy RK. U.S. board-certified pain physician practices: uniformity and census data of their locations. *J Pain.* 2007;8:244–250.

86. Day MA, Thorn BE. The relationship of demographic and psychosocial variables to pain-related outcomes in a rural chronic pain population. *Pain*. 2010;151:467–474.

87. Wood FG. Health literacy in a rural clinic. *Online J Rural Nurs Health Care*. 2005;5:9–18.

88. Cheong PH, Feeley TH, Servoss TJ. Understanding health inequalities for uninsured Americans: a population-wide survey. *J Health Commun*. 2007;12:285–300.

89. Smalley KB, Yancey CT, Warren JC, et al. Rural mental health and psychological treatment: a review for practitioners. *J Clin Psychol*. 2010;66:479–489.

90. Jones AR, Cook TM, Wang J. Rural-urban differences in stigma against depression and agreement with health professional about treatment. *J Affect Disord*. 2011;134:145–150.

91. Pederson KJ, Lutfiyya MN, Palombi LC, et al. Cross-sectional population based study ascertaining the characteristics of US rural adults with mental health concerns who perceived a stigma regarding mental health issues. *Health*. 2013;5:695–702.

92. Robinson JP, Leo R, Wallach J, et al. Rehabilitative treatment for chronic pain. In: Stannard C, Kalso E, Ballantyne JC, eds. *Evidence-Based Chronic Pain Management*. Oxford, UK: Blackwell Publishing; 2010:407–423.

93. Currie SR, Hodgins DC, Crabtree A, Jacobi J, Armstrong S. Outcome from integrated pain management treatment for recovering substance abusers. *J Pain*. 2003;4:91–100.

94. Wilson RD, Lewis SA, Murray PK. Trends in the rehabilitation therapist workforce in underserved areas: 1980–2000. *J Rural Health*. 2009;25:26–32.

95. Bigbee JL. The relationship between nurse to population ratio and population density: a pilot study in a rural/frontier state. *Online J Rural Nurs Health Care*. 2007;7:36–43.

96. Mwachofi A. Rural access to vocational rehabilitation services: minority farmers' perspective. *Disabil Rehabil*. 2007;11/12:891–902.

97. Eberhart MS, Ingram DD, Makuc DM, Pamuk ER, Freid VM, Harper SB. *Urban and Rural Health Chartbook*. Hyattsville, MD: National Center for Health Statistics; 2001.

98. Hummer RA, Pacewicz J, Wang S, Collins C. Health insurance coverage in nonmetropolitan America. In: Glasgow N, Morton LW, Johnson NE, eds. *Critical Issues in Rural Health*. Ames, IA: Blackwell Publishing; 2004:197–209.

99. Havens JR, Talbert JC, Robert W, Cynthia L, Leukefeld CG. Trends in controlled-release oxycodone (OxyContin®) prescribing among Medicaid recipients in Kentucky, 1998–2002. *J Rural Health*. 2006;22:276–278.

100. Rigg KK, Kurtz SP, Surratt HL. Patterns of prescription medication diversion among drug dealers. *Drugs*. 2012;19:144–155.

101. Helman C. Doctor–patient interaction. In: Helman C, ed. *Culture, Health, and Illness*, 4th ed. Boston: Butterworth Heineman; 2006:79–107, 179–201.

102. Committee for the Accreditation of Rehabilitation Facilities. Interdisciplinary Pain Rehabilitation Programs—Outpatient. http://www.carf.org/advancedProviderSearch.aspx. Accessed June 14, 2013.

103. Mitchinson AR, Kerr EA, Krein SL. Management of chronic noncancer pain by VA primary care providers: when is pain control a priority? *Am J Manag Care*. 2008;14:77–84.

104. Dorfman D, Papagallo M. Patients with chronic pain: a care model. *Top Pain Manag*. 2010;26:1–6.

105. Hines A, Fraze T, Stocks C. *Emergency Department Visits in Rural and Non-rural Community Hospitals, 2008*. Rockville, MD: Agency for Health Care Policy and Research; 2011.

106. Wilsey BL, Fishman SM, Crandall M, et al. A qualitative study of the barriers to chronic pain management in the ED. *Am J Emerg Med*. 2008;26:255–263.

107. Jonas AB, Young AM, Oser CB, et al. OxyContin® as currency: OxyContin® use and increased social capital among rural Appalachian drug users. *Soc Sci Med*. 2012;74:1602–1609.

108. Courtwright DT. The hidden epidemic: opiate addiction and cocaine use in the South, 1860–1920. *J South Hist.* 1983;49:57–72.

109. Courtwright D. *Dark Paradise: Opioid Addiction in America Before 1940.* Cambridge, MA: Harvard University Press; 1982.

110. Savage SR. Long-term opioid therapy: assessment of consequences and risks. *J Pain Symptom Manage.* 1996;11:274–286.

111. Joseph H, Appel P. Historical perspectives and public health issues. *State Methadone Treatment Guidelines.* Rockville. MD: U.S. Department of Health and Human Services; 1991.

112. Porter J, Jick H. Addiction rare in patients treated with narcotics. *N Engl J Med.* 1980;302:123.

113. Okifuji A. Interdisciplinary pain management with pain patients: evidence for its effectiveness. *Sem Pain Med.* 2003;1:110–119.

114. Bosy D, Etlin D, Corey D, Lee JW. An interdisciplinary pain rehabilitation programme: description and evaluation of outcomes. *Physiother Can.* 2010;62:316–326.

CHAPTER 11

PAIN MANAGEMENT ASSESSMENT BEYOND THE PHYSICIAN ENCOUNTER

Urine Drug Monitoring and Patient Agreements

Anand C. Thakur

INTRODUCTION

Over the past two decades, the use of opioids to relieve moderate to severe pain and improve quality of life has been associated with widespread inappropriate use of these drugs.[1] Urine drug monitoring (UDM) provides a biologic assessment of medication adherence (presence of prescribed drugs) and/or inappropriate use (absence of prescribed drugs, or presence of nonprescribed drugs or illicit substances).[2] Although screening of other biologic elements exists (serum, oral fluids, perspiration, and hair), urine is the most familiar and widely used, and is the only fluid specimen collected by some laboratories for toxicology testing of patients taking opioid.[3,4]

Published articles and guidelines recommend UDM, and some suggest that both random UDM and continuous UDM have been demonstrated to curtail use of illicit drugs.[5-7] Peppin et al., in providing recommendations for UDM, stated that all patients who are prescribed short- or long-term opioids for pain lasting more than 3 months should be tested.[8] They noted that drug testing should be considered one of a variety of evaluation tools, including patient history, physical examination, and psychological screening. A 2007 audit of services at a neuroscience practice in Kentucky showed that the use of UDM in adherence monitoring played a role in the referral of 40% of patients to behavioral health services.[9] Retrospective analysis of UDM showed that 45% of 470 patients presented abnormal results (absence of the prescribed medication, presence of an unprescribed medication, or presence of an illicit drug), with 20% of the patients testing positive for illicit drugs.[10]

Urine testing offers good specificity and sensitivity, can be easily administered, and is cost-effective.[11] It has been called a "first vital step towards establishing and maintaining the safe and effective use of opioid analgesics in the treatment of chronic pain."[3]

Though highly valuable and recommended, UDM is often underutilized, used inconsistently, or not used at all. In 2001, Adams et al. found that only 8% of chronic pain patients in a primary care setting had undergone urine toxicology screening.[12] A 2006 survey of 248 primary care physicians reported that 7% of physicians performed UDM prior to treating patients with opioids, and 15% of respondents conducted tests for patients already taking opioids.[13] Other reports put the use of UDM as high as 30% and as low as 18%.[8,14] Between 2005 and 2008, the use of UDM to monitor pain medication appeared to be on the rise, with one institution seeing a 33% average annual increase in its use.[15] However, recent data suggest that many primary care providers have poor skills in interpreting UDM results and thus underutilize UDM.[16] Use of drug testing may be related to specific patient and clinic factors.[17] Morasco et al. found that patients on high doses of opioids were tested more frequently than those on lower doses (26% vs. 20%, respectively).[18] Others have reported a demonstrated increase in the use of UDM when patient tracking systems were in place or an opioid risk reduction initiative was established.[13,17]

While UDM can be helpful in educating and guiding patients on the proper use of prescribed medication, results of tests are subject to misinterpretation. Other clinical indicators are needed before determining if a patient is nonadherent.[19] UDM results can be affected by differences in metabolic drug conversions, an individual's metabolism of medications, variations in testing sensitivity and specificity of a drug or its metabolite, and factors that may intentionally or unintentionally interfere with the test.[20] It is vital, therefore, that initial testing is deemed preliminary and followed with confirmatory testing before making patient treatment decisions.[21]

In the pain care setting, the goal of UDM is "backward" from forensic testing. Forensic testing tests for the presence of illicit drugs, usually in the workplace. Since this needs to be financially viable, high sensitivity and lower specificity are required. However, in pain management the questions are focused mainly on compliance with a medical regimen and only secondarily on drugs of abuse.[22] It is useful in demonstrating drug use in the beginning phases of or prior to treatment, in establishing a baseline by which to gauge compliance, and in detecting use of illegal or nonprescribed medications during therapy.[2,22]

Various urine testing methods exist, and they can be used alone, in combination, or in addition to other monitoring tools. Proper understanding of these tests is needed for optimal use and interpretation and for individualizing appropriate testing to the specific clinical need.[22] Accurate interpretation of results—including understanding false negatives and false positives—is vital for effective guidance of treatment decisions.[1] Considerations exist for the practical application of UDM in the clinical pain practice, especially in preserving the doctor–patient relationship and cost-effectiveness.

METHODS

There are two recognized testing groups, borrowed from a forensic model, which are often used in combination.[23,24] The first is a screening test, accomplished via either in-laboratory or point-of-care (POC) immunoassay.[25] Immunoassay testing that produces a result inconsistent with prescribed therapy should be followed by more specific confirmatory testing.[8] These screening tests have high specificity, so the false-positive rate is higher and the specificity is lower than confirmatory testing. Confirmatory tests include in-laboratory thin-layer chromatography (TLC)[4,23] and in-laboratory mass spectrometry (MS) testing, used with either gas chromatography (GCMS or GC/MS/MS) or liquid chromatography (LCMS).[20,21,26,27]

SCREENING

Immunoassays may be used as a first line of clinical action with regard to UDM. This testing is generally referred to as a screening, despite its inability to detect the presence of all drugs (generally implied by the term "screening").[2] It is thought, however, to be a simple way to test for multiple drugs cost-effectively and quickly and can signal a need for more thorough testing.[28] Few data exist to support its cost-efficacy.[26] Immunoassays use a competitive binding process. A known amount of antibody is introduced into a urine sample, along with an enzyme-labeled amount of the drug for which the sample is being tested. The drug, if present in the sample, will compete with the enzyme-labeled drug, which binds to the antibody to form antibody–antigen complexes. Once the process is complete, the amount of enzyme-labeled antigen in the sample will be inversely proportional to the amount of the actual drug or metabolite(s) present in the sample.[22,28]

The specific antibodies used in immunoassays vary based on laboratory and test manufacturer.[4] Some immunoassays test for classifications of drugs (class assays), while others test for specific substances, such as the parent drug or metabolite(s) (analyte-specific assays).[28,29] Class assays—which include amphetamines, barbiturates, benzodiazepines, and opiates—are limited in that they do not provide specific drug identification; instead, they offer either a "present" or "absent" reading. Thus, a patient may test positive for an opiate because he has taken his hydrocodone prescription appropriately or because he has injected street heroin. Even analyte-specific assays—which can test for (or metabolite), cannabinoids, methadone (or metabolites), oxycodone, buprenorphine, and fentanyl—still require confirmatory testing in most cases, as individual tests may be more or less sensitive to semisynthetic opioids (e.g., hydromorphone, hydrocodone, oxycodone).[29]

Another limitation is that immunoassays provide results based on a predetermined assay rate. Concentrations above the cutoff rate yield positive results, while those below are deemed negative. This means that the drug can be present in the sample, but if it is in levels below the cutoff rate, the test will read negative. If the test's cutoff limits are not calibrated to the patient's prescription, a patient may take his medications properly yet will still test negative, making it appear as if he is not taking his prescription appropriately. Forensic cutoff rates for opioids are around 2,000 ng/mL, but this is not appropriate for the clinical setting. Gourlay et al. stated it is important that cutoff levels for initial opiate screening remain at 300 ng/mL or below.[21]

Cross-reactivity is also common in immunoassay testing, meaning that an antibody might react differently with drugs that are in the same class.[29] Cross-reactivity can occur because specificities in immunoassays are imperfect,[20,30] A positive test for cocaine is predictive of cocaine use; however, a test designed for amphetamine/methamphetamine may be prone to cross-reactivity, detecting ephedrine/pseudoephedrine or other sympathomimetic amines, and thus it will lack reliability and diagnostic or predictive benefit.[2] Ultimately, no single test result should be the basis of a treatment decision.[36] Peppin et al. recommended that clinicians manage discrepancies in test results by first verifying them with the lab, then documenting the findings, and finally meeting with the patient for an open conversation, without judgment or accusations, before establishing next steps.[8] Cross-reactants can be a problem, yielding false positives in both kinds of urine testing, although confirmatory testing is much less prone to these problems. Box 11.1 lists cross-reactants for opioids.

POC immunoassay testing has grown rapidly in response to the demand for fast, cost-effective urine test results; this has led to the development of a variety of single-use noninstrumented and instrumented tests from various manufacturers.[22] Although this may benefit large clinics by helping them manage sizable caseloads quickly and at low costs, it also brings unique challenges in terms of incorporating test results into clinical practice. On the one hand, these tests offer rapid results and require minimal staff training; on the other hand, they lack specificity regarding particular opioids, may not be able to detect other common analgesics, are often performed without quality control, and are subject to error.[28,32] For example, a recent study looking at the sensitivity and diagnostic accuracy of immunoassays in the detection of cannabinoids yielded results of 8% and 51%. Table 11.1 compares POC and other urine drug testing methods.

POC testing with noninstrumented devices ("dipstick" or cup testing) generally involves immunochromatography with a visual readout.[34] Most of these tests rely on a competitive binding process; in the absence of a drug in the body, a dye-conjugated antibody binds to a drug conjugate and creates a colored line or bar, signifying a negative test.[35] Conversely, if

TABLE 11.1 UDM methods

Test	Method	Advantages	Limitations	Considerations
Screening				
Immunoassay	Competitive binding	Easy way to test for multiple drugs Cost-effective Fast	Specificity (positive or negative result only) Predetermined cutoff rates Cross-reactivity	Interpreting results requires understanding of metabolites. False-positive/false-negative results can be due to lab or human error.
Point-of-care (POC)	"Dipstick" immunoassay	Rapid Minimal staff training Low cost	Lack quality control	Sometimes has counterintuitive readout
Confirmatory				
Thin-layer chromatography (TLC)	Involves moving the sample in solvent(s) over a plate with a thin layer of adsorbant	Specific drug identification	Requires expensive equipment and may have to be outsourced	Has been replaced by immunoassays for the most part
Gas chromatography/mass spectrometry (GCMS)	Various chromatography techniques	Highly specific Very accurate	Higher cost Requires expensive equipment and may have to be outsourced	Impractical for routine clinical use
Liquid chromatography/mass spectrometry (LCMS) (also called high-performance liquid chromatography [HPLC])	Advanced chromatography technique using smaller particles	Better compound separation than GCMS Can identify specific drugs	Requires expensive equipment and may have to be outsourced	Highly advanced test but expensive and impractical for routine clinical use

there is a detectable amount of drug in the body (above the cutoff rate), the drug will saturate the antibody, preventing it from binding with the drug conjugate, resulting in no visual line or colored bar. These readings can be counterintuitive, and some newer devices now offer more logical readings (i.e., a colored bar or line indicates a positive result).[22,28]

Instrumented POC helps to eliminate the issue of visual readings through the use of small analyzers.[36] These instruments offer additional capability in terms of automation, software for additional quality control, and connectivity to electronic medical records, which may shorten test time; however, these tests are still subject to some of the limitations inherent with immunoassays.[22]

Despite their drawbacks—low specificity, variations in tests among manufacturers, differing cutoff rates, and susceptibility to cross-reactivity—immunoassay tests can be an effective tool.[2,33,35,37] In a single-site study (n = 1,000) comparing immunoassay (index test) with liquid chromatography and tandem mass spectrometry (LC/MS/MS]), Manchikanti et al. found that in 33% of cases requiring confirmatory tests.[35] The difference in accuracy in detecting prescribed opiates was 9% between the index and reference tests (80% vs. 89%, respectively).[36] That said, immunoassay results should be deemed presumptive; a positive or negative rest result should never be used to define treatment.[33] Results serve as an indicator for potential nonadherence and should be followed with additional testing, discussions with the patient and/or family members, and counseling, as applicable.[8]

CONFIRMATORY TESTING

Confirmatory tests are generally warranted when an immunoassay test turns up unexpected results that could alter the prescriber's treatment decisions. They are also useful when a false positive during screening could result in potentially serious consequences for the patient.[4] When appropriately designed and executed, confirmatory tests virtually eliminate false-positive results, offering legally defensible outcomes. Clinical labs, however, do not have to function at the same evidentiary level as forensic toxicology labs.[20] One survey showed that the percentage of physicians who always used confirmatory tests (LCMS) to verify findings from a less precise test was equal to the percentage of those who never used them (14% vs. 14%).[28] Confirmatory tests, such as GCMS, LCMS, or LC/MS/MS are more costly, more complex, and more time-intensive than screening tests; however, they are useful in verifying the presence of a specific drug, identifying a drug outside the scope of other testing methods, or addressing a contested result.[22,35,38]

Kim et al. demonstrated the importance of confirmatory testing in a case report of a 48-year-old man whose inpatient pain management for suspected—later confirmed—pancreatic carcinoma was impacted by a false-positive urine cocaine screening.[39] The patient was being followed by an outpatient clinic for chronic opioid therapy and had a remote history of drug abuse. The false-positive immunoassay test prompted the clinical team to question the use of opioids during treatment; however, confirmatory GCMS testing showed no evidence of cocaine or its metabolite. The authors reinforced that all unexpected urine drug screening results should be followed by a nonjudgmental conversation with the patient, follow-up testing, consultation with knowledgeable experts and, lastly, a clinical determination of next steps, along with appropriate documentation in the medical record.[38]

THIN-LAYER CHROMATOGRAPHY

TLC has been used historically in both forensic and clinical toxicology. While cost-effective and useful in screening for a range of drugs, for the most part it has been replaced by immunoassay techniques due to the latter's higher detection limits for most drugs.[32] TLC, as the name states, is based on the principle of chromatography (separating out components of a mixture) using a stationary phase (featuring a solid or liquid on a solid) and a mobile phase (featuring a liquid or gas). In all chromatography, the mobile phase passes through or over the stationary phase, and, because the different components of the mixture travel at different rates (due to molecular size), they are absorbed differently. TLC uses a thin layer of adsorbant (silica gel or alumina) that uniformly coats a piece of metal, glass, or hard plastic. The sample—consisting of drugs extracted from the biologic matrix into an organic solvent, and then evaporated and concentrated—is added to the plate and a solvent or mixture of solvents draws the sample up the plate in a capillary action.[32] The rates at which the components of the sample move up the plate differ depending upon their molecular makeup and mobile and stationary phase interactions. After the solvent moves up the plate to a specific height, the plate is removed from the solvent and the residual solvent is evaporated. The coated plate is then exposed to chemicals that will react with the drugs to develop colors. Specific drugs are identified based on their color development. If the substances being tested are colorless, a fluorescent indicator that appears under UV light may be added.[39] Table 11.1 compares TLC and other urine drug testing methods.

GAS CHROMATOGRAPHY MASS SPECTROMETRY

GCMS, a very sensitive and specific test for identifying individual drugs, involves visualizing a compound under electron ionization spectrometry.[40] A sample is extracted from the specimen, vaporized, and passed through a column that is bombarded with electrons. This causes the molecular bonds in the vapor to fracture and create patterns. The patterns are then compared with standard patterns for known drugs. GCMS has a very low incidence of false positives; errors using GCMS most often relate to data transcription or human visualization.[41] A 1991 study, however, showed that ingesting poppy-seed streusels or Danish pastries could led to positive test results for morphine and codeine using confirmatory GCMS.[42] A more recent study, however, stated that the morphine content in poppy-seed foods is reduced up to 90% during processing. Because no markers exist to differentiate poppy-seed ingestion from heroin or pharmaceutical morphine, further study is needed to determine if today's poppy-seed foods remain a concern with regard to false-positive test results.[43] In 1998, the US Department of Health and Human Services changed cutoff levels for morphine from 300 ng/mL to 2,000 ng/mL to help avoid false-positive readings for patients who have ingested poppy seeds. Most labs, however, still use 300 ng/mL, a standard cutoff rate for opioids.[11,30] Table 11.1 compares GCMS and other urine drug testing methods.

LIQUID CHROMATOGRAPHY/MASS SPECTROMETRY

With improved technology and more affordable equipment, LCMS, also called high-performance liquid chromatography (HPLC), is being used more often.[45] This test applies the principles of TLC and a form of column chromatography, a technique used in biochemistry and analytic chemistry.[28] The test uses a stationary phase (generally hydrophobic saturated carbon chains) densely packed in a stainless steel column. A pump moves the mobile phase (generally a buffer and organic solvent mixture) and analyte through the column at high pressure, while a detector (ultraviolet light, electron capture or mass spectrometer) reveals compounds passing through the column.[28,46] Smaller particles can be used in the stationary phase with this process, which results in better compound separation than GCMS, and, when used with several mass spectrometers (LC/MS/MS), this becomes a highly useful means by which to identify and quantify drugs in biologic specimens.[28] Table 11.1 compares LCMS and other urine drug testing methods.

Citing the propensity of many to adopt a "screen and reflex" approach, meaning the sample is screened and automatically sent for confirmatory testing if it is deemed positive for a certain class of drugs, McMillin et al. explored a "hybrid" approach to UDM.[47] Because of the proposed potential for unnecessary testing, increased costs, and the slowed results of a traditional two-step process, the authors used a combination of liquid chromatography and time-of-flight mass spectrometry with homogeneous enzyme immunoassays performed at the same time. They found that this hybrid approach offered simplified and specific testing that reduced the need for secondary testing and minimized the time to results.[47]

NON–URINE-BASED TESTING METHODS

Although urine is the preferred sample medium for screening for opioids, other tests exist, such as serum, oral fluid, hair, and perspiration analysis.[1,4] Reisfield et al. concluded that some of these other testing methods hold usefulness not in replacing the use of urine but in complementing it, due to the limitations of the latter (e.g., a small drug-detection window and tampering vulnerability).[48] Although serum (blood) can be used to determine opioid levels, it has been seen as unnecessary in the clinical setting and is not provided by most laboratories offering toxicological analysis. Serum testing offers insight into only the most recent drug use, so it does not provide an adequate picture of the patient's long-term adherence behaviors. In most cases, it is impractical to place patients on strict dosing regimens, requiring them to have precisely timed blood draws for optimal blood concentrations. Also, detailed pharmacokinetic data about many parent drugs and metabolite(s) are lacking in opioid serum testing.[4]

Nonetheless, serum testing may be developing into a helpful tool in managing patients on daily chronic opioid therapy. Deer and Gunn pointed out that serum testing does not need to be performed as often as UDM.[49] They suggest that semiannual testing can follow an initial baseline test once the patient has been on the medication long enough to achieve stable concentration levels.[46] Serum testing also offers a more objective approach for compliance monitoring. It helps to determine if the patient is taking the medication as prescribed, taking other medications that could contribute to an overdose, or developing a tolerance to the medication.[49]

In the last several years there has been an increase in the use of oral fluids in drug testing due to advances in collection techniques, the availability in POC devices, and the development of screening and confirmation testing methods.[50] Results of oral fluid testing have been found to be comparable to UDM, with the exception of minor differences in some drug class detection rates.[51] The testing of oral fluid has advantages over urine testing in that it can be collected under supervision with little opportunity for sample adulteration. Further, oral fluid is not vulnerable to some of the same result-altering activities as urine, such as diluting drug concentrations below the cutoff levels or adding common household products to produce false-negative results.[52] Further, it does not require elaborate bathroom features or laboratory relationships to reduce potential tampering. There are two primary ways in which oral fluids (consisting mostly of saliva but also including bacteria, residual particles from ingested products, buccal and mucosal transudates, and gingival crevice fluid) are tested, and they are similar in methodology to urine testing.[53] The first method involves collecting the sample via expectoration or by using a specialized device and then sending it for laboratory-based immunoassay followed by chromatographic confirmation. The second involves POC testing at the collection site, followed by laboratory-based confirmatory testing at a later time.[54] Oral fluid can be affected by absorptive devices, which can be used for fluid collection, can affect recovery of drugs/metabolites.[53,55] Further studies are needed to better understand the use of oral fluid drug testing.[56]

Hair and perspiration are also noninvasive and effective ways to test for opioids.[57,58] The benefit of sweat testing is that the patches used for sweat collection can be put in place for 1 week, extending the amount of time to obtain samples; however, one study found that weekly sweat testing may be less sensitive than frequent (thrice weekly) urine testing in detecting opioids.[54] Hair testing extends the detection of drug use from weeks to months, but the drug has to be extracted from the hair matrix prior to analysis, increasing the possibility of contamination from environmental exposure.[1,59]

ADJUNCT MONITORING

While other testing methods are available, UDM remains the standard at this time. However, regardless of the type of UDM used, UDM *alone* should not guide clinical decisions. UDM is an important element of an overall opioid-compliance program, but it should never represent the entire monitoring process. For that reason, adjunct monitoring is required.

Healthcare providers should combine UDM with the use of patient agreements for chronic opioid therapy that attempt to set forth in clear terms the expectations related to taking prescribed medications.[8] While clinicians are sometimes ambivalent about these so-called treatment agreements, they are now standard-of-care practice; they serve as an important tool for patient education and are useful in underscoring both the risks and benefits of chronic opioid therapy.[60] It is unclear if such treatment agreements and UDM (either alone or in combination) will reduce the inappropriate use of opioids, but they are recommended by government agencies, professional organizations, and industry experts.[5,8,60,71] Clinicians need to decide how to use these tools and how to balance them with other evaluation methods. While clinicians are most comfortable with patient self-reports alone, the nature of substance use disorders and the regulatory climate necessitate the use of confirmatory measures.

An important element in adjunct monitoring involves including spouses, family members, caregivers, and other people close to the patient who may be able to provide insight into the patient's activities.[63] While consent must be obtained to involve others in the patient's care, doing so, at times, may be beneficial. All decisions to confer with others must be carried out according to the Health Insurance Portability and Accountability Act privacy rules, and this should be done only if deemed appropriate for the individual patient.[8] To the extent possible, patient education efforts should also include caregivers and family members. Prescription monitoring services, if available, can also be helpful.

BOX 11.2 ABERRANT BEHAVIORS OF OPIOID USERS

- Testing positive (urine drug test) for nonprescribed controlled substances
- Testing negative (urine drug test) for prescribed medications
- Requesting early refills
- Reporting lost or stolen prescriptions
- Appearing for visits without appointments
- Making frequent telephone calls
- Taking more medication than prescribed
- Multiple drug intolerances or allergies
- Multiple unsanctioned drug increases
- Requesting specific drugs by name
- Using drug to treat other symptoms without permission
- Complaining aggressively about the need for higher dosages
- Stealing or borrowing another patient's drugs
- Demonstrating violence

Source: references 41, 63, 75, 76.

Behavioral monitoring can be another important adjunct technique. The healthcare provider and all clinicians should observe and monitor the patient's behavior and should be alert to specific triggers that indicate aberrant drug-taking behaviors (Box 11.2). Not all patients who have suspicious results from a urine test exhibit other aberrant drug-taking behaviors, and vice versa, but behavioral triggers warrant closer scrutiny, and patients with unexpected results from UDM should be interviewed about their drug-taking behaviors. All behavioral cues, however, must be taken in context and evaluated in light of other patient information.

For patients on chronic opioid therapy, the combination of UDM with behavior monitoring has been promising. In a retrospective study of 122 patients on chronic opioid therapy for noncancer pain, Katz et al. found that 53 (43%) had either a positive urine test or one or more deviant drug-related habits.[63] Twenty-six patients (21%) showed positive urine toxicology for a nonprescribed substance or an illicit drug but no other behavioral triggers. Seventeen (14%) had negative urine tests but displayed one or more aberrant practices.[63]

In another retrospective review, when presented with patients' aberrant behaviors (the most common of which is an abnormal urine screen, often showing a positive result for an illicit drug), most providers sought to "give the patient another chance."[47] The decision to discontinue therapy was more likely after a second occurrence and increased with each additional instance of aberrant behavior.

Aberrant drug-related behaviors can be due to a number of reasons, including misunderstanding prescription instructions or using medication to deal with anxiety, sleep issues, or an untreated mental conditions, as cited by the Substance Abuse and Mental Health Services Administration. A strong relationship between the patient and the prescriber can facilitate the sometimes difficult conversations that are needed for appropriate identification and treatment of underlying causes of aberrant behavior.[64]

UNDERSTANDING UDM RESULTS

To interpret UDM results, the prescriber must understand the complex biotransformations of parent drugs to metabolites.[65] Knowledge of metabolites plays a vital role in determining if a urine drug test result is normal or abnormal and if a patient is adhering to therapy. Historically, less informed clinicians have accused patients of inappropriate drug use when that was not the case.[2] For example, if a patient taking morphine has a urine drug test result that is positive for hydromorphone, he may still be adhering to his prescribed morphine therapy, as hydromorphone has been shown to be a minor metabolite of morphine.[66] Codeine can metabolize to morphine, so a compliant patient on codeine therapy may present with a urine drug test positive for morphine. Normetabolites (norcodeine, norhydrocodone, and noroxycodone) are unique metabolites that can appear in urine drug tests without the presence of the parent drugs (codeine, hydrocodone, oxycodone), indicating a patient's adherence to therapy.[64] More details about the metabolites formed by commonly prescribed opioid analgesics are given in Table 11.2.

TABLE 11.2 Parent drugs and metabolites

Parent Drug	Metabolite	Retrograde Metabolite
Weak Opioids		
Codeine	Codeine Hydrocodone Morphine Morphine-3-glucuronide Morphine-6-glucuronide Norcodeine,	
Tramadol	o-desmethyltramadol, Tramadol Nortramadol	
Strong Opioids		
Buprenorphine	Buprenorphine-3-glucuronide Norbuprenorphine Norbuprenorphine-3-glucuronide	
Fentanyl	Fentanyl Norfentanyl	
Hydrocodone	Dihydrocodeine Hydrocodol Hydrocodone Hydromorphol Hydromorphone Norhydrocodone Normorphine	Morphine
Hydromorphone	Dihydromorphine Hydromorphone Hydromorphone-3-glucuronide	
Meperidine	Merperidine, normerperidine	
Morphine	Hydromorphone Morphine-3-glucuronide Morphine-6-glucuronide Normorphine	
Oxycodone, oxycontin	Oxycodols Oxycodone Oxymorphone Noroxycodone	Morphine (potentially)

Source: reference 28.

INCORPORATING UDM INTO A CLINICAL PAIN PRACTICE

Even though there is agreement that UDM is an important component in clinical pain practice, it is not used by all clinicians consistently; in fact, its use is highly variable, and some healthcare providers opt not to incorporate it at all.[28] This decision may be due to some of its limitations or potential pitfalls, such as testing accuracy, potential for human error and mishandling of samples, false negatives/positives, and cost. UDM requires both knowledge of opioid metabolism and the awareness of the limitations and sensitivity of a particular tests.[1,3,67,68]

Although UDM may not be appropriate for all patients, decisions about its applicability should be determined globally for the practice rather than on an ad hoc basis. Patients on chronic opioid therapy for chronic pain should be considered appropriate candidates regardless of whether they have had prior substance abuse problems or exhibit aberrant drug-taking behaviors. Patients who might not be good candidates for UDM are those on short-term opioid therapy, patients receiving palliative care, and those with severe pain from terminal cancer.

As with any therapy or intervention, patients should be educated about the potential side effects and risks of this therapy prior to its initiation. They must be counseled that compliance with the prescription is essential for their therapy and well-being. Patients should be informed that random UDM will be carried out to ensure that they are taking their prescribed medication appropriately. The use of a written treatment agreement is recommended to confirm that the patient understands the nature of the therapeutic relationship and the prescription(s).[69] UDM should be presented as something that protects the patient and helps the clinical team provide optimal therapy.

UDM may be administered on a schedule known to the patient or at random. Scheduled tests offer the patient the opportunity to attempt to "defeat" the test, which can be accomplished by adhering to the prescription for 3 or 4 days prior to the test itself; this will allow those most eager to mislead the clinic the opportunity to do so. Random UDM is thus more effective, but it can be perceived as punitive by the patient or may undermine the trust on which the therapeutic relationship is based.[28] To give the patient a bit more sense of control over random UDM, patients can be asked to flip a coin at certain appointments to determine if the drug test is to be administered. This simple step can help preserve the patient's dignity and offer a sense of fairness.

The treatment agreement can also help to provide an important foundation for the patient–provider relationship. At the outset, as early as the patient evaluation, the provider should introduce the monitoring policy, explaining the reasons for monitoring, the methods of monitoring, and how the results will support future therapeutic decisions.[8] Further, gaining the patient's informed consent should be a fluid process that enables the practitioner and patient to form a collaborative relationship allowing open dialogue about the benefits and risks of chronic opioid treatment.[70]

Clinics that adopt regular UDM as part of their practice must then be prepared to perform and interpret these tests. Unexpected results should be discussed with the patient before any changes to treatment are made. Confirmatory tests may be required if the patient cannot adequately explain the unexpected results. As noted earlier in the chapter, unexpected results must always be considered inconclusive because UDM is subject to contamination, human error, and lack of specificity/sensitivity to specific agents. However, unexpected results should not be dismissed; they require investigation.

Absence of the prescribed agent, a common unexpected result, may be due to noncompliance (the patient prefers not to take the medicine or has had several "good days"), diversion (the patient is dispensing the drug outside of legitimate channels),[59] or overuse (the patient takes more than he should and runs out by the end of the prescription).

Another common unexpected result is the presence of nonprescribed drugs and/or illicit drugs. Some patients may be taking prescribed drugs appropriately but also indulging in other drugs, including illegal drugs. Patients may also fail to disclose that they have prescription drugs from other providers. If a patient is taking prescription pain relievers prescribed by more than one provider, contact with the other provider is an important step to prevent patients from getting multiple opioid prescriptions from clinicians who are unaware of each other. There is, of course, also the possibility that the test results were in error.

In discussing unexpected results and confirmatory testing with the patient, it is important to emphasize education rather than jump to the conclusion that the patient is abusing the drug. On the other hand, prescription opioid diversion and abuse are not uncommon. If opioid abuse is involved, it should be first addressed in the clinical setting. In the event of drug abuse, the clinical team should partner with the patient in finding solutions rather than transitioning abruptly to an adversarial relationship. Patients can be prescribed alternative drugs or alternative therapies to manage their pain. In some cases, an accelerated UDM schedule and closer monitoring may suffice.

Clinicians who prescribe opioids should be familiar with local substance abuse counselors and centers and should make appropriate referrals when necessary. A good knowledge of local laws and regulations is important; in the United States, these laws vary by state.[71] Most clinicians prefer to trust rather than suspect their patients, but there are situations when the greater risk is to be too trusting. Clinicians treating patients on long-term opioids must be cautious, ask a lot of questions, and monitor their patients closely. However, even in the presence of a good relationship with the patient, repeated positive results for nonprescribed opioids may indicate a need to refer the patient to a substance abuse specialist.[31]

Clinicians must also consider the possibility of opioid tolerance and pseudoaddiction. Opioid tolerance occurs when the patient must take escalating doses of the opioid to achieve the same level of analgesia. Opioid tolerance is not the same as addiction; in fact, it is the expected result of chronic opioid treatment. Some patients develop opioid tolerance to the point that their usual dose of medication provides inadequate analgesia; these patients may develop drug-seeking behaviors that mimic those of a drug addict but are actually an attempt to get better pain relief (this is termed "pseudoaddiction").[72] Opioid tolerance may develop early in therapy and is sometimes abrupt in onset. The proper response to pseudoaddiction is to increase the dose of the opioid agent, if deemed appropriate, or to rotate the patient to another opioid or pain regimen.

PRESERVING THE PROVIDER–PATIENT RELATIONSHIP

Patients are already under stress due to their chronic pain and can feel uneasy with chronic opioid therapy; the prospect of UDM might heighten their alarm still further. In a clinical setting, increased reliance on laboratory results or inappropriate testing can have a negative impact on the physician–patient relationship. As we have stressed repeatedly, clinical decisions should never be made solely on the basis of laboratory results.[28,31] Instead, it is important for the clinical team to be appropriately educated on the strengths and limitations of tests and how to use them appropriately. Likewise, staff should be reminded that urine testing is for the patient's benefit and is not a punitive act. Patients with a history of substance abuse might feel singled out and persecuted if asked to undergo UDM.[28] Patients should be informed that UDM is a normal part of treatment for all patients on chronic opioids, regardless of their history. Furthermore, UDM should be framed in the context of the patient's welfare: UDM is conducted to protect patients from opioid misuse.

COSTS

With modern cost-containment pressures, adding or expanding lab testing seems counterintuitive. From a global perspective, UDM may reduce inappropriate opioid use and, thus, reduce overall costs to the healthcare system and society at large. However, such "big picture" thinking does not always benefit the small clinic. Therefore, clinicians should consider the cost factor of UDM for their patients on chronic opioid therapy. The cost of urine drug testing ranges from $5 for a dipstick test to $200 for laboratory-based analysis. These costs can vary widely by location, service provider, and volume. Insurance providers differ in their coverage of testing costs; having an upfront discussion with the patient or including payment responsibility in the treatment agreement may be needed to address these factors. Other cost-related considerations include the speed with which results are received, their interpretation, and their clinical utility and reliability.[26] In-sourcing services may offer an attractive cost-saving alternative for practitioners. Brigham and Women's Hospital was able to save a reported $1 million in the 3 years after establishing on-site screening immunoassays and confirmatory LC/MS/MS testing.[15]

RECOMMENDATIONS

We propose a number of considerations for clinicians seeking to use UDM in clinical practice:

1. Recognize that UDM is an important part of adherence but should never be used in isolation.[4] UDM should be performed along with other evaluation methods, including the patient's history, physical examination, and psychological screening.[8]
2. Educate the patient on the risks and benefits of opioid therapy. Explain the role of UDM in the context of clinical supervision of the drug therapy. Share responsibility with the patient.[3] As much as possible, include the patient's caregivers and family in treatment decisions.
3. Determine what will be included in a treatment agreement. Make sure all of the clinical team understand and can explain the agreement to patients, their caregivers, and families. Both the patient and the practitioner should sign the treatment agreement, and a copy should be given to the patient, with another retained in the patient record. It should be emphasized that the intent of the agreement is to improve health outcomes.[8]

4. Define a testing protocol. Such decisions should be made globally for the practice rather than on an ad hoc basis; the latter might make certain patients feel singled out or persecuted.[73] Determine the frequency of follow-up based on risk factors; the Screener and Opioid Assessment for People with Pain Revised (SOAP-R) tool can help to assess patient risk by assigning a low-, medium-, or high-risk score.[8]

5. Develop a rapport with the lab to ensure that all questions and/or issues related to testing and results interpretation can be addressed.[2]

6. Educate the clinical team about the various options to be taken in case opioid misuse or abuse is detected, including accelerated UDM, change in medications, and referrals to counselors.

7. Handle every case individually; there is no "one size fits all" in opioid therapy. Patients intent on diverting drugs will most likely be able to pass the UDM, while patients who are "mostly compliant" may fail the test because they inadvertently missed a dose of medication.

8. Use adjunct monitoring as much as possible, in that the clinical team should be observant for aberrant behaviors and attitudes. In fact, these can sometimes be more telling than a UDM.

9. Discuss all unexpected results from UDM and any concerns about the patient's therapy directly with the patient first. Avoid adversarial relationships, if possible, even if it is clear that the patient is using the drug inappropriately.

Clinicians should always consider the patient's history and get to know the patient as well as they can. Preserving a functioning therapeutic relationship can be essential in preventing or ending inappropriate opioid use. Further, clinicians should not let preconceived ideas about substance abusers or drug diversion color their treatment of patients. Although many drug tests are performed based on a history of addiction or aberrant behavior, others patients who may not arouse suspicions might be using nonprescribed or illicit drugs.[73]

CONCLUSION

UDM is a familiar and important element in a comprehensive monitoring program for patients receiving chronic opioid treatment. Nevertheless, currently UDM is used inconsistently by pain physicians. Guidelines advocate its use, particularly when it is part of a wider program including patient treatment agreements, patient education, and monitoring. Regulatory agencies and professional societies advocate using both UDM and treatment agreements.[61,71] UDM by POC testing is an inexpensive, good frontline test, but its vulnerability to error means that unexpected results should always be confirmed. TLC, GCMS, and LCMS (or HPLC) are more accurate but more expensive and are probably best reserved for confirmatory testing. Patients should be advised about the benefits of UDM and given the opportunity to "flip a coin" at certain visits to determine when the random tests are to be administered. Unexpected results should always be discussed with the patient, and clinicians should make every attempt to preserve a good therapeutic relationship with the patient so that inappropriate opioid use can be addressed early.

REFERENCES

1. Milone MC. Laboratory testing for prescription opioids. *J Med Toxicol*. 2012;8:408–416.

2. Manchikanti L, Atluri S, Trescot AM, Giordano J. Monitoring opioid adherence in chronic pain patients: tools, techniques, and utility. *Pain Physician*. 2008;11(2 Suppl):S155–180.

3. Christo PJ, Manchikanti L, Ruan X, et al. Urine drug testing in chronic pain. *Pain Physician*. 2011;14:123–143.

4. Fishman SM, Wilsey B, Yang J, Reisfield GM, Bandman TB, Borsook D. Adherence monitoring and drug surveillance in chronic opioid therapy. *J Pain Symptom Manage*. 2000;20(4):293–307.

5. Chou R, Fanciullo GJ, Fine PG, et al. Clinical guidelines for the use of chronic opioid therapy in chronic noncancer pain. *J Pain*. 2009;10:113–130.

6. Manchikanti L, Manchukonda R, Pampati V, et al. Does random urine drug testing reduce illicit drug use in chronic pain patients receiving opioids? *Pain Physician*. 2006;9:123.

7. Pesce A, West C, Rosenthal M, et al. Illicit drug use in the pain patient population decreases with continued drug testing. *Pain Physician*. 2011;14:189–193.

8. Peppin JF, Passik SD, Couto JE, et al. Recommendations for urine drug monitoring as a component of opioid therapy in the treatment of chronic pain. *Pain Med*. 2012;13:886–896.

9. Gilbert JW, Wheeler GR, Mick GE, et al. Urine drug testing in the treatment of chronic noncancer pain in a Kentucky private neuroscience practice: the potential effect of Medicare benefit changes in Kentucky. *Pain Physician*. 2010;13:187–194.

10. Michna E, Jamison RN, Pham LD, et al. Urine toxicology screening among chronic pain patients on opioid therapy: frequency and predictability of abnormal findings. *Clin J Pain*. 2007;23:173–179.

11. Manchikanti L, Malla Y, Wargo BW, et al. Protocol for accuracy of point of care (POC) or in-office urine drug testing (immunoassay) in chronic pain patients: A prospective analysis of immunoassay and liquid chromatography tandem mass spectometry (LC/MS/MS). *Pain Physician*. 2010;13:E1–E22.

12. Adams NJ, Plane MB, Fleming MF, Mundt MP, Saunders LA, Stauffacher EA. Opioids and the treatment of chronic pain in a primary care sample. *J Pain Symptom Manage*. 2001;22(3):791–796.

13. Bhamb B, Brown D, Hariharan J, Anderson J, Balousek S, Fleming MF. Survey of select practice behaviors by primary care physicians on the use of opioids for chronic pain. *Curr Med Res Opin*. 2006;22(9):1859–1865.

14. Boulanger A, Clark AJ, Squire P, Cui E, Horbay GL. Chronic pain in Canada: have we improved our management of chronic noncancer pain? *Pain Res Manag*. 2007;12(1):39–47.

15. Melanson SE, Tanasijevic MJ, Snyder ML, Darragh A, Quade C, Jarolim P. Significant cost savings achieved by in-sourcing UDM for monitoring medication compliance in pain management. *Clin Chim Acta*. 2013;422C:10–14.

16. Ceasar R, Chang J, Zamora K, et al. Primary care providers' experiences with urine toxicology tests to manage prescription opioid misuse and substance use among chronic noncancer pain patients in safety net health care settings. *Substance Abuse*. 2016;37:154–160.

17. Turner JA, Saunders K, Shortreed SM, et al. Chronic opioid therapy risk reduction initiative: impact on urine drug testing rates and results. *J Gen Intern Med*. 2014;29:305–311.

18. Morasco BJ, Duckart JP, Carr TP, Deyo RA, Dobscha SK. Clinical characteristics of veterans prescribed high doses of opioid medications for chronic non-cancer pain. *Pain*. 2010;151(3):625–632.

19. Matteliano D, Chang YP. Describing prescription opioid adherence among individuals with chronic pain using UDM. *Pain Manag Nurs*. 2015;16(1):51–59.

20. Reisfield GM, Salazar E, Bertholf RL. Rational use and interpretation of UDM in chronic opioid therapy. *Ann Clin Lab Sci*. 2007;37:301–314.315.

21. Nafziger AN, Bertino JS, Jr. Utility and application of UDM in chronic pain management with opioids. *Clin J Pain*. 2009;25(1):73–79.

22. Gourlay DL HH, Caplan YH. UDM in Clinical Practice: The Art and Science of Patient Care. 2012. http://www.pharmacomgroup.com/udt/udt5.pdf. Accessed May 21, 2017.

23. Pesce A, West C, Egan City K, Strickland J. Interpretation of UDM in pain patients. *Pain Med*. 2012;13(7):868–885.

24. St John A, Price CP. Existing and emerging technologies for point-of-care testing. *Clinic Biochemist Rev*. 2014; 35: 155.

25. Sáiz J, García-Ruiz C, Gómara B. Comparison of different GC-MS configurations for the determination of prevalent drugs and related metabolites. *Anal Meth*. 2017;9:2897–2908.

26. Pecoraro V, Germagnoli L, Banfi G. Point-of-care testing: where is the evidence? A systematic survey. *Clin Chem Lab Med*. 2014; 52: 313–324.

27. Bertholf RL, Sharma R, Reisfield GM. Predictive value of positive drug screening results in an urban out-patient population. *J Anal Toxicol*. 2016;40(9):526–731.

28. Pergolizzi J, Pappagallo M, Stauffer J, et al. The role of urine drug testing for patients on opioid therapy. *Pain Practice*. 2010;10:497–507.

29. Magnani B, Kwong T. UDM for pain management. *Clin Lab Med*. 2012;32:379–390.

30. Moeller KE, Lee KC, Kissack JC. Urine drug screening: practical guide for clinicians. *Mayo Clin Proc*. 2008;83:66–76.

31. Tellioglu T. The use of UDM to monitor patients receiving chronic opioid therapy for persistent pain conditions. *Medicine and Health, Rhode Island*. 2008;91:279–280, 282.

32. O'Kane MJ, McManus P, McGowan N, Lynch PL. Quality error rates in point-of-care testing. *Clin Chem*. 2011;57:1267–1271.

33. Franz F, Angerer V, Jechle H, et al. Immunoassay screening in urine for synthetic cannabinoids—an evaluation of the diagnostic efficiency. *Clin Chem Lab Med*. 2017;55(9):1375–1384.

34. Saitman A, Park HD, Fitzgerald RL. False-positive interferences of common urine drug screen immunoassays: a review. *J Anal Toxicol*. 2014;38:387–396.

35. McMillin GA, Slawson MH, Marin SJ, Johnson-Davis KL. Demystifying analytical approaches for UDM to evaluate medication adherence in chronic pain management. *J Pain Palliat Care Pharmacother*. 2013;27:322–339.

36. Manchikanti L, Malla Y, Wargo BW, Fellows B. Comparative evaluation of the accuracy of immunoassay with liquid chromatography tandem mass spectrometry (LC/MS/MS) of urine drug testing (UDT) opioids and illicit drugs in chronic pain patients. *Pain Physician*. 2011;14:175–187.

37. Shaw JL. Practical challenges related to point of care testing. *Practical Lab Med*. 2016;4:22–29.

38. Kim JA, Ptolemy AS, Melanson SE, Janfaza DR, Ross EL. The clinical impact of a false-positive urine cocaine screening result on a patient's pain management. *Pain Med*. 2015;16:1073–1076.

39. Thin-layer chromatography. 2007. http://www.chemguide.co.uk/analysis/chromatography/thinlayer.html. Accessed May 15, 2017.

40. Shaw JL. Practical challenges related to point of care testing. *Practical Lab Med*. 2016;4:22–29.

41. Gupta A, Patton C, Diskina D, Cheatle M. Retrospective review of physician opioid prescribing practices in patients with aberrant behaviors. *Pain Physician*. 2011;14:383–389.

42. Selavka CM. Poppy seed ingestion as a contributing factor to opiate-positive urinalysis results: the Pacific perspective. *J Forensic Sci.* 1991;36:685–696.

43. Lachenmeier DW, Sproll C, Musshoff F. Poppy seed foods and opiate drug testing—where are we today? *Therapeutic Drug Monitoring.* 2010;32:11–18.

45. Marquet P, Lachatre G. Liquid chromatography-mass spectrometry: potential in forensic and clinical toxicology. *J Chromatogr B Biomed Sci Appl.* 1999;733:93–118.

46. High-performance liquid chromatography. 2007. http://www.chemguide.co.uk/analysis/chromatography/hplc.html. Accessed May 15, 2017.

47. McMillin GA, Marin SJ, Johnson-Davis KL, Lawlor BG, Strathmann FG. A hybrid approach to UDM using high-resolution mass spectrometry and select immunoassays. *Am J Clin Pathol.* 2015;143:234–240.

48. Reisfield GM, Goldberger BA, Bertholf RL. "False-positive" and "false-negative" test results in clinical UDM. *Bioanalysis.* 2009;1:937–952.

49. Deer TR, Gunn J. Blood testing in chronic pain management. *Pain Physician.* 2015;18:E157–161.

50. Bosker WM, Huestis MA. Oral fluid testing for drugs of abuse. *Clin Chem.* 2009;55:1910–1931.

51. Heltsley R, DePriest A, Black DL, et al. Oral fluid drug testing of chronic pain patients. II. Comparison of paired oral fluid and urine specimens. *J Anal Toxicol.* 2012;36:75–80.

52. Allen KR. Screening for drugs of abuse: which matrix, oral fluid or urine? *Ann Clin Biochem.* 2011;48(Pt 6):531–541.

53. Cone EJ, Huestis MA. Interpretation of oral fluid tests for drugs of abuse. *Ann NY Acad Sci.* 2007;1098:51–103.

54. Huestis MA, Cone EJ, Wong CJ, Umbricht A, Preston KL. Monitoring opiate use in substance abuse treatment patients with sweat and UDM. *J Anal Toxicol.* 2000;24:509–521.

55. Cummings OT, Morris AA, Enders JR, McIntire GL. Normalizing oral fluid hydrocodone data using calculated blood volume. *J Anal Toxicol.* 2016;40:486–491.

56. Shaparin N, Mehta N, Kunkel F, Stripp R, Borg D, Kolb E. A novel chronic opioid monitoring tool to assess prescription drug steady-state levels in oral fluid. *Pain Med.* 2017;18(11):2162–2169.

57. Moore C, Feldman M, Harrison E, et al. Disposition of hydrocodone in hair. *J Anal Toxicol.* 2006;30:353–359.

58. Chawarski MC, Fiellin DA, O'Connor PG, Bernard M, Schottenfeld RS. Utility of sweat patch testing for drug use monitoring in outpatient treatment for opiate dependence. *J Subst Abuse Treat.* 2007;33:411–415.

59. Romano G, Barbera N, Lombardo I. Hair testing for drugs of abuse: evaluation of external cocaine contamination and risk of false positives. *Forensic Sci Int.* 2001;123:119–129.

60. Starrels JL, Becker WC, Alford DP, Kapoor A, Williams AR, Turner BJ. Systematic review: treatment agreements and UDM to reduce opioid misuse in patients with chronic pain. *Ann Intern Med.* 2010;152:712–720.

61. Federation of State Medical Boards of the United States I. Model policy for the use of controlled substances for the treatment of pain. *J Pain Palliat Care Pharmacother.* 2005;19:73–78.

62. Rolfs RT, Johnson E, Williams NJ, Sundwall DN, Utah Department of Health. Utah clinical guidelines on prescribing opioids for treatment of pain. *J Pain Palliat Care Pharmacother.* 2010;24:219–235.

63. Katz N, Fanciullo GJ. Role of urine toxicology testing in the management of chronic opioid therapy. *Clin J Pain.* 2002;18(Suppl):S76–82.

64. Center for Substance Abuse Treatment. *Managing Chronic Pain in Adults With or in Recovery From Substance Use Disorders.* Substance Abuse and Mental Health Services Administration Report No.: (SMA) 12-4671. SAMHSA/CSAT Treatment Improvement Protocols. Rockville, MD; 2012.

65. Cone EJ, Zichterman A, Heltsley R, et al. Urine testing for norcodeine, norhydrocodone, and noroxycodone facilitates interpretation and reduces false negatives. *Forensic Sci Int.* 2010;198:58–61.

66. Wasan AD, Michna E, Janfaza D, Greenfield S, Teter CJ, Jamison RN. Interpreting urine drug tests: prevalence of morphine metabolism to hydromorphone in chronic pain patients treated with morphine. *Pain Med*. 2008;9:918–923.

67. Compton P. The role of urine toxicology in chronic opioid analgesic therapy. *Pain Manage Nurs*. 2007;8:166–172.

68. Vadivelu N, Chen IL, Kodumudi V, Ortigosa E, Gudin MT. The implications of UDM in pain management. *Current Drug Safety*. 2010;5:267–270.

69. Dowell D, Haegerich TM, Chou R. CDC guideline for prescribing opioids for chronic pain—United States, 2016. *JAMA*. 2016;315:1624–1645.

70. Cheatle MD, Savage SR. Informed consent in opioid therapy: a potential obligation and opportunity. *J Pain Symptom Manage*. 2012;44(1):105–116.

71. Twillman RK, Gilson AM, Duensing KN. State policies regulating the practice of pain management: statutes, rules, and guidelines that shape pain care. *Anesthesiol Clin*. 2016;34(2):409–424.

72. Passik SD, Kirsh KL, Webster L. Pseudoaddiction revisited: a commentary on clinical and historical considerations. *Pain Manag*. 2011;1(3):239–248.

73. Heit HA, Gourlay DL. Urine drug monitoring in pain medicine. *J Pain Symptom Manage*. 2004;27(3):260–267.

74. Owen GT, Burton AW, Schade CM, Passik S. Urine drug testing: current reocmmendations and best practices. *Pain Physician*. 2012;15:ES119–133.

75. Kirsh KL, Whitcomb LA, Donaghy K, Passik SD. Abuse and addiction issues in medically ill patients with pain: attempts at clarification of terms and empirical study. *Clin J Pain*. 2002;18:S52–S60.

76. Katz NP, Sherburne S, Beach M, et al. Behavioral monitoring and urine toxicology testing in patients receiving long-term opioid therapy. *Anesthesia Analgesia*. 2003;97:1097–1102.

EPILOGUE

John F. Peppin, John J. Coleman, and Kelly K. Dineen

In planning this book, the authors and contributors sought to provide a plethora of professions with a reference for many facets of modern pain management, including the appropriate use of scheduled medications. The book also includes the dark side of drug diversion and abuse—factors that are sometimes ignored by authors writing in this genre. It is possible that no other field of medicine or science is as constrained by regulatory controls as pain management. That constraint is usually based on fairly rare patient misuse or drug diversion and even rarer provider misprescribing.

Yet prescription opioid–related mortality and morbidity continue to increase at unprecedented levels. This suggests that a new paradigm is needed to address modern-day pain management. Given the complexity of the practice of pain management, the "opioid crisis" cannot be solved, nor can conditions for pain patients be improved, using only simple and direct approaches: one medication, one regulatory policy, one law, or one injection will not be the answer for our chronic pain patients. Rather, we need a multidisciplinary, multimodal approach that involves all stakeholders, including regulators and legislators. We hope that this book reflects this approach by bringing together specialists in the areas of regulation, legislation, law enforcement, pain medicine, addiction, and psychiatry/psychology. We must disabuse ourselves of the notion that we are on "opposite sides" and "at war." We each have contributions to make toward solving this problem, and history should teach us that without using interdisciplinary insights, even the best efforts are destined to fail. Moreover, patients with disorders associated with opioids—chronic pain, substance use disorders, or both—are ill served by adversarial positioning.

Our authors in the first half of the book discuss the government controls that have been placed on the commerce in opioids, beginning in 1914 with the passage of the Harrison Narcotic Tax Act. Since 1914, government strategies have focused on restricting access to opiates and other regulated drugs for medical and scientific purposes only. This control paradigm was at the core of domestic and international drug policy for many decades and remains dominant today. In the beginning, the pathophysiology of opiate addiction was poorly understood, and well-intended treatment protocols were brutal and largely ineffective. It would take decades before the disease model of addiction would prevail and lead to improved treatments. Even today, a number of cultural, social, and educational barriers prevent many providers from accepting the chronic disease model of addiction, and these barriers keep far too many people with substance abuse disorders from accessing adequate treatment.

By the final decades of the 20th century, the rising morbidity and mortality associated with the misuse of prescription drugs, particularly opioids, would breach the regulatory barriers set up to prevent drug diversion and abuse. Perhaps the most effective of these was the Controlled Substances Act of 1970 (CSA). The authors in the first half of this book offer varying interpretations of the CSA: some praise its regulatory schema for keeping the diversion of controlled substances within manageable parameters, but others argue that rigorous enforcement of the CSA may have produced more harm than good. For example, some patients with pain who benefit from opioid therapy have described that they have had difficulty finding compassionate providers or continuing their opioid therapy because of the government's crackdown on unlawful diversion. To avoid this, some policymakers have championed the principle of a balance between regulatory enforcement and appropriate access to regulated medications. However, as one of the authors points out, a strict policy of balance may actually have the unintended consequence of worsening divisions between the medical and regulatory communities because the concept of balance means that neither side can be more than half-satisfied at any time.

In Chapter 1, the authors provide a brief history of opiates from the earliest of recorded time to the present, showing, for example, how some of today's problems with misuse of these drugs were present in antiquity. Included is a chronology of the opiate treatment field, beginning with "narcotic farms," which represented the world's first therapeutic approach to addiction and provided the foundation for some of today's treatment protocols. The authors discuss some of the benefits and risks of opioid therapy for pain, stressing the need to reduce the associated morbidity and mortality.

In Chapter 2, the authors provide an overview of the regulatory regime around prescription opioids, focusing on the regulation of health professionals involved in the distribution and prescribing of opioids. Also addressed are the various legal entanglements that a provider may face for inappropriate prescribing of opioids or after a patient's bad outcome related to opioid use. To implement effective policies, the authors discuss the need to carefully define misprescribing and offer refined definitions of over- and underprescribing. They also provide an updated categorization of misprescribers that reflects existing evidence. The authors also discuss the relationship between the policy and legal focus on opioids overall relative to the harms of particular opioids and concurrent use of other medications and substances, such as benzodiazepines and alcohol. The authors offer some suggestions for appropriate legal scrutiny of opioid prescribing.

In Chapter 3, the author discusses the roles of manufacturers and distributors and how their business activities are tightly regulated by the CSA. Also discussed are regulatory investigations initiated by the US Drug Enforcement Administration (DEA) and the Department of Justice against registered wholesale drug distributors and one drug manufacturer accused of failing to identify and report to DEA—as the law requires—suspicious orders for controlled substances involving hundreds of millions of dosage units of opioids and other drugs. Chapter 3 also discusses state and federal efforts to address the prescription opioid abuse problem by a series of proposed changes that would expand the use of prescription drug monitoring program (PDMP) data to permit access by private-sector third-party payers. The interests of third-party payers, such as curtailing waste, fraud, and abuse, coincide with the government's interests in reducing "doctor shopping" and other prescription frauds, which account for a sizable portion of diverted pharmaceutical substances. The role of the prescription benefits manager (PBM) as it interfaces with that of the dispensing pharmacy is discussed, and the author recommends adding the PBM's business activities involving controlled substances to those already regulated by the CSA and DEA. This would indemnify PBMs when they identify and report suspicious prescriptions in a manner now required only of manufacturers and distributors when they receive suspicious orders from their customers.

In Chapter 4, the author discusses how the regulatory misdeeds of Purdue Pharma LP and others in the pharmaceutical industry muddied the national efforts to improve pain care. The *Decade of Pain Control and Research,* established by congressional action, was heralded by the pain community and was intended to highlight the need for improved pain treatment and the development of new treatment modalities for chronic pain. However, at the end of the decade, instead of hailing improvements in pain management, public health officials were warning about the "epidemic" of prescription drug abuse and proposing new guidelines to curtail the use of opioids for treating nonmalignant chronic pain. Further, it should be noted that no public funds were appropriated to achieve the ambitious goals of the *Decade of Pain Control and Research.* No discussion in this book would be complete without noting the emergence in 1996 of OxyContin, an extended-release oxycodone drug whose sponsor, Purdue Pharma LP, aggressively promoted it in ways that would result in federal criminal fraud convictions for the company and its three top executives. Chapter 4 describes how this happened and the impact that it has had on the industry, individual pain specialists, the public, and, ultimately, the *Decade of Pain Control and Research.*

In short, the first half of this book emphasizes the need for, and the importance of, the regulatory community in protecting the public's health against the harmful effects of controlled substances taken for nonmedical purposes. The authors present a chronology of how and when prescription drugs, particularly opioids, began to dominate the categories of substances most frequently abused. They provide an overview of the regulatory and legal frameworks intended to balance deterring diversion with allowing access to appropriate care and critically evaluate the success of those efforts. They show how government strategies to contain diversion and abuse had a negligible effect on reducing the mortality and morbidity associated with their diversion and abuse. They discuss why they believe this was so and what might be done to improve future strategies and outcomes. To be sure, there are small but significant emerging signs that suggest the "epidemic" of prescription drug abuse may have peaked and now is in decline.

The second half of the book addresses the substantive issue of pain management. In Chapter 5, the evaluation and assessment of the pain patients is described. As mentioned above, these cases are not simplistic and linear, but rather very complex. While the benefits of opioids used to treat chronic pain still outweigh their risks, as noted by the US Food and Drug Administration (FDA), it is also true that the risks associated with their use have increased significantly in the past several decades. For that reason alone, healthcare providers need to weigh the risks and benefits when proposing treatment plans for their chronic pain patients.

Understanding the pharmacology of controlled substances may aid clinicians in assessing these risk factors. In Chapter 6, a comprehensive analysis of sedative-hypnotics and stimulants is given. The authors discuss how the necessity of prescribing these drugs for disorders for which they have established efficacy heightens the risk that occasionally they will be misused.

In Chapter 7, the author describes the importance of considering the patient's mental status when assessing the pain threshold and when weighing the use of appropriate treatment protocols. The author uses a very effective case history to demonstrate the need to incorporate the patient's past medical record with a psychiatric and habit history for all chronic pain patients.

As a group, chronic pain patients sometimes are considered difficult to manage. This may be the result of numerous factors, including many that are beyond the control of providers. Perhaps the most difficult chronic pain patient is the one who has a comorbid substance use disorder. The patient whose substance use disorder involves opioid abuse presents a unique risk profile that greatly complicates the clinician's task. Chronic pain is prevalent among patients with substance use disorder; indeed, self-medicating to relieve pain may have facilitated the substance use disorder in the first instance. The author of Chapter 8 discusses ways in which the clinician may reduce risks when treating a chronic pain patient who has an substance use disorder while at the same time providing adequate and effective pain relief for the patient.

Similarly, as the author of Chapter 9 explains, there are certain populations of patients with chronic pain whose care is especially complicated and may be subject to clinical decision making errors and biases. The author discusses ways to provide effective pain management services for individuals in some of these special populations, such as those with sickle cell disease. Whether treating a special-population patient or one with a comorbid substance use disorder or psychological problem, the objective is always the same: provide effective and safe treatment.

In Chapter 10, interdisciplinary pain management is discussed. The author argues that bringing back into vogue this form of treatment may help reduce the overall volume of opioids in use. The author describes the interdisciplinary approach to pain treatment as an earlier and more successful method of dealing with chronic pain. Over time, however, third-party payers began to deny claims for this type of treatment, which has partly led to its demise. Because it was cheaper to pay for drug therapy, including opioids, third-party payers have favored drug therapy for treating chronic pain. The author speculates that this bias inadvertently may have contributed to today's "epidemic" of opioid abuse by increasing the volume of opioids being prescribed and dispensed—and diverted—and recommends returning to the interdisciplinary approach not only to achieve improved outcomes for patients, but also to stem the epidemic of opioid abuse.

In our concluding chapter, the author discusses the utility of urine drug monitoring (UDM) performed either at random or at planned encounters to determine whether the patient is taking the prescribed drugs and/or taking nonprescribed drugs. The author details the usefulness of UDM along with some of its limitations, such as the metabolic processes that may create false-positive results and otherwise confound test results. When they are used appropriately and the results are correctly interpreted, UDM can serve several useful purposes, especially in ensuring that patients placed on prescription opioids are compliant with the instructions of their prescriber.

The sequencing of these chapters was designed to provide the reader with a basis for understanding the regulatory schema surrounding the medications used primarily for treating chronic pain and for the application of these medications in the clinical setting. Much attention over the years has been given to the stigmatization of pain patients and their medications. Some pain patients in dire need of relief have even been known to turn down opioid therapy out of fear of being labeled a "dope fiend" or worse. Legitimate pain patients in some cases have had their integrity challenged openly by pharmacists and others in the healthcare profession who may doubt their need for the drugs they have been prescribed. Similarly, prescribers of opioids are viewed by some as contributing to the problem by failing to weed out the "doctor shoppers" and other frauds who use them to obtain supplies of controlled substances. Many of these unfair characterizations can be traced back to the public's fear of addiction and stigmatization of individuals with substance use disorders. This fear approaches phobic levels among some and at times may cast the entire field of pain management in a bad light when, in fact, only a very small fraction of the many millions of pain patients and their caregivers are at fault. Education is a good antidote for fear. The contributing authors and editors of this book hope that the educational content found herein helps to dispel some of that fear and the stigmatization that it produces.

INDEX

Page numbers followed by *f, b,* and *t* refer to figures, boxes, and tables, respectively.

diagoras, 2
diathesis/stress model, 163
diazepam, 139t
DiBella, Roberto D., 95
diethylpropion, 144t
Dinan, James H., 93
disciplinary actions, 28–29
disease-based biases, 196
disorders, 156–57, 159–65, 169t. *See also* substance
    use disorder
"doctor shoppers," 41, 61, 63, 67
Dole, Vincent, 6
dopamine, 137
Doremus, Charles T., 5
dronabinol (Marinol), 146, 147t
Drug Abuse Warning Network (DAWN), 67,
    80–81, 136
drug distributors, 40–41, 87–92
Drug Enforcement Administration. *See* US Drug
    Enforcement Administration (DEA)
drug enforcement agencies, 30
drug interactions, deaths from, 8
drug manufacturers, 53–54
drug safety, 21–24
DSM, See *Diagnostic and Statistical Manual of Mental
    Disorders*
dual process theory, 192
Duke University School of Medicine, 40
Dunbar, S., 182
Durham-Humphrey Amendments (1951), 21–22
dysphagia, 116–17

East India Company, 1
economic medicalization, 210
ED (emergency department) visits, 39–40, 136–37,
    194–95, 211
electronic records, 47–48
emergency department (ED) visits, 39–40, 136–37,
    194–95, 211
endocrinopathy, 122–23
Engel, G. L., 153
Ensuring Patient Access and Effective Drug
    Enforcement Act (2016), 92–93
Ephedra (ma huang), 145
Erasistratus, 2
euphoria, from benzodiazepines, 138
Europe, chronic pain in, 112
Express Scripts Holding Company, 63–65

FDA. *See* US Food and Drug Administration
FDCA (Federal Food, Drug, and Cosmetic
    Act), 11, 21
Federal Bureau of Narcotics, 6

Federal Food, Drug, and Cosmetic Act (FDCA), 11, 21
Federation of State Medical Boards of the United
    States, 9
fentanyl, 230t
Ferrell, B. R., 111
Florida, prescription monitoring in, 44–45, 52
Foley, Kathleen M., 80
Food and Drug Administration. *See* US Food and
    Drug Administration (FDA)
Forbes, 98
forensic testing, 220
forfeiture, asset, 53
Fortune, 94
4D model of misprescribers, 26
fraud, 61–62
funding, 51–54, 53t, 100

gabapentin, 125, 141, 147t
gabapentinoids, 125
Galen, 2
Gallagher, R. M., 206
GAO (Government Accountability Office), 43,
    62, 66, 96
gas chromatography/mass spectrometry (GCMS),
    223t, 224, 225–26
gate control model, 163
GCMS (gas chromatography/mass spectrometry),
    223t, 224, 225–26
generic drug distributors, 89–92
genetic polymorphism, 194
Gil, M., 120
goals, in chronic pain management, 113
Goggin, Wendy H., 96
Goldbaum, Jacob, 5
Gorelick, Jamie S., 93–94
Government Accountability Office (GAO), 43,
    62, 66, 96
Grants, Rogers, 45, 57–58
"Great American Fraud, The " (Adams), 3–4
Great Britain, in opium wars, 2
Green, T. C., 49
Gressler, L. E., 126
Guardian, 93
"Guidelines for Prescribing Opioids for Chronic
    Pain" (CDC), 185
Gunn, J., 227
Gwira Baumblatt, J. A., 50

Haddox, J. D., 84
hair, drug testing using, 227
hallucinogens, 146, 147t
Harold Rogers Prescription Drug Monitoring
    Program (HRPDMP), 45–46

Loeser, John, 207
Los Angeles Times, 51–52, 97
Lyrica (pregabalin), 141

Madadi, P., 200
major depressive disorder (MDD), 159–60, 169*t*
Mallinckrodt plc, 89–92, 94
marijuana, 115–16
Marinol (dronabinol), 146, 147*t*
Massachusetts General Hospital Pain Center's Pain
    Assessment Form (MGH-PCPAF), 158
Masters Pharmaceuticals, 90
MAT (medication-assisted therapy), 20–21, 183–85
Maughan, B. C., 50
Maurer, D., 20–21
McAdam-Marx, C., 62
McGill Pain Questionnaire (MPQ), 158
McKesson, 87, 90, 94
McLellan, A. T., 179
McMillin, G. A., 226
MDD (major depressive disorder), 159–60, 169*t*
media, investigating opioid abuse, 86–87
Medicaid, 61–62
medical malpractice cases, 27–28
Medicare, 55–56
medication-assisted therapy (MAT), 20–21, 183–85
meperidine, 230*t*
metabolites, 229, 230*t*
methadone, 6, 8, 43, 120–22, 183–84
methylphenidate, 142, 144*t*, 145–46
MGH-PCPAF (Massachusetts General Hospital
    Pain Center's Pain Assessment Form), 158
Milione, Louis J., 96
Millennium Laboratories, 52
Miller, Steve, 63
Milwaukee Journal Sentinel, 86
misprescribing, 24–32
    defined, 25
    models of, 25–27
    remedies for, 27–32
Mississippi, litigation in, 84
misuse, defined, 178
MITRE Corporation, 57
modafinil (Provigil), 144*t*, 145–46
Model Guidelines for the Use of Controlled
    Substances for the Treatment of Pain, 9
monitoring, 227–29, 228*b*
monitoring prescriptions, 39–68
    and bulk distributions, 40–41
    in Florida, 44–45
    with health insurers, 54–56
    in hospitals/clinics, 41
    importance of, 39–40

for opioid diversion, 43–44
    in pharmacies, 41
    to prevent waste/fraud/abuse, 61–62
    private-sector initiatives for, 58–61
    as public health vs. public safety, 51
    through PBMs, 62–68
    through PDMPs, 45–51, 51–54, 54–56
mood disorders, 169*t*
mood stabilizers, 168
Morasco, B. J., 220
Morford, Craig S., 93–94
morphine, 229, 230*t*
mortality, 7–8, 98–99
Moy, Jin Fuey, 5
MPQ (McGill Pain Questionnaire), 158
Mulrooney, John J., II, 95–96
multi-class misprescribing, 25
Mundipharma International, 98
muscle relaxants, 125–26, 183
Musto, D. F., 3
myoclonus, 118

NA (Narcotics Anonymous), 182
nabilone (Cesamet), 146, 147*t*
NABP (National Association of Boards of
    Pharmacy), 58–59
"narcotic farms," 5–6
Narcotics Anonymous (NA), 182
Narcotics Division, of Treasury Department, 20
NAS (neonatal abstinence syndrome), 121–22
NASMDL (National Alliance of State Model Drug
    Laws), 46, 48, 51, 60
NASPER (National All Schedules Prescription
    Electronic Reporting Act), 45–46, 57
National Academy of Medicine, 85
National Alliance of State Model Drug Laws
    (NASMDL), 46, 48, 51, 60
National All Schedules Prescription Electronic
    Reporting Act (NASPER), 45–46, 57
National Association of Boards of Pharmacy
    (NABP), 58–59
National Council for Prescription Drug Programs
    (NCPDP), 58, 63
National Institutes of Health, 100
National Institutes of Health (NIH), 154
National Practitioner Data Bank, 29
National Prescription Drug Take-Back Day, 9
National Research Council, 101
nausea, 116
NCPDP (National Council for Prescription Drug
    Programs), 58, 63
negative loading, 192
neonatal abstinence syndrome (NAS), 121–22

neuropathic pain, 155–56, 196
neuroplastic changes, 155–56
New England Journal of Medicine, 80, 212
New York State, PDMPs in, 46
NIH (National Institutes of Health), 154
nociceptive pain, 155
nonbenzodiazepine sedatives, 140
nonopioids, 136–48
    as chronic pain treatments, 124–27
    and CNS pharmacology, 137
    other/hallucinogens, 146, 147t
    sedative-hypnotics, 138, 139t, 140–42
    stimulants, 142, 143t–45t, 145–46
    use of, 136–37
nonsteroidal anti-inflammatories (NSAIDs),
    125, 182–83
non–urine-based drug monitoring, 226–27
norepinephrine, 137
NPR, 199–200
NSAIDs (nonsteroidal anti-inflammatories),
    125, 182–83
Nuvigil (armodafinil), 145–46, 145t
Nyswander, Marie, 6

Obamacare, 85
obesity, 113
O'Connor, S., 195
Office of Diversion Control (DEA), 95
Office of Inspector General (OIG), 65–66, 81
Office of National Drug Control Policy
    (ONDCP), 55, 59
Ohio, PDMPs in, 60
OIG (Office of Inspector General), 65–66, 81
OIH (opioid-induced hyperalgesia), 122
Okifuji, A., 205
older patients, biases against, 197–98
ONDCP (Office of National Drug Control
    Policy), 55, 59
opiate, defined, 1
opioid abuse
    behaviors of, 228b
    history of, 82, 212
    and IPMP decrease, 209–10
    and pain, 177
    prevalence of, 178–79
    See also substance use disorder
opioid-induced androgen deficiency, 123
opioid induced constipation, 117
opioid-induced hyperalgesia (OIH), 122
opioid-induced respiratory depression, 118–19
opioids
    abuse of (*see* opioid abuse)
    cross-reactants for, 222b

current perception of, xiii
diversion of, 43–44, 96, 210–12
history of, 1–7, 78–79
increase in use of, 8–10
long term use of, xiv, 115–24
morbidity and mortality with, 7–8
side effects of, 115–24
tolerance to, 232
treatments of addiction to, 3–6, 20
opioid use disorder. *See* opioid abuse
opium poppy, 136
"opium wars," 2
oral fluids, drug testing using, 227
Oregon, PDMPs in, 47
Osler, William, 2
overdose, 28, 39, 100f
overprescribing, 3, 25
oversimplications, 190–91, 200
Ower, K., 120
oxycodone, 230t
OxyContin', xiv, 11, 230t
    in Appalachia, 211
    history of, 78–83
    use abroad, 97–98

pain
    acute, 194–95
    cancer, 10–11, 110
    classifications of, 155–56
    definitions of, 154
    imagined vs. real, 156
    neuropathic, 196
    substance use disorder and, 177–79
    See also chronic pain
Pain Beliefs Questionnaire (PBQ), 157
pain centers, 185
pain clinician, defined, 111
pain community, 8–9
pain-control era, 80–81
Pain Disorder, 157
pain management teams, 167
Pain Medicine, 49, 208
Pain Quality Assessment Scale (PQAS), 156
pain scales, 157–58
Pain Self-Efficacy Questionnaire (PSEQ), 158
palliative care, 10–11, 197–98
panic disorder, 160–61
Papaver somniferum, 136
paracetamol (APAP), 125, 182
Parente, S. T., 49
Passik, Steven, 84
Patient Protection and Affordable Care Act, 85
patient–provider relationships, 231–33

in healthcare, 17
legal (*see* legal regulations)
state vs. federal, 11
for wholesale drug distributors, 87, 88*t*, 89
Reifler, L. M., 49–50
Reisfield, G. M., 226
Reisman, R. M., 49
relationships, patient-provider, 231–33
relaxants, muscle, 125–26, 183
"Relieving Pain in America: A Blueprint for Transforming Prevention, Care, Education, and Research" (IOM), 85, 110
REMS (Risk Evaluation and Mitigation Strategy), 11, 23
respiratory depression, opioid-induced, 118–19
Ringwalt, C., 50
Risk Evaluation and Mitigation Strategy (REMS), 11, 23
risks, 113–14, 121, 121*t*
Rite Aid Corp., 63
Rogers grants, 45, 57–58
ROME group, 117
Rosenberg, Chuck, 96

Sackler, Arthur, 98
Sackler, Mortimer, 98
Sackler, Raymond, 98
safety, public, 51
Safety and Innovation Act, 56
SAMHSA (Substance Abuse and Mental Health Services Administration), 67
Saunders, K. W., 117
Savage, S. R., 212
scar hypothesis episodes, 160
SCD (sickle cell disease), 193–97
scheduled urine drug monitoring, 229
Screener and Opioid Assessment for People with Pain Revised (SOAP-R), 234
screening, in UDM, 221–22, 223*t*
scrutiny, legal, 17–18
secobarbital, 139*t*
sedation, as side effect, 117
sedative-hypnotics, 136, 138, 139*t*, 140–42, 139*t*
Self-administered Leeds Assessment of Neuropathic Symptoms and Signs (S-LANSS), 156
self-management, 164–65, 206
Sentinel, 86–87
serotonin, 137
serotonin antagonists, 116
serum testing, 226–27
sexual function, 123–24
SF-MPQ (short-form McGill Pain Questionnaire), 158

sickle cell disease (SCD), 193–97
side effect(s), 115–24
cardiac, 119–20
of methadone, 120–22
nausea as, 116
sedation as, 117
treating, 124
vomiting as, 116
S-LANSS (self-administered Leeds Assessment of Neuropathic Symptoms and Signs), 156
sleep, 113, 118, 161–62, 169*t*
sleep apnea, 119
SOAP-R (Screener and Opioid Assessment for People with Pain Revised), 234
social support, 181–82
somatic pain, 155
somatoform disorders, 156–57
"special K," 146
special populations. *See* stigmatized/special populations
stabilizers, mood, 168
state professional boards, 19, 28–29
stepped-care model, 166–67
stigmatized/special populations, 190–200
chronic pain patients, 198–200
palliative care/hospice, 197–98
provider decision-making in, 192–93
sickle cell disease patients, 193–97
stimulant nonopioids, 142, 143*t*–45*t*, 145–46
Substance Abuse and Mental Health Services Administration (SAMHSA), 67
substance use disorders, 162–63, 165–66, 176–86
barriers to care with, 185
managing pain in patients with, 177–82, 180*f*
and medication-assisted therapy, 183–85
and pharmacotherapy, 182–83
and suicide, 185
See also opioid abuse
suicide, 185, 199–200
Sumerians, 1
support, social, 181–82
System Theory (Engels), 153

Tang, N. K., 185
TBI (traumatic brain injury), 112
teams, pain management, 167
technophilic approaches, to chronic pain, 209
testing
confirmatory, 223*t*, 224–25
forensic, 220
immunoassay, 221–22, 223*t*
serum, 226–27
therapies, 114, 126

thin-layer chromatography (TLC), 223t, 225
third-party payers, 54–55
3C model of misprescribers, 26
thyroids, 124
TLC (thin-layer chromatography), 223t, 225
Tompkins, D. A., 78
torsades risk, 121, 121t
To the Ends of the Earth (film), 6
Towne, Charles B., 3
Towns Cure, 3
tramadol, 230t
traumatic brain injury (TBI), 112
Treasury Department (U.S.), 5, 20
treatments
  opioid addiction, 3–4
  psychiatric, 152, 165
  psychopharmacologic, 167–68
Tversky, A., 192
twelve-step programs, 181–82
type 1 decisions, 192
type 2 decisions, 192

UDM. *See* urine drug monitoring
underprescribing, 25
United States v. Feingold, 31
United States v. Katz, 30
Universal Precautions, 115, 198
University of Wisconsin, 80, 86
UN Office of Drugs and Crime, 1
urine drug monitoring (UDM), 219–34
  adjunct monitoring with, 227–29
  and chromatography, 225–26
  confirmatory testing for, 224–25
  considerations for, 233–34
  costs of, 233
  importance of, 219–20
  interpreting results of, 229–32
  methods for, 221–24
  methods of, 220–21, 223t
  non–urine-based methods vs., 226–27
  and provider–patient relationship, 232–33
USA Today, 86
US Congress, 4, 81, 92–93
US Drug Enforcement Administration (DEA), 7, 9
  and the Decade of Pain Control and
    Research, 93–96
  and drug classification, 22–23

on legal scrutiny, 17–18
monitoring prescriptions, 41–42
registering with, 65–66
regulations for distributors by, 88t
and wholesale drug distributors, 87–89
on willful blindness, 31
US Food and Drug Administration (FDA), 9
  and buprenophine formulations, 184
  creation of, 21–24
  and *Decade of Pain Control and Research*, 85–86
  on opioid diversion, 43–44
  on OxyContin, 79–80
  and Safety and Innovation Act, 56
US Pain Foundation, 97
US Public Health Service, 5
US Supreme Court, 5, 20, 24

Veterans Administration hospitals, 197
visceral pain, 155
Vogel, V. H., 20–21
Volkow, N. D., 179
vomiting, 116
Vyvanse (lisdexamfetamine), 142, 143t

Wailoo, Keith, 191
Walker, J. M., 119
Wall Street Journal, 82
Washington Post, 91, 93–97
Washington University, 97
waste, monitoring prescriptions to prevent, 61–62
Webb, W. S., 5
Webster, Lynn, 199
Weissman, D. E., 84
WHO (World Health Organization), 10–11, 152–53
wholesale drug distributors, 40–41, 87–92
willful blindness, 31
Wilsey, B. L., 49
Wilson, Woodrow, 4
Woolf, Clifford J., 100, 101
Workers' Compensation Institute (California), 54
World Health Organization (WHO),
    10–11, 152–53
Wright State University School of Medicine, 84
wrongful death lawsuits, 28

Xanax (alprazolam), 138, 139t
xerostomia, 116